The Relational Self

The Relational Self

Theoretical Convergences in Psychoanalysis and Social Psychology

Edited by
REBECCA C. CURTIS
Adelphi University

THE GUILFORD PRESS
New York   London

To my family and friends,
who are always there for me.
—R. C. C.

© 1991 The Guilford Press
A Division of Guilford Publications, Inc.
72 Spring Street, New York, NY 10012

Printed in the United States of America

This book is printed on acid-free paper.

Last digit is print number: 9   8   7   6   5   4   3   2   1

Library of Congress Cataloging-in-Publication Data

The Relational self: theoretical convergences in psychoanalysis and
    social psychology / edited by Rebecca C. Curtis.
        p.   cm.
    Based on papers presented at a conference held at Adelphi
University on March 23–24, 1990.
    Includes bibliographical references and index.
    ISBN 0-89862-558-0
    1. Self. 2. Self—Social aspects. I. Curtis, Rebecca C.
    [DNLM: 1. Psychology, Social—congresses. 2. Self Concept—
congresses. BF 697.5.S43 R382 1990]
BF697.R418   1991
155.2—dc20
DNLM/DLC
for Library of Congress   90-15734
                                                                  CIP

Contributors

RICHARD D. ASHMORE, PhD, Department of Psychology, Rutgers, The State University of New Jersey, New Brunswick, New Jersey

ROY F. BAUMEISTER, PhD, Department of Psychology, Case Western Reserve University, Cleveland, Ohio

REBECCA C. CURTIS, PhD, Gordon F. Derner Institute of Advanced Psychological Studies, Adelphi University, Garden City, New York

KAY DEAUX, PhD, Social–Personality Doctoral Program, Graduate School and University Center, City University of New York, New York, New York

SEYMOUR EPSTEIN, PhD, Psychology Department, University of Massachusetts, Amherst, Massachusetts

STEFAN E. HORMUTH, PhD, Psychologisches Institut, University of Heidelberg, Heidelberg, Germany; present address: FB 06 Psychologie, University of Giessen, Giessen, Germany

LAWRENCE JOSEPHS, PhD, Gordon F. Derner Institute of Advanced Psychological Studies, Adelphi University, Garden City, New York

MICHAEL R. LEIPPE, PhD, Department of Psychology, Adelphi University, Garden City, New York

SHAWN E. McNULTY, AB, Department of Psychology, University of Texas at Austin, Austin, Texas

DANIEL M. OGILVIE, PhD, Department of Psychology, Rutgers, The State University of New Jersey, New Brunswick, New Jersey

ALAN ROLAND, PhD, Psychoanalyst in private practice, New York, New York; faculty and board of directors, National Psychological Association for Psychoanalysis, New York, New York

ROBERT D. STOLOROW, PhD, Southern California Psychoanalytic Institute, Beverly Hills, California; Institute for the Psychoanalytic Study of Subjectivity, New York, New York

WILLIAM B. SWANN, JR., PhD, Department of Psychology, University of Texas at Austin, Austin, Texas

KATE SZYMANSKI, PhD, Department of Psychology, Adelphi University, Garden City, New York

ABRAHAM TESSER, PhD, Institute for Behavioral Research, University of Georgia, Athens, Georgia

DREW WESTEN, PhD, Department of Psychology, University of Michigan, Ann Arbor, Michigan

GARRY ZASLOW, BA, Department of Psychology, Adelphi University, Garden City, New York

Preface

We have reversed the usual classical notion that the independent "elementary parts" of the world are the fundamental reality and that the various systems are merely particular contingent forms and arrangements of these parts. Rather, we say that inseparable quantum interconnectedness of the whole universe is the fundamental reality, and that relatively independently behaving parts are merely particular and contingent forms within this world.
> —BOHM AND HILEY (*Foundations of Physics*, 1975, Vol. 5, p. 102)

There is no such thing as a baby.... A baby cannot exist alone, but is essentially part of a relationship.
> —WINNICOTT (*The Child, the Family, and the Outside World*, 1964, p. 88)

In this century the view of reality apparent in the "new physics" has also permeated our view of the self and of social reality. Just as it is no longer possible to conceive of nonorganic objects as isolated particles, it makes no sense to try to observe an organic "self" except in interaction with other systems.

Heinz Pagels in *The Dreams of Reason*, citing the work of Charles Bennett at IBM Research, described self-organizing systems as systems that lower their entropy (a measure of their degree of disorganization) by expelling entropy into their environment and hence avoiding deterioration. Certainly this is an apt description of the self systems studied by psychologists, which expel from immediate awareness information and affect that their current organization is unable to tolerate.

The recognition of the interaction of the self-organization with the social and physical environment has led the contributors to this volume to focus on the changing sense of the "self with others" instead of a self with autonomy as the ultimate stage of development. This focus recognizes the importance of the submersion of the self in the goals of a group as well as the individuation of the self. Such submersion implies a choice of co-operative as opposed to individualistic or competitive goals but does not necessarily mean a lack of differentiation of self from others as some psychoanalysts or clinical psychologists might infer.

How is the self different from the personality? Personality is a word that is frequently used to mean the relatively enduring dispositions of an individual. The "self," on the other hand, derived from a word meaning "the same," requires recognition, that is, awareness of sameness. It has been this focus on self-awareness, self-recognition, and "mirroring" by such recent theorists as diverse as Lacan and Kohut, both psychoanalysts, to Stuss, a neuropsychologist, Gallup, a comparative psychologist, and Duval and Wicklund, experimental social psychologists, that has accelerated the differentiation of "self processes" from the whole of personality research.

Although social psychologists had long been interested in the interaction of situational and dispositional variables and theories of the self had burgeoned since the 1940s, the publication in 1972 of Duval and Wicklund's *A Theory of Objective Self-Awareness* marked the beginning of a new surge of research regarding the self in experimental social psychology. In the same year Bem's model of self-perception also appeared, making "the self" a topic of experimentation even among behaviorally oriented psychologists. By this time, psychoanalysts had witnessed the publication in 1971 of Kohut's *The Analysis of the Self* and the development of relational models of human beings no longer primarily focused on inborn drives and conflicts, but examining the deficits in development that new interpersonal relationships might supply.

Both psychoanalysts and social psychologists have seen the representation of self and others, and their maintenance and change, become the subject of much theory, investigation, and many publications in the past two decades. As social psychologists have pursued their study of "how the thoughts, feelings, and behavior of the individual are influenced by the actual, imagined, or implied presence of others" (Allport, 1968), as psychoanalysts have engaged in their endeavor of making the unconscious conscious, and as personality psychologists have studied the sum total of the ways an individual characteristically reacts to others (Ferguson, 1970), the work of all three groups in recent years has focused increasingly on the individual's reflection upon the processes by which thoughts, feelings, and behaviors are organized in interactions with others and how stimuli leading to disorganization are frequently excluded from conscious awareness. This reflection upon the organizing processes of one's own conscious awareness has become the dominant use of the term "self" (cf. Hall & Lindzey, 1957), in contrast to the broader sense of the word, referring to the totality of one's being.

In spite of this convergence in focus, there has been little cross-fertilization between experimental social psychologists and psychoanalysts. Although there has been some integration of work between social psychologists and clinical researchers with a cognitive–behavioral viewpoint, and also between psychoanalytic theory and developmental psychology, the theory of social–personality psychologists has been informed largely by research limited to verbal reports and the theory of psychoanalysts drawn from little other than the case study. In social psychology the dominant model of the self has remained that of a cognitive structure, that is, an information-processor analogous to a conscious computer. The role of affect and motivation is frequently absent and, when considered, remains secondary. Many models of the self in psychoanalytic theory have stressed the resistance to change, with causality frequently attributed to relatively enduring personality dispositions—these models representing examples of the fundamental attribution error in their lack of attention to the influence of current situational variables, including the therapist's expectations, on maintaining the current self-organization and behavior. Social-psychological research would benefit from knowledge about the rigidity of self-organizational processes when anxiety interferes with their functioning, knowledge about the effects on behavior of experiences not included in conscious awareness, and knowledge of nonverbal experiences and images; psychoanalysts would benefit from investigations of theoretical assumptions by methods other than the case study including more controlled studies of situational variables such as therapists' responses and variables affecting representations of self and others, and the particular defensive maneuvers used to maintain the self-organization.

With these possibilities in mind, a conference was organized and held at Adelphi University on March 23–24, 1990. The first 13 chapters in this volume are based on papers presented at that conference. (A portion of the data reported in the final chapter, by Ogilvie and Ashmore, was presented at the Nags Head conference on the Self and Identity, June 20–25, 1990.) The purpose of both the Adelphi conference and the current volume was to begin an attempt to explore similarities and differences in working assumptions about self-processes, to help researchers and clinicians become more aware of both situational and dispositional variables related to self–other interactions, and, it is hoped, to further the scientific study of our "quantum interconnectedness."

REBECCA C. CURTIS

REFERENCES

Allport, G. W. (1968). The historical background of modern psychology. In G. Lindzey & E. Aronson (Eds.), *The handbook of social psychology* (Vol. 1, 2nd ed.). Reading, MA: Addison-Wesley.

Ferguson, L. R. (1970). *Personality development.* Belmont, CA: Brooks/Cole.

Hall, C. S., & Lindzey, G. (1957). *Theories of personality.* New York: Wiley.

Contents

I. CURRENT PERSPECTIVES FROM PSYCHOANALYTIC
SELF PSYCHOLOGY   1

1. Character Structure, Self-Esteem Regulation, and the
   Principle of Identity Maintenance   3
   Lawrence Josephs

   Introduction   3
   The Psychodynamic Model of Character Structure   3
   The Psychology of Self-Esteem Regulation   7
   The Principle of Identity Maintenance   10
   Conclusion   15
   References   15

2. The Intersubjective Context of Intrapsychic Experience,
   with Special Reference to Therapeutic Impasses   17
   Robert D. Stolorow

   Psychoanalysis as a Theory of the Mind   17
   Psychoanalysis as a Research Method   21
   Psychoanalysis as a Form of Therapy   23
   An Intersubjective Analysis of a Therapeutic Impasse   25
   Acknowledgments   30
   References   31

II. CURRENT PERSPECTIVES FROM SOCIAL PSYCHOLOGY   35

3. A Self-Image Analysis of Persuasion and Attitude
   Involvement   37
   Michael R. Leippe

   The Relevance of Relevance   38
   Goals, Selves, and Message Elaboration: Conceptual
     Background   39

Persuasion and the Two Selves   43
Implications for the Would-Be Persuader   54
Conclusion   58
Acknowledgments   59
References   59

**4. The Potency and Fragility of Self-Evaluation in Reducing
the Social Loafing Effect**   **64**
Kate Szymanski

The Social Loafing Effect and Its Mediator—Evaluation   64
Implications of the Self-Evaluation Effect   68
Group Evaluation as a Form of Self-Evaluation   71
Conclusions   74
References   74

5. Social Identities: Thoughts on Structure and Change   **77**
Kay Deaux

The Concept of Identity   77
Dimensions and Categories of Identity   79
Structure and Hierarchy   80
Descriptive Work on Identity   81
Salience of Identities   84
Identity and Change   86
Constructing Social Identities   90
Concluding Thoughts   91
Acknowledgments   91
References   91

6. An Ecological Perspective on the Self-Concept   **94**
Stefan E. Hormuth

Definition and Theoretical Development of the Self   94
The Social–Ecological Approach   95
Overview of the Research Program   96
Conditions for Stability and Change: Commitment   98
Operationalizations of Commitment   99
Summary of the Theory   101
The Role of Things in Self-Concept Change   102
Pictures of the Ecology of the Self: Autophotography   103
Variability of Behavior   106
Predictors of the Course of Adaptation   106
Conclusion   107
References   108

III. INTEGRATIVE APPROACHES FROM CLINICAL PSYCHOLOGY AND PSYCHOANALYSIS 109

7. Cognitive–Experiential Self-Theory: An Integrative Theory of Personality 111
Seymour Epstein

Introduction 111
Comparison of Basic Assumptions in CEST and
 Psychoanalysis 113
The Basic Theory 117
Evidence for the Existence of a Separate Experiential
 Conceptual System 124
Implications 133
Acknowledgments 135
References 136

8. Seeing with the Third Eye: Cognitive–Affective Regulation and the Acquisition of Self-Knowledge 138
Rebecca C. Curtis and Garry Zaslow

Knowledge of the Physical Self: Self-Recognition 140
Knowledge of the Aware Self: "Objective"
 Self-Awareness 140
Knowledge of One's Strengths and Weaknesses 142
Knowledge of One's Emotional States 145
Self-Knowledge in Psychoanalytic and Experiential
 Psychotherapies, Existential Philosophy, and Zen
 Buddhism: The Disintegration of the Self 149
The Magical Apples of the Human Psyche 152
References 154

9. The Self in Cross-Civilizational Perspective: An Indian–Japanese–American Comparison 160
Alan Roland

Comparative Conceptualizations of the Self 160
Psychosocial Dimensions of Hierarchical
 Relationships 163
Suborganizations of the Familial Self 165
The Spiritual Self 174
The Expanding Self 176
Acknowledgment 178
References 178

10. Cultural, Emotional, and Unconscious Aspects of Self   181
Drew Westen

The Multiple Meanings of "Self": Distinguishing Conscious
   and Unconscious Aspects of Self   183
Affect, Discrepancies, and Self-Schemas: The Motivational
   Properties of the "Self"   195
Methodological Implications   201
Culture, Self, and the Role of Technological
   Development   203
References   206

IV. INTEGRATIVE APPROACHES FROM SOCIAL AND
PERSONALITY PSYCHOLOGY   211

11. Psychotherapy, Self-Concept Change, and Self-Verification   213
Shawn E. McNulty and William B. Swann, Jr.

The Pleasure Principle and Self-Enhancement Processes   214
Self-Defeating Behavior and Self-Consistency Strivings   215
Self-Verification Theory   218
Therapy: Eluding the Crossfire between Self-Enhancement
   and Self-Verification   222
Summary and Conclusions   232
Notes   232
References   233

12. The Self against Itself: Escape or Defeat?   238
Roy F. Baumeister

Roots of Self-Defeating Behavior   239
The Burden of Self   242
Varieties of Escape   246
Conclusion   252
References   253

13. Social versus Clinical Approaches to Self Psychology:
The Self-Evaluation Maintenance Model and Kohutian
Object Relations Theory   257
Abraham Tesser

The Basic Assumptions and Processes   258
Dynamics   268
The Awareness Issue   273
Questions of Epistemology   274
Clinical Implications   275

A Concluding Observation   276
Acknowledgments   277
Notes   277
References   278

14. Self-with-Other Representation as a Unit of Analysis in Self-Concept Research   282

Daniel M. Ogilvie and Richard D. Ashmore

Introduction   282
An Overview of Modern Research on the Self   283
Self-with-Other as a Unit of Analysis   286
Toward a Theory of Self-with-Other Representations   289
Methods and Procedures   291
Purposes behind Sessions 1 through 4   296
Structural Representations of Matrices   299
Beyond Case Studies: Nomothetic Prospects   308
A Brief Recapitulation   310
Acknowledgment   311
Notes   311
References   312

Index   315

Current Perspectives from Psychoanalytic Self Psychology

The first contributions to this volume present the point of view of two contemporary theorists in self psychology. The chapter by Josephs provides a review of psychoanalytic theories of character "structure." Josephs focuses upon the maintenance of an identity theme and, like many thinkers in clinical psychology, upon the resistance to change. He sees the therapist as able to facilitate variations around the theme, using as an example the tendency of the obsessive–compulsive personality to be obedient and self-controlled in order to obtain love. As has been the tradition in psychoanalytically oriented clinical psychology and psychiatry, Josephs emphasizes relatively stable and enduring personality dispositions, which become more rigid when threats to identity are triggered.

Stolorow provides a more interactional view of the self, closer in this respect to the viewpoints of the other authors in this volume. As Stolorow describes the self-psychological theory of the mind, experience is composed of relational configurations and is constituted in the infant by the interplay of differently organized subjectivities. Motivation is viewed as depending upon the affective interchanges between infants and caregivers, not upon instinctual drives. According to this perspective on the self, unintegrated affect states are experienced as threats to the self-organization and become the source of lifelong conflicts. Stolorow presents the traditional point of view of psychoanalysts that the in-depth case study will continue to be the primary method of research regarding analytic theory. His "intersubjective" approach recognizes, however, that the self-organization of the therapist must change in order for the affect in the patient to become integrated—an acknowledgment that may seem long overdue by those outside the psychoanalytic community, but one that apparently differs enough from the orientation of some Freudians to warrant comment. The example Stolorow provides of a therapeutic "impasse" demonstrates how the therapist had to learn to tolerate his own painful feelings, in order to enable his patient to integrate hers.

Current Perspectives from Psychoanalytic Self Psychology

Character Structure, Self-Esteem Regulation, and the Principle of Identity Maintenance

LAWRENCE JOSEPHS

INTRODUCTION

The term "character" possesses a psychological, a literary, and a moral meaning in everday discourse. From the psychological perspective, "character" is synonymous with the term "personality" and refers to those distinguishing attributes that comprise a person's individuality. The assumption is that individuals display temporal stability and cross-situational consistency in their personal conduct. Stability and consistency at the level of overt behavior are presumed to reflect the operation of underlying organizational principles that account for the inner logic and coherence of personal conduct. From a literary perspective, "character" reflects a role in a storyline; the assumption is that individuals never act out of character, whether they are heroes or villains. Character is a predictor of one's fate or destiny, as character is the driving force that shapes the unfolding narrative. From a moral perspective, the term "character" refers to one's sense of personal integrity or lack of it, one's inner strength or weakness. Whether character portraiture is a crude caricature reflecting personal prejudice or an astute description with empathy for human imperfection, there appears to be a human tendency to approach the understanding of human individuality in terms of the notion of character.

THE PSYCHODYNAMIC MODEL OF CHARACTER STRUCTURE

Freud illustrated his view of human character in his clinical case histories. He often worried that his case histories read more like novellas than scientific investigations. Yet he believed that only the case history format could do justice to his findings, which required the elucidation of the private life of the individual in great detail. Freud attempted to demonstrate that neurotic symptoms are not so much aberrant manifestations of an otherwise normal personality, but rather that they are disguised expressions of the person's deepest wishes and fears, and in that sense not out of character at all. Freud (1900) believed that human character possesses a surface dimension that is accessible to conscious awareness and a depth dimension that is inaccessible to conscious awareness. The dynamic unconscious includes those aspects of oneself that are considered unacceptable and are therefore repudiated, disavowed, and disclaimed. In contrast, those aspects of oneself that are judged to be socially acceptable are accessible to consciousness. Freud (1900) hypothesized that an inner censor edits one's thoughts, feelings, and fantasies, so that what is accessible to conscious awareness is only the news that is fit to print, so to speak—those items not subject to repression.

Those thoughts, feelings, memories, fantasies, and wishes that have been banished from awareness nevertheless strive for expression, so that there is a perennial intrapsychic conflict between the censor and the representatives of free speech attempting to evade censorship. The final result is a compromise in which even the most repudiated aspects of ourselves partially evade censorship and are expressed in a disguised and concealed manner—what Freud (1900) called the "return of the repressed." Unconscious psychic content may slip past the censor if it is expressed in symbolic form. Symbolization allows meaning to be concealed from the literal-minded but revealed to those open to the metaphorical meaning of the symbol.

To illustrate the Freudian theory of character structure, the obsessive–compulsive personality is used as a case example. The obsessive–compulsive personality has been described as someone who is characteristically overly organized, dutiful, work-oriented, conscientious, disciplined, perfectionistic, rule-bound, detail-oriented, and concerned with propriety, control, and achievement. Privately, such individuals are likely to be fault-finding, self-doubting, self-critical, worrying, needy of approval, fearful of disapproval, guilt-ridden, and frightened of expressing hostility. Interpersonally, they tend to be inflexible, formal, pedantic, dogmatic, serious, and lacking in spontaneity.

Freud (1908) suggested that this overt display of compliance, orderliness, and dutifulness is in fact a disguised expression of the polar opposite trend—an unconscious defiance, resentment, hostility, and sadism. The censor, judging defiance and hostility to be unacceptable for open expression, attempts to repudiate these attitudes and in fact replaces them with their opposites, as if to say, "I am not a defiant person—look how obedient and eager to please I really am." Nevertheless, excessive obedience to the rules can become irritating and exasperating to others. Rigidity in the name of doing things the right way imposes a harsh and impersonal discipline on those who are expected to go by the book. The perfectionistic imposition of rules, though overtly presented as for the others' own good, may covertly express an intolerant and abusive attitude. Thus Freud painted a multidimensional picture of the obsessive–compulsive personality: Though overtly a model citizen, a paragon of conscientiousness, and a humble person always trying to do better, at an unconscious level the obsessive–compulsive person is defiant, sadistic, domineering, and controlling. The overt persona is a false self disguising the person's true intent, which is hidden from himself as well as from others.

If the obsessive–compulsive person were to be confronted with this picture of himself, he would be shocked and hurt, and would rise in protest of an unfair character assassination as if to say, "Me a sadist? I'm only trying to be helpful. Me defiant? I always obey the letter of the law, no matter how burdensome a chore it is. Me bent upon domination and control? I'm always meeting the expectations of others rather than my own." For Freud, the conscious and unconscious aspects of the personality reflect a dialectic—a dynamic tension between aspects of the self in polar opposition to each other. For the obsessive–compulsive person, the core dialectic is the conflict between compliance and defiance. Freud believed that character description remains superficial as long as it focuses only upon overt behavior and conscious experience. To understand a person in depth, one must grasp unconscious motivation and conflict. Nevertheless, many if not all individuals struggle with conflicts between compliance and defiance. Some individuals are open rebels, whereas others engage in sit-down strikes. Some individuals become mindless conformists or subservient slaves, but do not display any obsession with following the rules or a compulsion to be perfectionistically well organized. It is unique to the obsessive–compulsive personality to resolve the conflict between defiance and compliance with the paradoxical solution of turning complete self-control into the highest virtue.

In the 1920s Freud moved from id psychology, the study of unconscious motivation, to ego psychology, the study of unconscious defense mechanisms. According to Freud (1923), the id appears to be universal, more or less the same from individual to individual: Love, sexuality, dependency, competitiveness, aggression, and so on appear to constitute universal human passions. Everyone seems to share the same needs, desires, and fears in common. What distinguishes one individual from another is not so much the underlying conflict as the particular manner of defending against the intrapsychic conflicts that constitute the human condition. Everyone has conflicts about defiance and compliance, but perhaps only the obsessive–compulsive personality defends against that conflict through such a heightened emphasis upon self-control.

Wilhelm Reich (1933) coined the term "character armor" to capture the notion that character reflects an overarching strategy of defense. "Character armor" is a holistic concept because what is protected is the whole person. The word "armor" as a metaphor suggests a hard protective covering that protects the whole person from head to toe, so to speak. Reich proposed that character armor is a narcissistic defense of the ego— that character armor protects the sense of self. Perhaps what distinguishes one character type from another is the nature of the overarching strategy of defense through which each type protects this sense of self.

Reich (1933) viewed character armor as multilayered. The surface dimension of character armor is reflected in the person's verbal self-presentation, whereas the deeper dimensions of character armor are reflected in nonverbally conveyed attitudes—what has come to be known as "body language." If we return to our example of the obsessive–compulsive personality, we can see that the obsessive–compulsive's overarching strategy of self-defense is to maintain complete self-control. If the obsessive–compulsive is frightened of his competitiveness, he controls himself; if he is frightened of his sexuality, he controls himself; if he is frightened of his hostility, he controls himself; and if he is frightened of his dependency needs, he controls himself. No matter what the conflict or anxiety, it is defended against through improved and intensified efforts at self-control. Reich called obsessive–compulsive characters "living machines." Total self-control to the obsessive–compulsive person is an all-purpose solution to the problems of living, a sort of philosophy of life. As a consequence, the obsessive–compulsive person puts all his energies into constantly anticipating worst-case scenarios and continually planning as preparation for potential disaster management, so that he will never be surprised or taken off guard by something beyond his control, whether that "something" consists of his own feelings and needs or of unforeseen external events.

In 1939, when Heinz Hartmann published *Ego Psychology and the Problem of Adaptation*, ego psychology shifted from a predominant focus on unconscious defense mechanisms to a focus on the ego as an agency of adaptation to external reality. Prior to the adaptive viewpoint, character formation was understood as an essentially reactive, defensive, and compensatory process. Character structure was thought to emerge in reaction to frustration, in avoidance of anxiety, and in compensation for perceived deficiencies. From the adaptive point of view, character formation could be conceptualized as a progressive and goal-directed process. The goal of character development is to adapt to the demands of external reality, progressively achieving higher levels of adaptive fit to the environment. Ego functions such as judgment, planning, anticipation, reality testing, problem solving, abstraction, symbolization, and so on constitute some of the cognitive operations through which the person adapts to external reality. Character style could be reconceptualized as the particular strategy of adaptation to external reality. Since adaptation is reliant upon the cognitive operations through which adaptation transpires, character style could be construed as a cognitive style. This is the point of view that Shapiro adopted in his 1965 classic, *Neurotic Styles*.

Shapiro (1965) portrayed the obsessive–compulsive personality as possessing a cognitive style characterized by the persistent tendency to deploy an intense, sharp focus of attention that concentrates upon the fine details of experience. The obsessive–compulsive person is perennially examining details. The obsessive–compulsive experiences a continuous sense of tense deliberateness and a constant sense of effort, of constantly trying. Such an intense focus of attention gives rise to a style of thinking that tends to be analytical, reductionistic, critical, and dogmatic; a style of affective experience that is constricted, controlled, and lacking in spontaneity; and a style of relating to others that is overly formal, rigid, and concerned with rules of propriety. This characteristic mode of adaptive functioning can result in a high capacity for achievement, stubborn perseverance in the face of adversity, superior analytical problem-solving skills, and a capacity to assume a considerable burden of responsibility and execute it successfully in a highly organized and disciplined manner. This mode of functioning may prove maladaptive if perfectionism leads to excessive self-doubt and indecision, if being rule-oriented becomes rigid inflexibility, and if over-formality stifles the spontaneous give and take of normal social discourse. Under conditions of stress, such a style of adaptation could be deployed self-protectively as a defensive style. If the obsessive–compulsive person feels overwhelmed by the anxiety of keeping everything under control, then the defensive solution is just to keep trying even harder until everything is totally under control.

THE PSYCHOLOGY OF SELF-ESTEEM REGULATION

Ego psychology looked at the problem of adaptation without much specification of the nature of the particular external reality or environment to which the person must adjust. Harry Stack Sullivan (1953) suggested that the fundamental reality to which humans must adapt is the particular sociocultural environment into which they are born. Character formation is a particular type of adaptation; specifically, it is an interpersonal adaptation designed to help one fit into the social organization of which one is a part. Character style is then always an interpersonal style, a strategy of relating to others so that one will fit in and be accepted. Presumably, the obsessive–compulsive person is raised in a family that emphasizes obedience, compliance, following the rules, and self-control. The child becomes the sort of obedient, compliant, dutiful, and self-controlled person the parents expect the child to be, in order to please them and win their approval. For Sullivan, the basis of self-esteem is being approved of and accepted by others. As an adult, the obsessive–compulsive person hopes to gain status and acceptance in the adult world through obedience, compliance, and dutiful execution of the rules of proper conduct.

Karen Horney (1950) also assumed an interpersonal view of character structure, but with a slightly different emphasis from Sullivan's. Horney did not view the child as quite so accommodating and eager to fit in, but rather as possessing a unique, "real self" with innate potentialities whose actualization constitutes the purpose of life. The child cannot actualize its potentialities on its own, but requires parents who recognize the child's innate talents, encourage those talents, and facilitate their development. If the parents fail to appreciate the child's innate potentialities and expect the child to conform to their expectations instead, the child's real self will fail to develop naturally and wholesomely, and innate potentialities will remain unrealized. In response to the injury to the child's real self, the child develops neurotic self-idealization, as if to say, "If I can't be accepted for being the real me, I'll get even by being superior to everyone, for whom I'll have contempt." If the parents fail to validate the child's real self, neurotic self-hatred develops, as if to say, "If my parents don't love me, than I must be a really terrible person."

From the Horneyian point of view, the obsessive–compulsive person is someone with a strong innate capacity to master external reality. The real self of the obsessive–compulsive person is bright, curious, and questioning; is eager to find solutions to problems; and delights in the pleasure of mastery. As such, the real self of the obsessive–compulsive appears to constitute a healthy, wholesome, and adaptive potential. When the parents fail to cultivate such a real self, whether through neglect or through overly strict discipline to which the child must conform, the real self becomes impoverished and a compensatory false self takes its place. Brightness is turned into the need to be omniscient. Curiosity is turned into the need never to be taken by surprise and to figure everything out in advance. A questioning attitude is turned into relentless finding of faults. An orientation toward problem solving turns into constant worrying in anticipating the worst and planning for every conceivable disaster. Pleasure in mastery is turned into a quest for omnipotent control. Failure to be omniscient and omnipotently self-controlled leads to feelings of self-hatred for being weak, helpless, impotent, and out of control.

Josephs (1991) has suggested that Sullivan and Horney, taken together, highlight a dialectical tension in the interpersonal maintenance of self-esteem. On the one hand, self-esteem is based upon fitting in, being accepted, pleasing others, and gaining approval for meeting the expectations of others. On the other hand, self-esteem is based upon realizing one's unique potentialities; being an individual in one's own right; and having others recognize, respect, affirm, support, and encourage one's personal talents and individual uniqueness. Self-esteem based predominantly upon fitting in can lead to a sense of mindless conformity, false-self compliance, and overdependency on others for guidance and approval. Self-esteem based predominantly upon cultivating one's individuality may lead to a feeling that one is so completely unique that one is unlike anyone else. This results in feelings of social alienation. There is an inability to achieve mutuality in relationships, which requires an acknowledgment of commonality with the other; consequently, there is resentment of the world for insufficient provision of adoration and admiration. A balance must be achieved between fitting in and being an individual in one's own right. The obsessive–compulsive person has significant difficulty in achieving stable self-esteem regulation because of an inability to achieve a dynamic balance between these two trends. The obsessive–compulsive tries to fit in and gain approval through obedience and compliance, yet feels humiliated by the loss of self-respect in being so ingratiating, obsequious, and submissive. Yet when the obsessive–compulsive person feels defiant, wanting to stand up to authority in order to express individuality and self-respect, there is a terrible sense of guilt, fear of hurting the other, and loss of approval. To be successfully self-assertive may mean to risk ending a relationship with someone whose approval was highly valued.

Heinz Kohut (1977), the founder of psychoanalytic self psychology, integrated these two dimensions of self-esteem regulation in his theory of the "bipolar self." The two poles of the self are "nuclear ambitions" on the one side and "nuclear ideals" on the other. Nuclear ambitions derive from the fundamental need to experience oneself as a unique individual in one's own right, whereas nuclear ideals derive from a fundamental need to feel an integral and valued part of someone or something greater than oneself. Kohut described a developmental progression of those two fundamental needs. The fundamental need to be an individual in one's own right is expressed in childhood in illusions of omnipotence and grandeur. The acquisition of realistic mastery is experienced as if one were all-powerful without limits. The acquisition of knowledge is experienced as if one were all-knowing without areas of ignorance. The possession of the love of others is experienced as though one were the most lovable person in the world without imperfection.

In normal development, such grandiose illusions about oneself are gradually relinquished in favor of a more realistic self-assessment. In pathology, such illusions are maintained and become the basis for a pathological form of self-esteem regulation based upon the notion of one's intrinsic superiority and entitlement to special treatment. The fundamental need to be a valued part of someone greater than oneself is experienced in childhood in the form of viewing one's parents as the most powerful, knowledgeable, loving, and wonderful parents in the world, and believing that to be cared for by these perfect parents provides the greatest bliss, security, protection, and guidance. In normal development, one gradually becomes disillusioned with one's parents, learns to love them despite their flaws, and learns to recreate the sense of being part of something greater than oneself in living by one's ideals. In pathology, the archaic idealization of authority figures is maintained and forms the basis of a pathological form of self-esteem regulation based upon selfless surrender and mindless conformity to the expectations of domineering, controlling, and abusive others.

The obsessive–compulsive person can be understood as continuing to live in a world of archaic illusions. The belief that obedient, compliant, and dutiful submission to the expectations of idealized authority figures will gain security and love proves to be rather naive, as others are likely either to exploit or to have contempt for someone as obsequious as the obsessive–compulsive person. The obsessive–compulsive person's belief in his superior critical faculties, his superior capacity for self-control, and the admiration that these abilities should earn also proves naive, because others become exasperated and irritated with the obsessive–compulsive's relentless finding of faults and attention to minor details, as well as his inflexible, rigid, and controlling manner of relating. Thus, illusions of gaining the approval of idealized authority figures and of proudly exhibiting one's superior critical faculties and self-control are continually punctured and deflated, resulting in a traumatic loss of self-esteem.

The obsessive–compulsive experiences narcissistic decompensation in the form of tortured self-doubts, relentless worry about future catastrophes, and fears of suffering a humiliating defeat at the hands of punitive authority figures. This traumatic blow to the obsessive–compulsive's illusory sense of self also results in narcissistic rage, which takes the form of defiance, vindictiveness, and hatred. Yet, since such hostility provokes considerable guilt out of a fear of hurting those whose approval is desperately required, such hostility is repudiated and expressed covertly. Despite the suffering that holding on to illusions about the self entails, the obsessive–compulsive person nevertheless attempts to restore a sense of self-esteem through intensified efforts (1) to restore illusions of gaining love through obedience, and (2) to restore pride in the self through exhibition of superior critical faculties and superior self-control. The obsessive–compulsive person does not seem to learn from experience.

THE PRINCIPLE OF IDENTITY MAINTENANCE

Why is it that self-defeating illusions are reinstated so reflexively and that there seems to be a failure to learn from experience, despite the fact that the obsessive–compulsive person regularly fails to obtain the interpersonal approval and admiration he so eagerly seeks? If obsessive–compulsive behavior constitutes an interpersonal strategy for fitting in, and if it fails miserably at that task, then why doesn't the person simply switch to a more adaptive strategy that is more finely attuned to the interpersonal demands of the current life situation? Freud (1920) called this phenomenon of constantly repeating self-defeating patterns of behavior the "repetition compulsion." The repetition compulsion perplexed Freud, for he believed that human behavior is organized according to two principles: (1) the pleasure principle and (2) the reality principle. The repetition compulsion appears to be beyond the pleasure principle. Why should someone constantly repeat a pattern of functioning that brings pain rather than pleasure and proves to be maladaptive in terms of adjustment to external reality? Freud (1920) speculated that perhaps there is a death instinct in which aggression is regularly unleashed upon the self. Though human beings show abundant evidence of self-destructiveness in their conduct, most psychoanalysts have found Freud's theory of a death instinct to be untenable.

What is it that preserves the stability of human character at different times and in different places, even when that character style proves maladaptive in terms of the current interpersonal reality? Freud used the term "resistance" to describe the difficulty of changing human character. If one never acts out of character, how can one's character be changed? Freud's (1905) first theory of resistance was the theory of psychosexual fixation points. According to this theory, if one is either overly gratified or overly frustrated at any point in development, one becomes fixated on the pleasures and attachments characteristic of that stage of development. Presumably, the obsessive–compulsive is fixated at the anal stage of psychosexual development. Overly strict toilet training was thought to result in outwardly excessive obedience to authority, which masks underlying defiance. Freud's (1926) second theory of resistance was that people resist change because change is anxiety-arousing. According to this theory, character structure reflects a defensive attitude in the service of anxiety avoidance. For example, as long as the obsessive–compulsive person can feel sure of following the rules and being in full self-control, then the anxiety of losing control, of being punished for breaking the rules, and of suffering a humiliating defeat can be avoided.

Nevertheless, clinging to infantile gratifications and anxiety avoidance do not seem to account fully for the phenomenon of repeating self-defeating characterological patterns. After all, self-defeating patterns of behavior are not particularly gratifying and arouse considerable anxiety. What would make someone hold on to a pattern of behavior that is unpleasurable and anxiety-arousing, given that there is clearly a human tendency to be pleasure-seeking and anxiety-avoiding? What human tendency may be more powerful than pleasure seeking and anxiety avoidance? Bowlby's (1969) studies of human attachment in the first years of life suggested that the need to be related and attached to a primary caretaker is a fundamental human need. Fairbairn (1952) suggested that children would rather maintain an attachment to a depriving or abusive parent than have no parent at all to whom to be attached. Though the obsessive–compulsive person may have resented the parent's authoritarian child-rearing practices, the obsessive–compulsive person nevertheless maintains a loyal attachment to such authoritarian parents rather than have no parents at all to whom to relate.

Resistance to change, then, is like preserving a family tradition out of a sense of loyalty to old attachments, no matter how unhappy those attachments may have been. One recreates the past in the present; no matter how unpleasant that recreation may be, at least it is familiar. It is the sense of familiarity, of stability, and of constancy that provides the sense of security, for which a certain degree of deprivation, suffering, and anxiety will be willingly endured. To the degree that one can choose the interpersonal environment in which one will live, one can recreate the past in the present by choosing to live in an interpersonal environment that recreates the family of origin. Thus, obsessive–compulsive individuals tend to choose careers (e.g., accounting, law, computer programming, scientific research, etc.) that are exceedingly rule-bound, recreating the rule-bound atmosphere of their childhoods. The rule orientation of the workplace reinforces and sustains obsessive–compulsive character traits.

Despite the obsessive–compulsive's effort to recreate the past in the present through selecting familiar interpersonal environments in which to live and provoking others to treat him as his parents treated him, more often than not he must learn to adapt to an environment quite dissimilar to the one in which he was raised, given that people's control over their environment is quite limited in many ways. Especially in the modern world, the culture in which a person was raised is likely to seem quite outdated in the culture 20 to 50 years later, to which that person must adapt as an adult. Despite the interpersonal pressure to change with the changing times, character structure tends to resist such change as though it were a form of selling out, of betraying the family tradition. The need to maintain a sense of self-sameness, to remain in touch with one's roots, represents a conservative force in personality organization.

This sense of self-sameness, self-continuity, self-stability, self-consistency, and self-cohesiveness is what Erik Erikson (1959) called the sense of "identity." For Erikson, identity formation and identity maintenance constitute the superordinate organizers of personality functioning. Experiencing oneself as a whole person rather than as divided and fragmented, and experiencing oneself as possessing some familiar sense of self-sameness despite changing times and changing situational contexts, capture that phenomenological thread of experience within the stream of consciousness that constitutes the sense of identity.

Lichtenstein (1975) hypothesized that the principle of identity maintenance is the crucial organizing principle in personality functioning:

> Psychoanalytic evidence makes it also probable that the maintenance of identity in man has priority over any other principle determining human behavior, not only the reality principle but also the pleasure principle. (p. 59)

> Identity establishment and maintenance must be considered basic biological principles—principles defining the concept of living matter itself. As soon as a living organism ceases to maintain its identity we speak of its decay. (p. 114)

From the perspective of the principle of identity maintenance, the obsessive–compulsive person remains obsessive–compulsive because that is who he is. The obsessive–compulsive person is one whose sense of identity is to be loved for being obedient and admired for being self-controlled.

The dynamic organization of the particular character style is based upon what Lichtenstein (1975) calls an "identity theme" (p. 78), which evolves out of the mother–infant interaction in the first years of life.

> The child is the organ, the instrument for the fulfillment of the mother's unconscious needs. Out of the infinite potentialities within the human infant, the specific stimulus combination emanating from the individual mother "releases" one, and only one, concrete way of being this organ. . . . The mother imprints upon the infant not an identity but an "identity theme." This theme is irreversible, but it is capable of variations, variations that spell the difference between creativity and a destiny neurosis. (p. 78)

An identity theme, like a musical theme, possesses a distinctive essence; yet almost an infinite number of variations on a theme could potentially be derived from a single identity theme.

The concept of identity points to the functioning of the whole person as an integrated unit, yet Freud demonstrated how deeply conflicted and divided humans tend to be. What is the relationship between the conscious yet prereflective sense of identity and the Freudian unconscious of conflicting passions? If the actualization and maintenance of the core identity theme constitute the organizing force in personality functioning, then the loss of the sense of identity is perhaps the most disorganizing force in the personality. It is apparent that the current interpersonal environment either supports or opposes the person's sense of identity. To the degree that the interpersonal surround undermines the sense of identity, there is a threat of identity loss. The anticipation of loss of identity, of becoming disorganized and disintegrated, triggers defensive and compensatory operations in order to ward off threats to the sense of identity and to repair whatever damage has occurred.

It is easy to see how external forces may oppose the sense of identity, but are there inner forces that undermine the establishment of a sense of identity from within? The establishment of an identity theme requires certain innate potentials to be selectively cultivated and other potentials to be selectively neglected and suppressed. The unconscious can be understood as all those aspects of the self that by virtue of being incompatible with the predominant identity theme are selectively repudiated, disavowed, and disclaimed (Josephs, 1991). If one's identity theme is to be a saint, then any aspect of the self that even faintly seems to be a sinner is a threat to that identity theme and therefore must be repudiated. Repudiated aspects of the self nevertheless may demand conscious representation, especially when environmental triggers provoke that aspect of self. It may be difficult to maintain an image of oneself as a saint in the face of temptations to be a sinner that evoke a less spiritual aspect of the self. Thus there is a threat of identity loss any time a repudiated aspect of self threatens to enter conscious awareness. Of course, the greater the degree to which repudiated aspects of self can be integrated into the consciously maintained identity theme, the greater the stability of the personality.

Let us return to our case example, the obsessive–compulsive character. If the identity theme of the obsessive–compulsive is to be loved for being obedient and admired for being self-controlled, then which aspects of the self would need to be repudiated by virtue of seeming irreconcilable with this predominant identity theme? Whatever trend proves to be in polar opposition to the predominant identity theme is what will prove irreconcilable with that identity theme necessitating repudiation. The polar opposite of being loved for being obedient is to be hated for being defiant, and the polar opposite of being admired for being self-controlled is to be held in contempt for being weak-willed and poorly controlled. Thus the unconscious trends that the obsessive–compulsive must disavow are aspects of the self that appear either defiant or weak. If self-assertiveness is construed as willful disobedience, and if needs for nurturance are construed as a shameful weakness of will, then self-assertiveness and needs for affection will be repudiated as well. To the degree that the obsessive–compulsive person can learn that self-assertiveness and desires for affection are not entirely incompatible with dutifulness and self-control, then the sense of identity can be enriched and expanded. To the extent that the obsessive–compulsive person can learn that occasional acts of overt defiance or the momentary exposure of a weakness of will do not completely undermine the predominant identity theme of being dutiful and self-controlled, then the person may function more flexibly and adaptively.

CONCLUSION

A model of character structure that highlights the principle of identity maintenance has implications for dynamic psychotherapy, which focuses on facilitating character change. If one never acts out of character, how is it that psychotherapy can effect a change in character? If a particular character style reflects a particular identity theme, and if that theme may be played out according to a number of variations, then the therapist may serve as a sort of co-composer who accepts the basic theme as a starting point but helps the patient learn to improvise around the identity theme in ever more creative ways, instead of playing out that theme in the most routine and repetitive manner. From this perspective, resistance to change results not so much from clinging to infantile ways in a refusal to grow up, or from a defensive, self-deceptive attitude that leads to a distorted view of reality. Rather, resistance to change is resistance to whatever opposes the actualization of the predominant identity theme. That identity theme may be relatively difficult to actualize, if not an impossible dream; however, perhaps it is not the therapist's role to stand in judgment upon the feasibility of realizing that particular identity theme. Instead, the therapist may empathize with the frustration and disappointment evoked in the patient's realization that he may be imprinted with an identity theme that proves impossible to actualize fully in real life.

In conclusion, the identity theme points toward an ideal—the ideal self one wishes to become in the future. Like all ideals, it gives meaning, purpose, and direction to life, regardless of whether or not it ever materializes in reality. In that sense, the ideal self dictated by the identity theme—the self one would be if all innate potentials were fully realized—stands as a guiding light that shapes and organizes personal conduct. Who one is in the moment is shaped by who one hopes to become in the future, and in this sense character is destiny.

REFERENCES

Bowlby, J. (1969). *Attachment and loss: Vol. 1. Attachment.* New York: Basic Books.

Erikson, E. (1959). *Identity and the life cycle.* New York: Norton.

Fairbairn, W. R. D. (1952). *Psychoanalytic studies of the personality* London: Routledge & Kegan Paul.

Freud, S. (1900). The interpretation of dreams. *Standard Edition, 4,* 1–338; *5,* 339–627.

Freud, S. (1905). Three essays on the theory of sexuality. *Standard Edition, 7,* 125–245.

Freud, S. (1908). Character and anal erotism. *Standard Edition, 9,* 169–175.

Freud, S. (1920). Beyond the pleasure principle. *Standard Edition, 18*, 3–64.

Freud, S. (1923). The ego and the id. *Standard Edition, 19*, 1–66.

Freud, S. (1926). Inhibitions, symptoms and anxiety. *Standard Edition, 20*, 77–175.

Hartmann, H. (1939). *Ego psychology and the problem of adaptation.* New York: International Universities Press.

Horney, K. (1950). *Neurosis and human growth.* New York: Norton.

Josephs, L. (1991). *Character structure and the organization of the self.* New York: Columbia University Press.

Kohut, H. (1977). *The restoration of the self.* New York: International Universities Press.

Lichtenstein, H. (1975). *The dilemma of human identity.* New York: Jason Aronson.

Reich, W. (1933). *Character analysis.* New York: Orgone Institute Press, 1949.

Shapiro, D. (1965). *Neurotic styles.* New York: Basic Books.

Sullivan, H. S. (1953). *The interpersonal theory of psychiatry.* New York: Norton.

CHAPTER TWO

The Intersubjective Context of Intrapsychic Experience, with Special Reference to Therapeutic Impasses

ROBERT D. STOLOROW

[A]nalysis . . . must turn from the study of Freud
to the study of man.
— KOHUT (1982, p. 405)

To my mind, the most important development in psychoanalysis in recent years has been the growing recognition that intrapsychic phenomena must be understood in the context of the larger interactional systems in which they take form. Evidence of this trend can be found in the increasingly frequent appearance in the psychoanalytic literature of such terms as *"self–selfobject relationship"* (Kohut, 1984), *"two-person psychology"* (Modell, 1984), *"relational matrix"* (Mitchell, 1988), *"mutual influence structures"* (Beebe & Lachmann, 1988a, 1988b), and *"intersubjective context"* (Atwood & Stolorow, 1984; Stolorow, Brandchaft, & Atwood, 1987). This recognition of the broader context of intrapsychic experience holds critical implications for each of the three interrelated psychoanalytic domains envisioned by Freud: psychoanalysis as a theory of the mind, as a research method, and as a form of therapy.

PSYCHOANALYSIS AS A THEORY OF THE MIND

In psychoanalytic theory, the ascension of "relational-model" theories of the mind has been aptly described by Mitchell (1988):

> In this vision the basic unit of study is not the individual as a separate entity whose desires clash with an external reality, but an interactional

field within which the individual arises and struggles to make contact and to articulate himself. *Desire* is experienced always *in the context of relatedness*, and it is that context which defines its meaning. Mind is composed of relational configurations. . . . Experience is understood as structured through interactions. . . . (pp. 3–4, emphasis in original)

This same vision has been captured succinctly by both Loewald (1988) and Kohut (1984): "The origin of individual psychic life . . . is a *transindividual field*, represented by the mother/infant matrix, not an individual unconscious and instincts residing in an individual" (Loewald, 1988, pp. 50–51, emphasis added); "self–selfobject relationships form the essence of psychological life from birth to death" (Kohut, 1984, p. 47).

Nowhere can the growing appreciation of the intersubjective context of intrapsychic experience be seen more clearly than in psychoanalytic developmental psychology, which is being profoundly influenced by findings and concepts emerging from contemporary infancy research. Atwood and I (1984), in a chapter written in collaboration with Brandchaft, summarized the intersubjective perspective on psychological development:

[B]oth psychological development and pathogenesis are . . . conceptualized in terms of the specific intersubjective contexts that shape the developmental process and that facilitate or obstruct the child's negotiation of critical developmental tasks and successful passage through developmental phases. The observational focus is the evolving psychological field constituted by the interplay between the differently organized subjectivities of child and caretakers. (p. 65)

An impressive body of research evidence has recently been amassed to document that the developing organization of the child's experience must be seen as a property of the *child–caregiver system of mutual regulation* (see Lichtenberg, 1983, 1989; Sander, 1985, 1987; Stern, 1985, 1988; Beebe & Lachmann, 1988a, 1988b; Emde, 1988a, 1988b). According to Sander (1985, 1987), the infant–caregiver system is what regulates and organizes the infant's experience of inner states. The development of self-regulatory competence, therefore, is a *systems competence*. Stern (1985) has described in great detail the formation of various senses of self from the child's interactions with "self-regulating others." Beebe and Lachmann (1988a, 1988b) have shown that recurrent patterns of mutual influence between mother and infant provide the basis for the development of self- and object representations. They argue that in the earliest representations what is represented is "an emergent dyadic phenomenon, structures of the interaction, which cannot be described on the basis of either partner alone" (1988a, p. 305). A similar view of the interactional basis of psychic structure formation is implicit in Lichtenberg's (1989) discussion of the schemas or "scripts" that underlie the experience of various motivational systems, and in Emde's (1988a) description of personality structures developing from the internalization of "infant–caregiver relationship patterns." Each of these authors, in different language, is describing how recurring patterns of intersubjective transaction within the developmental system result in the establishment of invariant principles that unconsciously organize the child's subsequent experiences (Atwood & Stolorow, 1984; Stolorow et al., 1987). These unconscious ordering principles, crystallized within the matrix of the child–caregiver system, form the essential building blocks of personality development (Stolorow & Atwood, 1989).

I wish to emphasize that the intersubjective view of psychological development should not be confused with a naive environmentalism. Rather, it embraces what Wallace (1985) felicitously terms "intersectional causation." At any moment, the child's formative experiences are understood to emerge from the intersection of, and to be codetermined by, his psychological organization as it has evolved to that point and by specific features of the caregiving surround.

Studies of the vicissitudes of the developmental system are giving rise to a radically altered psychoanalytic theory of motivation. It is no longer satisfactory to view motivation in terms of the workings of a mental apparatus processing instinctual drive energies. Instead, it has increasingly come to be recognized, as Lichtenberg (1989) aptly argues, that "motivations arise solely from *lived experience*" and that "the vitality of the motivational experience will depend . . . on the manner in which affect-laden exchanges unfold between infants and their caregivers" (p. 2, emphasis in original). Most important, in my view, has been the shift from drive to affect as the central motivational construct for psychoanalysis (see Basch, 1984; Demos & Kaplan, 1986; Jones, 1989). Affectivity, we now know, is not a product of isolated intrapsychic mechanisms; it is a property of the child–caregiver system of mutual regulation (Sander, 1985; Rogawski, 1987; Demos, 1988). Stern (1985) has described in exquisite detail the regulation of affective experience within the infant–caregiver dyad through processes of intersubjective sharing and mutual affect attunement. The "affective core of the self" (Emde, 1988a) derives from the person's history of intersubjective transactions. Early developmental trauma, from this perspective, is viewed not as an instinctual flooding of an ill-equipped mental apparatus. Rather, the tendency for affective experiences to create a disorganized or disintegrated self-state is seen to originate from early faulty affect attunements—breakdowns of the infant–caregiver system—leading to the loss of affect-regulating capacity (Socarides & Stolorow, 1984–1985). These are the rock-bottom dangers for which later states of anxiety sound the alarm.

The shift from drive to affect leads inevitably to an intersubjective view of intrapsychic conflict formation:

> The specific intersubjective contexts in which conflict takes form are those in which central affect states of the child cannot be integrated because they fail to evoke the requisite attuned responsiveness from the caregiving surround. Such unintegrated affect states become the source of lifelong inner conflict, because they are experienced as threats both to the person's established psychological organization and to the maintenance of vitally needed ties. Thus affect-dissociating defensive operations are called into play, which reappear in the analytic situation in the form of resistance. A defensive self-ideal is often established, which represents the self purified of the "offending" affect states that were perceived as intolerable to the early surround . . . and the inability to fully embody this affectively purified ideal then becomes a continual source of shame and self-loathing. *It is in the defensive walling off of central affect states, rooted in early derailments of affect integration, that the origins of what has traditionally been called the "dynamic unconscious" can be found.* (Stolorow et al., 1987, pp. 91–92, emphasis added)

From this perspective, the dynamic unconscious is seen to consist not of repressed, endogenously arising drive derivatives, but of affect states that have been evoked and faultily responded to within the child–caregiver system, and then defensively sequestered in an attempt to protect against retraumatization. The boundary between conscious and unconscious is thus revealed to be a fluid one, a product of the varying attunement of the surround to different regions of the child's experience (Stolorow & Atwood, 1989). The idea of a shifting boundary forming within an intersubjective field contrasts sharply with the traditional notion of the repression barrier as a fixed intrapsychic structure permanently separating conscious and unconscious contents.

Defensive activities of all kinds are evoked by perceptions of the surround that lend themselves to the person's fears and anticipations of retraumatization. This was well understood by Kohut (1984), who wrote:

> Defense motivation . . . will be understood in terms of activities undertaken in the service of psychological survival, that is, as the patient's attempt to save at least that sector of his nuclear self, however small and precariously established it may be, that he has been able to construct and maintain despite serious insufficiencies in the development-enhancing matrix of the selfobjects of childhood. (p. 115)

In his studies of family relationships, Lansky (1985–1986, 1987) has delineated a number of "transpersonal defenses" evoked by situations of intense narcissistic injury and vulnerability. These defenses (blaming, impulsive action, preoccupation, and overt shaming) serve to regulate the emotional distance among family members, thereby protecting against intolerable experiences of disorganization and shame. Lansky's studies demonstrate both the intersubjective contexts in which defensive activities arise and the function of such defenses in readjusting the intersubjective system so that a sense of safety can be restored.

To summarize, from the perspective of the "relational-model" concepts pervading psychoanalytic theorizing during the past decade, psychological phenomena, including even unconscious conflicts and defenses, are understood as properties of an intersubjective system and thus as taking form at the interface of interacting subjectivities. Inexorably, we are led to question the very concept of an isolated mind or psyche—a foundational assumption of traditional psychoanalysis. It is my view that the concept of an isolated, individual mind is a theoretical fiction or myth, which reifies the subjective experience of psychological *distinctness* (Stolorow & Atwood, 1989). According to the theory of mind that I have been developing here, even the experience of distinctness requires a nexus of intersubjective relatedness that encourages and sustains the process of self-delineation throughout the life cycle (Stolorow et al., 1987). The experience of differentiated selfhood, in other words, is always embedded in a "living system" (Sander, 1985).

PSYCHOANALYSIS AS A RESEARCH METHOD

Psychoanalysis, in its essence, is a hermeneutic and historical science whose principal research method is and seems assured of remaining the in-depth case study (Atwood & Stolorow, 1984; Wallace, 1985). Most psychoanalytic case studies are conducted in concert with an ongoing psychoanalytic treatment and thus take form within a patient–analyst system of *mutual*-interaction (Wolf, 1984), in which each participant is affecting and interpreting the other's experience (Hoffman, 1983). The increasing appreciation of the intersubjective nature of psychoanalytic research has a profoundly relativizing impact on our conception of psychoanalytic understanding and knowledge.

One of the most important contributions of psychoanalytic self psychology has been the heightened attention to the impact of the analyst/observer on the field that he observes. Kohut (1984) drew a parallel between the shift from traditional analysis to self psychology and the shift from Newtonian physics to the Planckian physics of atomic and subatomic particles, in which "the field that is observed, of necessity, includes the observer" (p. 41). Whereas, according to Kohut, traditional analysis "sees the analyst only as the observer and the analysand only as the field that the observer-analyst surveys," the self-psychological orientation "acknowledges and then examines the analyst's influence . . . as an *intrinsically significant human presence*" (p. 37, emphasis added). Schwaber (1983) regards this proposed change in the analyst's listening stance as Kohut's most creative contribution:

> It is my view that the crucial dimension here was . . . that the understanding of the resistance had shifted from being viewed as a phenomenon arising from internal pressures within the patient, from which the analyst, as a blank screen, could stand apart and observe, to that in which *the specificity of the analyst's contribution was seen as intrinsic to its very nature*. (p. 381, emphasis added)

Like Kohut, Schwaber (1983) advocates a listening stance that recognizes "the impact of the analyst-observer as *intrinsic* to the field of observation" (p. 386, emphasis in original; see Meissner, 1989, and Langs, 1989, for further discussions of this issue).

Atwood and I (1984) have spelled out the implications of this ever-present impact of the observer on the observed for conceptualizing the conduct of a psychoanalytic case study:

> The varied patterns of meaning that emerge in psychoanalytic research are brought to light within a specific psychological field located at the point of intersection of two subjectivities. Because the dimensions and boundaries of this field are intersubjective in nature, the interpretive conclusions of every case study must, in a very profound sense, be understood as *relative* to the intersubjective context of their origin. . . . An appreciation of this dependence of psychoanalytic insight on a particular intersubjective interaction helps us to understand why the results of a case study may vary as a function of the person conducting it. Such variation, an anathema to the natural sciences, occurs because of the diverse perspectives of different investigators on material displaying an inherent plurality of meanings. (p. 6, emphasis in original)

Psychoanalytic understanding evolves from a process of dialogue between two personal universes (Leavy, 1980). The understanding that crystallizes in the course of a psychoanalytic case study is intersubjectively derived, codetermined by the organizing activities of both participants in the dialogue. Hence, it is essential that analysts continually strive to expand their reflective awareness of their own unconscious organizing principles, including especially those enshrined in their theories, so that the impact of those principles on the analytic process can be recognized and itself become a focus of analytic investigation. The domain of a psychoanalytic case study must, of necessity, include the entire intersubjective field created by the interplay between the subjective worlds of patient and analyst: "Patient and analyst together form an indissoluble psychological system, and it is this system that constitutes the empirical domain of psychoanalytic inquiry" (Atwood & Stolorow, 1984, p. 64).

PSYCHOANALYSIS AS A FORM OF THERAPY

Gill (1984) has highlighted the importance for the theory of psychoanalytic technique of recognizing the interactional context of intrapsychic experience:

> The increasing recognition that *all aspects of the analytic situation are contributed to by both parties*, in however varying proportions, must be taken into account in conceptualizing crucial psychoanalytic concepts like transference, free association, regression and the role of the experience of the relationship. (pp. 176–177, emphasis added)

This point is well illustrated in Gill's (1982, 1984) extensive discussions of the analysis of transference, in which he has emphasized the necessity of acknowledging and investigating the analyst's contribution to the patient's transference experience:

> [T]he setting and the analyst's behaviour exert an influence . . . on the manifestations of the potential intrapsychically organized patterns of interpersonal interaction and in that sense *co-determine the transference.* (1984, p. 164, emphasis added)

> [I]n analysing the transference the analyst should first focus on his contribution to the patient's experience of the relationship in the patient's response both to interventions and to the features of the analytic setting. (1984, p. 167)

Both Gill (1982, 1984) and Schwaber (1986) have noted that attention to the analyst's contribution to the transference, which affirms the plausibility or perceptual validity of the patient's experience, can bring about a deepening of the analytic process in both its here-and-now and genetic-reconstructive dimensions.

Lachmann and I (Stolorow & Lachmann, 1984–1985) have also discussed the analyst's contribution to the transference. We have defined transference as referring "to all the ways in which the patient's experience of the analytic relationship is shaped by his own psychological structures— by the distinctive, archaically rooted configurations of self and object that unconsciously organize his subjective universe" (p. 26). So defined, transference is an instance of *unconscious organizing activity*: The patient assimilates the analytic relationship into the thematic structures of his personal subjective world. This concept of transference as organizing activity explicitly invites attention to *both* the activities of the analyst *and* the recurrent meanings that these acquire for the patient.

The contribution of the patient's transference to the production of the analyst's countertransference has long held a place within psychoanalytic clinical theory. According to the viewpoint being developed here, countertransference (broadly conceptualized as a manifestation of the analyst's psychological structures and organizing activity) also has a decisive impact in codetermining the transference (detailed clinical illustrations of this point can be found in Atwood, Stolorow, & Trop, 1989, and Thomson, 1989). Transference and countertransference together form an intersubjective system of reciprocal mutual influence (Stolorow et al., 1987).

In agreement with Gill (1982), my collaborators and I (Stolorow et al., 1987) have argued that resistance analysis is coextensive with the analysis of transference. In resistance, the patient's experience of the analytic relationship is organized by expectations or fears that his emerging affective states and needs will meet with the same traumatogenic responses from the analyst that they received from the original caregivers. Resistance, we have emphasized, is always evoked by some quality or activity of the analyst that for the patient heralds an impending recurrence of traumatic developmental failure. Thus, while the persistence of resistance reflects the continuing influence of pre-established organizing principles, the working through of resistance requires careful investigation of the specific intersubjective contexts in which the defensive reactions arise and recede.

A similar mode of investigation has been employed in an effort to reconceptualize such clinical phenomena as negative therapeutic reactions (Brandchaft, 1983; Atwood & Stolorow, 1984); therapeutic impasses (Atwood et al., 1989); and the appearance, in analysis, of borderline and psychotic states (Stolorow et al., 1987). Formerly seen as products of isolated intrapsychic mechanisms, negative therapeutic reactions and impasses are now comprehended as rooted in unrecognized conjunctions and disjunctions between the principles unconsciously organizing the experiences of patient and analyst. Similarly, borderline and even psychotic states are understood to result from disturbances in archaic selfobject transference bonds, to which both patient and therapist contribute. In each instance, the context of relatedness established between patient and analyst has been revealed to play a *constitutive role* in forming and maintaining the particular pathological constellations that emerge in treatment, just as the early patterns of intersubjective transaction established between child and caregivers can be shown to play a constitutive role in the genesis of psychopathology.

A similar constitutive role is played by the analytic dyad in determining the *mutative* potential of psychoanalytic treatment. It is increasingly becoming recognized, for example, that analyzability is a property not of the patient alone, but of the patient–analyst system—the goodness of fit between what the patient most needs to have understood and what the analyst is capable of understanding (see Kantrowitz, 1986, and Emde, 1988b).

There has been long-standing debate within psychoanalysis over the role of cognitive insight versus affective attachment in the process of therapeutic change. During the past decade the pendulum seems to have swung in the direction of affective attachment. A number of authors, each from his own theoretical vantage point, have emphasized the mutative power of new relational experiences with the analyst: For example, Kohut (1984) has done so in terms of the disruption and repair of selfobject transference ties; Modell (1984), in terms of the holding functions of the analytic setting; Emde (1988b), in terms of the emotional availability of the analyst correcting for early deficits; and Gill (1982, 1984) and Weiss, Sampson, and the Mount Zion Psychotherapy Research Group (1986), in terms of the new interpersonal experiences with the analyst disconfirming transference expectations. It is my view that once the psychoanalytic situation is recognized as an intersubjective system, the dichotomy between insight through interpretation and affective bonding with the analyst is revealed to be a false one. The therapeutic impact of the analyst's accurate transference interpretations, for example, lies not only in the insights they convey, but also in the extent to which they demonstrate the analyst's attunement to the patient's affective states and developmental longings (see also Ornstein & Ornstein, 1980, and Tolpin, 1987). The analyst's transference interpretations, in other words, are not disembodied transmissions of insight *about* the analytic relationship. They are an inherent, inseparable component *of* that very bond. As Atwood and I (1984) have stated it, "Every transference interpretation that successfully illuminates for the patient his unconscious past simultaneously crystallizes an illusive present—the novelty of the therapist as an understanding presence" (p. 60). The patient's insights into the nature and origins of his unconscious organizing activity go hand in hand with the establishment of new modes of affective bonding with the analyst, and both contribute to the patient's growing capacity to integrate conflictual, formerly dissociated experiential contents (Stolorow et al., 1987). Interpretations, I am contending, derive their mutative power from the intersubjective matrix in which they take form.

I conclude this chapter with some case material illustrating the intersubjective context of a severe therapeutic impasse. The clinical presentation demonstrates the new understandings and enhancements of the therapeutic process that can be achieved when the priniciples unconsciously organizing the experiences of patient and therapist in an impasse are successfully investigated and illuminated.

AN INTERSUBJECTIVE ANALYSIS OF A
THERAPEUTIC IMPASSE

Sarah, a 29-year-old physical therapist, entered treatment because of recurring experiences of herself as a small, vulnerable child lost in a threatening world of powerful grownups. This patient was in actuality a successful, well-respected professional, with many supervisees and disabled patients relying on her expertise. Subjectively, however, she was increasingly prey to feelings of extreme intimidation, as if she were a weak and inadequate little girl suddenly thrust into high-powered adult roles and responsibilities.

Sarah had made one earlier attempt at psychotherapy while she was in college, but this had ended disastrously after 2 years when her therapist had begun to use her for the fulfillment of his own sexual needs. She was devastated when, after finally expressing confusion and doubt concerning their physical intimacy, she was angrily told by him that he had made a mistake in believing she had become capable of "mature love." Never showing any understanding of her reactions, he made her feel completely deserted by him. The final result of this was that she resolved never to rely so deeply on another person again, and tried to block the entire episode out of her mind for the next several years.

A pattern of being emotionally neglected and exploited was actually characteristic of her whole life history. During her early years there was massive neglect by her depressed and alcoholic parents, who for the most part relied on her to take care of them. Being nurturant to her parents provided her only consistent means of experiencing a connection with them, and major aspects of her developing self became organized around the caregiving role. This role specifically excluded the showing of any direct need for care from her mother or father: Expressing such a need seemed invariably to make the parents resentful, and they reacted either by pressuring her to be grown-up or by angrily rejecting her for being a burden to them. Illustrative of this pattern were the patient's earliest memories, which were of times when she cried uncontrollably in her crib and her mother responded by screaming at her to be quiet and violently throwing a bottle into her bedding.

Among the long-range consequences of Sarah's early situation was an interpersonal style of giving to others but asking nothing directly for herself. This affected not only her career choice in the field of disability, but also her intimate relationships. Her history was one of a series of romances in which she played a nurturant role with men who gave little or nothing in return. She always reacted to the depriving quality of these relationships with upset and depression, but regarded such feelings as signs of something wrong with her rather than reflections of how she was being mistreated.

The first months of Sarah's new therapy seemed to unfold very smoothly. She told the long story of her life in all its sad detail, including the story of her relationship to her first therapist. Her new therapist listened sympathetically as she spoke, and although he noted the rapidity with which she seemed to be opening up the various areas of her experience, he did not anticipate the transference storms that were soon to arise. There was an early dream, symbolizing the process that was occurring, in which the patient traveled back to the town where she had grown up and approached a large house. Going in, she passed through room after room, and finally came to a small closet in which there was an infant covered with dirt, cuts, and bruises cowering against the wall. In discussing the dream, she and her therapist understood the imagery as a picturing of their developing discovery of the sequestered, deeply hurt child within her.

The impasse to be described crystallized around the therapist's telling Sarah of a 6-week interruption in their work that was to occur during the following summer. Recognizing that such a long separation might be exceptionally difficult for her, he explained that he would be only a phone call away. She showed no special reaction to the announcement for a few days, but then reported a dream of an old mangy animal left lying on its back in the wilderness. When her therapist suggested that perhaps the dream was related to his plans for the summer, she grew visibly frightened, haltingly saying that maybe she was experiencing an impending abandonment. At this point, the therapist repeated his reassurances that he could remain in touch with her by phone, and reminded her that they still had a number of months to decide how they would handle the separation. To his surprise, Sarah reacted to the intended reassurance by becoming still more upset and turning physically away from him. When asked what she had felt, she said that she could not bear being in the room for a moment longer and wanted to go home. Her therapist asked her not to leave, but rather to stay and tell him more of what she was feeling. Again she responded fearfully and was now unable to talk. The session continued essentially in a tense silence until the hour was finally over, at which point Sarah rushed out the door.

The patient now began coming late to their meetings, reported great difficulty restraining herself from running away once she had arrived, and otherwise had little to say. The therapist redoubled his efforts to understand the meaning of the impending separation and continued to seek ways to ameliorate its inexplicably growing disruptive impact. He told the patient he was *sure* they could find their way through this period by planning for it and having occasional contacts by telephone; he even offered to see her once during the middle of the 6-week interruption when he had to return briefly. With each of these efforts to explore and soften the effect of his departure, Sarah became still more frightened and unable to communicate her feelings to him. She then told of repeating nightmares in which she arrived at his building for a session, but somehow his office had vanished and she was unable to find him. As the situation worsened, the therapist began to feel more and more helpless, at times becoming consumed with anxiety on her behalf. Sarah noted her therapist's growing distress, and this added to her difficulties, for now she felt she had become a painful burden to him.

During the vacation itself, the patient refused to have ongoing contacts of any kind, rejecting her therapist's calls with what he experienced as icy hostility. Finally she sent a letter telling him that he had treated her with brutal insensitivity. She added that she felt completely betrayed by him and was therefore terminating treatment. Still not understanding what had transpired, he replied in writing that he regretted the ending of their relationship and hoped she would feel welcome to come back if she ever changed her mind. Sarah did finally return after several more weeks had passed, and their sessions continued. The impasse, however, persisted through a series of subsequent episodes and was only very slowly clarified over the next 18 months. These episodes had in common a crisis around a physical separation's interrupting their work or some other circumstance's dramatizing an aspect of the therapist's unavailability to the patient. In each instance Sarah again reacted to her therapist's attempts to understand and alleviate her pain by withdrawing, and the treatment was maintained during this interval only on the most precarious basis.

The illumination of the impasse occurred gradually and involved not only a new understanding of the patient, but also a concomitant change in the therapist's self-understanding. For Sarah, the crises pertained must fundamentally to her sense that her therapist showed no concern for the enormously frightened, vulnerable child she repeatedly experienced herself as being. His attempted reassurances that a way could be found to overcome the disruptions of occasional separations were perceived as implicit demands that she feel better and not become scared. This replicated early childhood scenes in which her parents expected her to withstand very trying circumstances, including sometimes long separations from them, and behave like the grown-up girl they needed her to be. Her first therapist had also told her he expected her to be "mature," and had made her feel she had lost all connection to him on account of her failure to do so.

A fundamental truth of Sarah's life was that she had never been allowed to be a child, and with her new therapist she was again experiencing this same disastrous situation. His expectation that she join with him in planning for a separation flew in the face of her feeling that such a long break in their contacts was utterly impossible to bear. What was most disruptive for her was not, it was later understood, the 6-week separation itself; the more central problem was that she felt her therapist could neither understand nor accept the paralyzing sadness and despair that his departure was triggering. His well-meaning efforts to arrange contacts to help her only dramatized this lack of understanding. She also had been experiencing his efforts as containing the implicit message that she should not be so upset, and thus as a rejection of her child-self. This self had originally been disavowed in consequence of repeated events making her believe that the expression of her needs threatened her ties to the people closest to her. The specific danger associated with the emergence of her long-suppressed childhood longing for understanding and loving care was that she would be rejected for imposing such a loathsome burden on anyone around her. This danger had seemed to materialize when her therapist first informed her of his summer plans.

The therapist, throughout the period of the impasse, did not clearly perceive the patient's child-self as a distinct part of her. He was aware of her intense suffering, but did not fully comprehend the nature of this suffering as the boundless despair of a small child. Instead, he tended to see the difficulty she was having in terms of the relationship between them and felt responsible for her pain. This feeling of magnified responsibility contributed to *his* intense distress and formed part of a vicious cycle by reinforcing her picture of herself as an intrinsically burdensome, rotten creature whom no one could ever love.

The changes in the therapist's self-understanding that contributed to the resolution of the impasse arose largely out of his personal analysis, which was occurring in parallel to the treatment being described. He was a person in whom there was also a disavowed child-self, but with a different background from the one of his patient. He had grown up in a family that had been profoundly affected by the sudden death of his mother when he was 8 years old. She had been the emotional center of family life, and her loss had been utterly shattering to all the family members. The therapist had as a child responded to this massive upheaval in part by forming an identification with his mother and assuming aspects of her nurturant, supporting role in relation to his grieving father and siblings. His own sense of inner desolation was hidden in this process, becoming buried, as it were, with his mother. The result was that much of his style of relating to others began to center around the themes of caretaking and rescue, which served to protect him from feelings of devastating powerlessness and solitude. His inability to rescue Sarah as she spiraled into despair had thus challenged a central part of his way of maintaining his own emotional equilibrium.

As a result of intensive analytic work, the therapist began to have the immediate experience of his own child-self, with all its attendant feelings. The gradual integration of this previously disavowed part of himself occurred within the bond to *his* analyst, which provided the holding, containing context that had been missing in the shattered family of his youth. A central theme in his analysis was in fact the recognition of how he had been hurt not only by the loss of his mother, but equally by the emotional unavailability into which his father and other family members had lapsed in the aftermath of her death. As this integration slowly took place, the therapist's perception of his patient also began to change. He now came to see her child-self as a much more distinct entity than had been apparent to him before. He understood also that within this part of her there was an indescribable depth of despair and loneliness—feelings that again and again had been triggered in the transference. He specifically grasped why all his efforts to ease Sarah's pain during their separations had failed: The separations were simply impossible for the child within her to manage, and she had needed from him a response showing his understanding and acceptance of this fact. His efforts to reassure her contained the expectation that she would do well while he was away, which was very far from how she felt. This expectation had made it seem that he was no longer available for contact with her, and this was symbolized by the dreams in which his office had disappeared. The reassurances were in addition felt as rejections of her child-self, which replicated the many traumatic interactions with her parents and first therapist.

With the therapist's increasing acceptance and tolerance of the catastrophically extreme emotions of his own childhood, he became able to tolerate and contain the correspondingly extreme feelings of his patient. No longer assimilating the circumstances of the treatment to the trauma of his early family situation, he no longer felt a compelling need to rescue his patient from her pain and despair. As he moved away from attempts to ameliorate her suffering and focused instead on conveying his understanding of what she felt, Sarah slowly began to relax in his presence. The changing intersubjective field then made it possible for her to tell of a wishful fantasy concerning what she most deeply yearned for from him—a fantasy that previously she would have been far too frightened to disclose. It was that she could be held protectively in her therapist's arms and fall gradually into a peaceful sleep. This imagery concretized a needed bond that was at this point crystallizing between them—a bond of holding and containment within which the patient could experience secure acceptance of her child-self and thus discover the possibility of her own emotional wholeness.

ACKNOWLEDGMENTS

The theoretical portion of this chapter is a modified version of "The Intersubjective Context of Intrapsychic Experience: A Decade of Psychoanalytic Inquiry" by R. D. Stolorow, 1991, originally published in *Psychoanalytic Inquiry*, *11*, 171–184. The clinical material was originally published in "Impasses in Psychoanalytic Therapy: A Royal Road" by G. Atwood, R. D. Stolorow, and J. Trop, 1989, *Contemporary Psychoanalysis*, *25*, 565–571.

REFERENCES

Atwood, G., & Stolorow, R. D. (1984). *Structures of subjectivity: Explorations in psychoanalytic phenomenology.* Hillsdale, NJ: Analytic Press.

Atwood, G., Stolorow, R. D., & Trop, J. (1989). Impasses in psychoanalytic therapy: A royal road. *Contemporary Psychoanalysis, 25,* 554–573.

Basch, M. (1984). Selfobjects and selfobject transference: Theoretical implications. In P. Stepansky & A. Goldberg (Eds.), *Kohut's legacy* (pp. 21–41). Hillsdale, NJ: Analytic Press.

Beebe, B., & Lachmann, F. (1988a). The contribution of mother–infant mutual influence to the origins of self- and object representations. *Psychoanalytic Psychology, 5,* 305–337.

Beebe, B., & Lachmann, F. (1988b). Mother–infant mutual influence and precursors of psychic structure. In A. Goldberg (Ed.), *Frontiers in self psychology* (pp. 3–25). Hillsdale, NJ: Analytic Press.

Brandchaft, B. (1983). The negativism of the negative therapeutic reaction and the psychology of the self. In A. Goldberg (Ed.), *The future of psychoanalysis* (pp. 327–359). New York: International Universities Press.

Demos, E. V. (1988). Affect and the development of the self: A new frontier. In A. Goldberg (Ed.), *Frontiers in self psychology* (pp. 27–53). Hillsdale, NJ: Analytic Press.

Demos, E. V., & Kaplan, S. (1986). Motivation and affect reconsidered. *Psychoanalysis and Contemporary Thought, 9,* 147–221.

Emde, R. (1988a). Development terminable and interminable: I. Innate and motivational factors from infancy. *International Journal of Psycho-Analysis, 69,* 23–42.

Emde, R. (1988b). Development terminable and interminable: II. Recent psychoanalytic theory and therapeutic considerations. *International Journal of Psycho-Analysis, 69,* 283–296.

Gill, M. (1982). *Analysis of transference* (Vol. 1). New York: International Universities Press.

Gill, M. (1984). Psychoanalysis and psychotherapy: A revision. *International Review of Psychoanalysis, 11,* 161–179.

Hoffman, I. (1983). The patient as interpreter of the analyst's experience. *Contemporary Psychoanalysis, 19,* 389–422.

Jones, J. (1989). *Affects as process.* Unpublished manuscript.

Kantrowitz, J. (1986). The role of the patient–analyst "match" in the outcome of psychoanalysis. *Annual of Psychoanalysis, 14,* 273–297.

Kohut, H. (1982). Introspection, empathy, and the semicircle of mental health. *International Journal of Psycho-Analysis, 63,* 395–407.

Kohut, H. (1984). *How does analysis cure?* (A. Goldberg, Ed.). Chicago: University of Chicago Press.

Langs, R. (1989). Models, theory, and research strategies: Toward the evolution of new paradigms. *Psychoanalytic Inquiry, 9,* 305–331.

Lansky, M. (1985–1986). Preoccupation as a mode of pathologic distance regulation. *International Journal of Psychoanalytic Psychotherapy, 11,* 409–425.

Lansky, M. (1987). Shame in the family relationships of borderline patients. In J.

Grotstein, M. Solomon, & J. Lang (Eds.), *The borderline patient* (Vol. 2, pp. 187–199). Hillsdale, NJ: Analytic Press.

Leavy, S. (1980). *The psychoanalytic dialogue.* New Haven, CT: Yale University Press.

Lichtenberg, J. (1983). *Psychoanalysis and infant research.* Hillsdale, NJ: Analytic Press.

Lichtenberg, J. (1989). *Psychoanalysis and motivation.* Hillsdale, NJ: Analytic Press.

Loewald, H. (1988). Psychoanalysis in search of nature: Thoughts on metapsychology, "metaphysics," projection. *Annual of Psychoanalysis, 16,* 49–54.

Meissner, W. (1989). A note on psychoanalytic facts. *Psychoanalytic Inquiry, 9,* 193–219.

Mitchell, S. (1988). *Relational concepts in psychoanalysis.* Cambridge, MA: Harvard University Press.

Modell, A. (1984). *Psychoanalysis in a new context.* New York: International Universities Press.

Ornstein, P., & Ornstein, A. (1980). Formulating interpretations in clinical psychoanalysis. *International Journal of Psycho-Analysis, 61,* 203–211.

Rogawski, A. (1987). A systems theoretical approach to the understanding of emotions. *Journal of the American Academy of Psychoanalysis, 15,* 133–151.

Sander, L. (1985). Toward a logic of organization in psychobiological development. In H. Klar & L. Siever (Eds.), *Biologic response styles* (pp. 20–36). Washington, DC: American Psychiatric Press.

Sander, L. (1987). Awareness of inner experience: A systems perspective on self-regulatory process in early development. *Child Abuse and Neglect, 11,* 339–346.

Schwaber, E. (1983). Psychoanalytic listening and psychic reality. *International Review of Psychoanalysis, 10,* 379–392.

Schwaber, E. (1986). Reconstruction and perceptual experience: Further thoughts on psychoanalytic listening. *Journal of the American Psychoanalytic Association, 34,* 911–932.

Socarides, D., & Stolorow, R. (1984–1985). Affects and selfobjects. *Annual of Psychoanalysis, 12–13,* 105–119.

Stern, D. (1985). *The interpersonal world of the infant.* New York: Basic Books.

Stern, D. (1988). The dialectic between the "interpersonal" and the "intrapsychic." *Psychoanalytic Inquiry, 8,* 505–512.

Stolorow, R. D., & Atwood, G. (1989). The unconscious and unconscious fantasy: An intersubjective–developmental perspective. *Psychoanalytic Inquiry, 9,* 364–374.

Stolorow, R. D., Brandchaft, B., & Atwood, G. (1987). *Psychoanalytic treatment: An intersubjective approach.* Hillsdale, NJ: Analytic Press.

Stolorow, R. D., & Lachmann, F. (1984–1985). Transference: The future of an illusion. *Annual of Psychoanalysis, 12–13,* 19–37.

Thomson, P. (1989, October). *Counter-transference in an intersubjective perspective: An experiment.* Paper presented at the 12th Annual Conference on the Psychology of the Self, San Francisco.

Tolpin, M. (1987). Discussion of "The analyst's stance," by M. Black. *Annual of Psychoanalysis, 15,* 159–164.

Wallace, E. (1985). *Historiography and causation in psychoanalysis*. Hillsdale, NJ: Analytic Press.

Weiss, J., Sampson, H., & the Mount Zion Psychotherapy Research Group. (1986). *The psychoanalytic process*. New York: Guilford Press.

Wolf, E. (1984). The inevitability of interaction. *Psychoanalytic Inquiry, 4*, 413–428.

PART TWO

Current Perspectives from Social Psychology

The chapters in this section reflect the perspectives of mainstream social psychology. The reader will note the shift from the largely unconscious intrapsychic self to the self as affected by situational variables. In Chapter Three, Leippe explores attitude change by considering the relationship between self-image and attitudes, traditionally conceptualized as a person's beliefs, affects, and dispositions toward action. He argues that the effectiveness of different types of persuasive messages depends upon whether the public or private self is made salient. He then suggests strategies for disengaging the self and using paradoxical techniques to obtain small but significant changes in self-image.

In Chapter Four, Szymanski addresses the phenomenon of "loafing" in groups and the prevention of this effect by opportunities for self-evaluation. Underlying this phenomenon is the assumption that people are motivated to obtain self-knowledge and to engage in social comparisons. Her chapter provides an example of how situational variables affect self-evaluation processes and how these processes in turn affect group life.

The chapters by Deaux and Hormuth present more of a "sociological" social-psychological approach to the self: Deaux examines the social categories people claim as important to their identity, and Hormuth reports the effects of physical relocation upon self-concept change. Hormuth also looks at the relationship between the material world of objects and the self-concept. His technique of autophotography represents a novel way of getting at potentially unconscious processes. This technique also provides data that are not dependent upon verbal reports, but instead rely upon visual images—a distinction both Epstein (Chapter Seven) and Curtis and Zaslow (Chapter Eight) highlight later.

CHAPTER THREE

A Self-Image Analysis of Persuasion and Attitude Involvement

MICHAEL R. LEIPPE

Persuasion, broadly defined, is a method of influence in which a change agent attempts to change the beliefs and knowledge of someone, in the hope that such changes will lead to changes in affect or attitudes and ultimately in behavior. Persuasive appeals are the most popular of influence techniques. In our highly verbal society, persuasion is often the influence tool of first resort. Research on naturally occurring compliance-gaining activities demonstrates that people most often identify persuasive appeals as the means by which they get others to do as they want. Before they "butter up," threaten, or bargain, they offer logical and personalized reasons, lend their expertise, and state the facts (Rule & Bisanz, 1987). Persuasion is also reported by marriage partners as a popular method of gaining control over their spouses, especially among partners most compelled to be controlling (Falbo & Peplau, 1980).

Of course, persuasive appeals are ubiquitous in our world of advertising, political campaigning, and public service announcements. Educators rely on persuasion—and so do therapists and counselors. Whereas advertisers seek to change or shape attitudes about cars, camcorders, and cigarette smoking, and editorialists address attitudes about sociopolitical issues, therapists often seek to change attitudes and beliefs about social situations (if clients are pathologically shy), about self-efficacy (if clients feel depressed or helpless), about skills and abilities (if clients feel insecure), or about other people's motives (if clients are paranoid). The science of persuasion has wide and deep relevance everywhere—including the clinic.

In this chapter, I concentrate mainly on social-psychological studies of attitude change and persuasion. The term "attitude" refers here to one's summary evaluation of an object (e.g., an issue, a person, an idea) based on experiences, beliefs, and past behaviors toward the object (cf. Fazio, 1986; Zanna & Rempel, 1988). Where possible, I relate the social-psychological research to clinical and other applied concerns. But my major intention is to attempt to understand the effectiveness of persuasion and the role of the multifaceted concept of "attitude involvement," in terms of recent research and theory about the self and self-presentation.

THE RELEVANCE OF RELEVANCE

It is a truism that different people are differently influenced by the same persuasive appeal. One factor that helps explain different reactions is the personal relevance of the message. Personal relevance has been considered a defining quality of attitude involvement (Johnson & Eagly, 1989). For example, a straightforward manipulation of relevance in the laboratory has a significant effect on cognitive responses to a message (Petty & Cacioppo, 1984, 1986; Leippe & Elkin, 1987). College students hear either a strong or a weak message advocating some unfamiliar policy such as mandatory senior comprehensive exams, delivered by either an expert or a nonexpert on the matter. Half the students are informed that the exams may take effect the following year; the other half are told that they will not take effect for another 6 years—long after the students have graduated. The former group (those for whom the message has suddenly assumed high relevance) are much influenced by the strength of message argumentation. They reject a weak message and accept a strong one, pretty much without regard to the source's level of expertise. In contrast, students for whom the message issue has low relevance do not discriminate between weak and strong messages; instead, they tend to accept any message delivered by an expert, and to reject any message of a nonexpert (Petty, Cacioppo, & Goldman, 1981).

Findings like these have been interpreted to mean that people are motivated to analyze message content systematically and effortfully when the message is relevant (Chaiken, 1980; Petty & Cacioppo, 1986). When the message is not relevant, they behave like "cognitive misers" (Taylor & Fiske, 1978) and decide whether or not to be influenced on the basis of peripheral cues outside of the message content that suggest a heuristic rule of thumb (e.g., "Experts can be trusted," "A message is valid if most people agree with it"). The notion that personal relevance—or involvement— spurs systematic processing is supported by studies showing that when relevance is high (as opposed to low), more message-relevant thinking occurs (Chaiken, 1980), covert counterarguing of weak messages is greater (Petty, Cacioppo, & Heesacker, 1981), memory for message arguments is better (Leippe & Elkin, 1987), attitude change persists longer (Chaiken, 1980), and attitude change is more predictive of changes in behavior (Leippe & Elkin, 1987; Sivacek & Crano, 1982).

But what makes a message issue relevant or involving? And cannot an issue be relevant for different reasons? A major thesis advanced here is that an issue is relevant if and only if it implicates self-images, or what Schlenker (1986) calls "self-identities" (see also Johnson & Eagly, 1989). And because the self is multifaceted, different aspects of the self may be implicated depending on the issue or attitude object at hand, the situational context in which the message occurs, and the recipient's history with the attitude object and the situation. In general, when confronted by a message that is relevant, people always have a *goal* of serving a particular self-image, and their processing of, or thinking about, the message is directed by that goal. A self-image framework for understanding the persuasion process yields some important theoretical insights, as well as some intriguing implications for the practice of persuasion.

Before delving squarely into this self-image analysis, I must review an important body of research on goals and on cognitive appraisals of social stimuli. This research establishes the psychological mechanisms by which concerns about self-identities drive reactions to persuasion.

GOALS, SELVES, AND MESSAGE ELABORATION: CONCEPTUAL BACKGROUND

Goals in Information Processing

Goals clearly influence how we think about incoming social information. For example, when we anticipate social interaction with someone we are watching only from a distance, so to speak, we presumably have the goal of learning things about the person that will help us plan the interaction. Consistent with this, Devine, Sedikides, and Fuhrman (1989) found that people remembered more about and had a more organized impression of a stimulus person they expected to work with later, compared to one they did not expect to ever meet. In a study by Higgins and McCann (1984), research participants were given the goal of describing a stimulus person in a way that would reveal his identity to an audience who knew him. When the audience was said to like the person, participants picked up on more positive traits of the person as they read about his behavior, compared to when the audience was said to dislike him. Finally, in the persuasion realm, when message recipients were given the explicit goal of critiquing an essay as a magazine editor would, they were less persuaded—and generated more counterarguments—than if they were given the goal of relating the message to their personal values (Leippe & Ferrari, 1985).

Carver and Scheier's (1990) control-process theory helps explain how people stay goal-directed and how goals permeate both their cognitive activity and overt behavior. These authors posit an ongoing feedback process in which people periodically compare what they are doing or thinking to their current goals, and if they discover discrepancies between intended and actual aspects of their behavior, they recalibrate their behavior to the goal. Hence, people pay at least unconscious attention to what they are doing, so that their behavior usually achieves their goals and their cognitions support the goal or contain traces of the goal-directed behavior.

Cognitive Responses and the Principle of Evaluative Consistency

This concept of feedback control over thought and behavioral processes concurs nicely with research on persuasion that suggests what might be called a "principle of evaluative consistency." Since the 1960s and earlier (e.g., Hovland, Janis, & Kelley, 1953), many persuasion researchers have assumed that the persuasive impact of communications depends on the thoughts they evoke in recipients (Greenwald, 1968; Petty, Ostrom, & Brock, 1981). This "cognitive-response" view suggests that message recipients actively relate message information to their own pre-existing attitudes and knowledge, and, through this process of cognitive elaboration, generate salient message-relevant thoughts that may or may not resemble the message arguments. In turn, the net *evaluative* tone of these elaboration-produced thoughts determines the amount and direction of persuasion.

When the message issue is self-relevant, as we have seen, people are motivated to do a lot of elaboration. They generate many cognitive responses. Interestingly, the initial cognitive responses people make to a message or less complex stimulus are usually good predictors of subsequent cognitive responses. Message-favorable responses give way primarily to more message-favorable responses. Unfavorable ones are followed primarily by more unfavorable ones. This principle of evaluative consistency is evident in several diverse lines of research. Tesser (1978) has observed that a consequence of simply thinking about an object is attitude polarization. If a person positively evaluates a novel stimulus (e.g., a painting) and then thinks about the stimulus in its absence, an even more positive evaluation is often given after the thought period. Conversely, initially negatively evaluated objects become even less desirable following thought. Tesser argues that polarization occurs because the initial attitude selectively directs thinking toward mental constructs that support it. This pattern of attitude polarization is also evident in repeated-exposure effects (e.g., Brickman, Redfield, Harrison, & Crandell, 1972; Grush, 1976). Grush (1976), for example, observed a positive, monotonic exposure–liking relationship for affectively positive stimuli (pleasant words) and a negative relationship for affectively negative stimuli (unpleasant words). In yet another paradigm, Hoch (1984) found evaluative consistency when people generated reasons for and against performing some future behavior and then estimated how likely they were to perform the behavior. People generated more reasons for whatever side of the issue they were instructed to think about first, and the side first considered had greater influence on their predictive judgments even when they were required to generate an equal number of "pro" and "con" reasons. Hoch concluded that initially generated reasons *inhibit* generation and retrieval of *opposing* thoughts—a process, of course, that results in evaluative consistency.

In the persuasion realm, I have found that the persuasive impact of a strong printed message increases monotonically as duration of exposure to the message increases from sufficient to more than sufficient for full comprehension (Leippe, 1979). Similarly, there is evidence that limited repeated exposure to appealing messages enhances persuasion (McCullough & Ostrom, 1974; Cacioppo & Petty, 1979).

Finally, in clinical situations, cognitive therapists have observed that the habitual negative thinking of depressed clients may exacerbate their depression and interfere with acceptance of reasonable and more optimistic insights offered by the therapist (Kendall, 1987; McNulty & Swann, Chapter Eleven, this volume). In fine evaluatively consistent fashion, negative explanations beget more negative explanations of one's life situation. Accordingly, one aspect of cognitive therapy for depression is to get clients to re-examine their beliefs. But the procedure works best if clients practice a new "mindset" of positive expectations and then are re-exposed to the situations that initiated their depression (Hollon & Garber, 1990). If this can be accomplished, the tendency toward evaluative consistency with the new perspective may lead to increasingly constructive appraisals of these situations.

The principle of evaluative consistency implies that whatever governs people's initial orientation to a persuasive message will play a large part in determining whether they accept or reject the message. The more people process a message, the firmer their disposition to oppose or agree will become. And involved people will do a lot of processing. But what determines the dominant orientation to the message? For one thing, goals do—in particular, goals associated with establishing, maintaining, or presenting a certain self-identity.

The Public and Private Selves as Sources of Processing Goals

Very often in life, goals relevant to presenting, protecting, or changing one's sense of self or self-identity become important. Practically all theoretical discussions of the self distinguish between the "private self" and the "public self" (Baumeister & Tice, 1986; Greenwald, 1982; Scheier & Carver, 1980; Schlenker, 1986; Tesser & Moore, 1986). The private self roughly corresponds to one's self-concept—beliefs about one's personality, the values one holds, and so on. In contrast, the public self is, in Baumeister and Tice's (1986) words, the "totality of how one is known to others" (p. 65). Both selves are important to most people. In fact, a basic assumption of contemporary theories of the self—one grounded in a rather large body of empirical research—is that much behavior is instigated by a desire to maintain either a positive self-image, a positive public image, or both. In other words, behavior, including cognition, is often undertaken with the *goal* of constructing or maintaining a certain private or public self-identity (Schlenker, 1982, 1986).

It is important to note that concern with the public self, with the impression one gives to others, does not necessarily instigate only disingenuous "facework." Schlenker (1986) has argued that self-identification—showing an audience that one is a particular type of person—is an *activity* involving thoughts, memories, and scripted plans. This is true whether the audience is oneself or other people. In the case of the public self, situational and contextual cues make salient the public identity that is most desirable, activating those aspects of the person that best serve the goal of attaining that identity. The individual genuinely presents himself or herself, but it is the "best-fitting" self. In essence, the self one presents to others (and the ongoing creation of that self-identity) is no less genuine than the private self-identity one creates for oneself.

In addition, even if the publicly presented self is somewhat far from the person's norm, the cognitions and self-reflections that are part of the self-presentational activity may influence subsequent self-identifications, thus creating a lasting change in the person. Finally, self-presentational activity may occur unconsciously, and thus without the controlled deliberateness implied by disingenuous impression management (Baumeister, Hutton, & Tice, 1989; Cialdini & Petty, 1981).

These considerations of self-relevant goals and message processing set the stage for a self-image analysis of persuasion and involvement. As noted, a persuasive message is relevant or involving if the message or the context in which it occurs instigates a "self-serving" goal. The equation of relevance with a self-serving goal should be easy to see. The information in any relevant message has possible implications for how one views the world, and therefore for who one is or should be to oneself and others. To put it differently, the message recipient basically has the task of deciding whether or not to incorporate the message information into his or her attitude and behavior—things that are part of the self.

PERSUASION AND THE TWO SELVES

A lingering mystery has been that some forms of involvement increase the persuasive impact of a strong message (as we have seen in the "senior exams" example), whereas others increase resistance to persuasion. At the same time, all forms of heightened involvement seem to be generally associated with greater levels of thinking about and elaborating message information. The mystery falls away somewhat when we consider that, across forms of involvement, it may be either the public self or the private self to whom the message is primarily relevant. In addition, the costs of changing in terms of implications for valued aspects of self may be higher or lower than the costs of not changing the attitude. We can thus identify two more or less dichotomous dimensions that conspire to create the specific self-relevant goals that, via evaluative consistency and feedback control, guide the cognitive and emotional reactions to any involving communication. First, the goal may be to advance either a private self-image or a public one. Second, the service of the self-image that is too costly to abandon may require, to use Fazio's (1979) terms, either *validating* one's existing attitude on the communication topic or *constructing* a new attitude. In the validating case, the individual is closed or resistant to persuasion. In the constructing case, the individual is open to influence. These two dimensions combine to create four forms of involvement, as depicted in Table 3.1.

Each involvement form is represented in the social-psychological research literature. "Ego involvement" is characterized by the goal of advancing a private self-image by validating an existing attitude. "Commitment" is an involvement state characterized by validating an existing attitude in the service of a public self-image. "Issue involvement" and "impression involvement" each involve a motivation to construct a new attitude—to advance a private self-image and a public self-image, respectively. Let us examine each in turn, with a theoretical bent, and then consider some possible applications.

Ego Involvement and Value Bonding

Perhaps the best-known form of involvement is ego involvement. This term initially was used by Sherif and Cantril (1947) and Sherif and Hovland (1961) to refer to the state in which there is a close bond between one's attitude toward some issue and one's self-defining reference groups (cf. Greenwald, 1982). Studies have shown that people who are ego-involved in an issue strongly resist attacks on their position; they counterargue and

TABLE 3.1. Four Forms of Attitude Involvement Based on Message Recipients' Self-Relevant Goals

Aspect of self to which message is more relevant	Goal regarding attitudes in question that best advances the relevant self-image	
	Construction	Validation
Private self-image	Issue involvement	Ego involvement
	• Message processing directed toward finding out how the issue relates to values, current needs, and other aspects of the private self.	• Message processing entails evaluating it against current values and self-identity that support an opposing attitude.
	• The person is *open* to persuasion.	• The person is *closed* to persuasion.
Public self-image	Impression involvement	Commitment
	• Message processing entails finding support from the message for an attitude that provides the most suitable public image.	• Message processing directed at counterarguing in order to maintain mental consistency with prior public acts.
	• The person is *open* to *some* persuasion.	• The person is *closed* to persuasion.

often distort the message or derogate the source. We all know that it does no good to talk to true believers whose social lives revolve around an issue—certain activists on either side of the abortion issue; members of gun clubs supported by the National Rifle Association; union activists; religious zealots; and the like.

At first glance, it would seem that for ego-involved people it is the public self that is relevant, or what Greenwald and Breckler (1985) refer to as the "collective self." One's self-image must be acceptable to the significant others in one's reference group. However, ego involvement would seem to be more closely related to the private self. Ego-involved people resist influence attempts when members of their reference groups are nowhere to be seen, as in psychological laboratories (C. Sherif, Kelly, Rogers, Sarup, & Tittler, 1973). Socialization into, or a long and rewarding association with, a reference group leads to *internalization* of its values (cf. Hormuth, Chapter Six, this volume). The values become one's own; they become *self-defining*—both in the company of others and when the person looks in the mirror. Sherif and Cantril (1947) put it aptly when they characterized ego-involved attitudes as those "that have been learned, largely as social values, that the individual identifies with, and makes part of himself" (pp. 126–127).

Why are ego-involved people resistant to persuasion? When one is confronted with a communication dealing with a self-defining attitude issue, one's attitude (Fazio, 1986; Zanna, in press), as well as the implicated self-definition or image, almost certainly will be activated from memory. There is extensive evidence that important and often used self-images, or "self-schemas," are readily activated by situational cues, and that by some form of spreading activation, they bring forth a host of intricately related self-knowledge (Fiske & Taylor, 1984; Markus, 1977; Schlenker, 1986). Hence, cued by the message, considerable information, values, and related beliefs will be activated from memory, with both motivational and cognitive consequences. Motivationally, the linkage of the challenged attitude to so many values and beliefs will highlight for the individual the consequences for self-esteem of accepting the message. Changing one's attitude would require major changes in one's entire value system and private self-identity, and would imply an existing lack of self-worth. The prospects of such costs instigate the goal of *validating*—protecting and reaffirming—the existing attitude, and thus preserving the positive private self-image. Cognitively, the individual's wealth of supportive beliefs and information will aid in reaching that goal. Resistance to persuasion increases as a function of how knowledgeable the individual is about the message issue (McGuire, 1964; Wood, 1982).

An experimental study by Ostrom and Brock (1968) demonstrates just how potent the linkage of an attitude to self-defining values can be in instigating the goal of validating an existing attitude that is closely tied to the private self. College students heard a speech advocating that Greenland should not be admitted to membership in the Pan-American Bank. Clearly this message is irrelevant to most college students, so the students went along with it and accepted its conclusion. The students then participated in a "value-bonding" task in which, in essence, they were asked to think about and rate how and to what extent excerpts from this trivial message related either to their central, self-defining values or to superficial ideas and values. Those who had made links to their central values were significantly more resistant to a later counterpersuasion attempt. Even attitudes newly incorporated into the larger, established private self resist change.

Commitment

Both social and clinical psychologists are well aware of the psychological properties of commitment. Verbal and behavioral commitments to a point of view or course of action increase the likelihood that people will stick to it. Therapy patients who choose their own therapy comply more readily with its regimens (Brehm & Smith, 1986). People who commit themselves in a small way to prosocial causes become more willing to make larger contributions to those causes (Freedman & Fraser, 1966). Of course, ego involvement implies a history of acts committing the individual to her or his stand. But in persuasion, commitments to an initial stand can be gained for attitudes that are anything but self-defining. Yet resistance to persuasion may be every bit as staunch as it is among the ego-involved. In laboratory experiments, message recipients who have indicated their attitude about an otherwise uninvolving issue to the experimenter before the message, by jotting down their thoughts or a numerical response to an attitude scale, are less persuaded by a counterattitudinal message than are uncommitted recipients (Pallak, Mueller, Dollar, & Pollack, 1972; Leippe, 1990; Rosnow & Suls, 1970).

The power of commitment may be drawn from concern for the public self. We all grow up in a society that values "keeping one's word" and looks down on wishy-washy, unpredictable "changes of heart." There is a well-learned social utility of being consistent (Tedeschi, Schlenker, & Bonoma, 1971). Commitment, then, may create the goal of validating one's initial stance in order to maintain a public appearance of integrity, or of presenting a public self-identity of a person who is consistent and not easily swayed from his or her beliefs by a single communication.

Commitment thus increases the self-relevance of the message. And, as the notion of heightened relevance implies, commitment is associated with greater levels of systematic message processing, not a simple superficial rejection of the message meant to impress one's audience. The "genuineness" and "deepness" of the effects of commitment are demonstrated by the observations that committed people engage in cognitive bolstering in anticipation of an attack on their attitude (Hass, 1981), and in considerable counterarguing as they receive the attack (Leippe, 1990). Though the public self is at issue, it is the public self-identity that one creates for *oneself*. People engage in consistent behavior and the necessary cognitive work behind it if they see consistency as reflective of a public identity that corresponds to their personal ideals (Baumeister, 1982). The immediate audience (e.g., an experimenter or therapist) may be incidental, except insofar, as Schlenker (1986) put it, as to "draw one's attention to a particular set of beliefs, behavioral prototypes, standards, and potential consequences relevant to the self-identification" (p. 31). In a related vein, Cialdini (1987) has posited a "consistency heuristic," a rule of thumb unconsciously triggered by a committing act that unconsciously directs cognitive activities that are consistent with the act. That commitment may involve a public self-identity constructed for oneself as an internalized audience is evident from research on cognitive dissonance. This research demonstrates that people will later express attitudes consistent with undesirable acts they believe they previously freely chose, even when those acts were entirely private—apparently invisible to the experimenter and other potential evaluating audiences (Baumeister & Tice, 1984; Elkin & Leippe, 1988). People feel accountable to an idealized public self-identity of consistency.

In sum, both ego involvement and commitment engage the goal of validating an existing attitude in order to satisfy a desired self-image. The goal initiates thinking about the message that results in antimessage thoughts, which should increase as thinking and appraisal of the message progress further. It is interesting to note that the resistance to new information suggestive of change by ego-involved and committed message recipients resembles the premature closure or attitudinal "freezing" observed when people experience time pressure to reach a decision. People with a deadline make a decision and then, relative to people without a deadline, avoid seeking new information (Mayseless & Kruglanski, 1987), including the bases of others' dissimilar opinions (Kruglanski & Mayseless, 1987); they are also more likely to reject a dissenting minority when their own decision represents the majority view (Webster & Kruglanski, 1990). In his theory of epistemic behavior, Kruglanski (1988) refers to such closed-mindedness as a need for specific structure—in this case, to accomplish a task. Ego involvement and commitment may be special cases of motivational states associated with maintaining or achieving structure. In the case of ego involvement and commitment, structure is preserved because "destructuring" will be unbecoming to valued qualities of the self.

Two other forms of involvement generate self-relevant goals that, unlike ego involvement and commitment, can be served by changing one's attitude—part of one's self-image—in response to the message. These involvement states arouse a construction motive, and we may refer to them as issue involvement and impression involvement.

Issue Involvement

Earlier in this chapter, I have described the "senior exams study"—an experiment representative of numerous ones conducted by Petty and Cacioppo and their colleagues. These studies show that message recipients who expect the issue discussed in a counterattitudinal message to have a personal impact on them are persuaded by a strong, compelling message but reject a weak, illogical one. Social psychologists refer to this as issue involvement, and the change by issue-involved people in response to a strong message is what contrasts with the effects of the involvement states I have discussed so far. Why are these personally involved people persuaded? The critical factor seems to be that the issue is a new one, or one that was not previously tied to central, self-defining values. Only now has the issue become important to a person's life. Under these circumstances, the message recipient has the goal of finding out how the issue relates to the private self, and then of *constructing* (or revising) an attitude on the issue that best fits the personal values, current needs, and other attributes characterizing his or her self-identity.

In Kruglanski's epistemic scheme, issue-involved people have a high "fear of invalidity." The "fear" in this case is of missing out on self-relevant knowledge or of assuming a position that does not fit the private self's best interests. The goal is to construct an attitude that is valid in terms of the self.

Such a goal is served by open-minded analysis of the message that is sensitive to how well the message argues its case in a fashion that connects positively to one's private self-identity. If the message strikes a chord, continued active analysis will yield increasing reasons why its position is a good one vis-à-vis the private self. Importantly, in the process of changing one's attitude *because* the message fits with the self-concept, at least a small part of the self-concept may change as well. The new attitude has its own implications that may permeate self-identity through self-perception and inconsistency resolution processes (Bem, 1972; Cooper & Fazio, 1984). For example, postmessage contemplation of one's agreement with a message advocating senior comprehensive exams may yield thoughts such as "I believe senior exams are good; thus I value higher standards in education and a meritocracy based on comparative academic achievement." In addition, the principle of evaluative consistency suggests that once the recipient is thinking positively about the message's position, only selectively supportive aspects of the private self will be accessed, and the less supportive aspects of self that do get accessed may be themselves counterargued.

Impression Involvement

My own research, like Petty and Cacioppo's, has found that issue-involved message recipients are indeed persuaded by strong messages that connect well to self-identity (Leippe & Elkin, 1987). My colleagues and I have also found that this persuasive impact can be dampened when issue involvement is overridden by a fourth and final basis for self-relevance in persuasion—what social psychologists have referred to as "response involvement" (Zimbardo, 1960) and, more recently, "impression-relevant involvement" (Johnson & Eagly, 1989) or simply "impression involvement."

College students in the Leippe and Elkin (1987) study listened to a strong or weak message on an issue such as senior comprehensive exams, after learning that they would discuss the message issue with a professor. Anticipated public presentation of one's attitude to the professor was the manipulation of impression involvement, which conveys a concern with the significance for the public self of one's response to a persuasive message. Other participants were issue-involved, but not impression-involved. Participants' agreement with the message and other facets of their attitude were assessed within minutes following the message. The attitude results are summarized in Figure 3.1. As can be seen, participants who were not impression-involved (i.e., who anticipated no discussion) were highly persuaded by a strong message, but roundly rejected a weak one. This agreement difference between strong and weak messages, however, was attenuated among impression-involved participants who anticipated a postmessage discussion. Instead of polarizing in the direction of message strength, these impression-involved subjects expressed relatively moderate attitudes, regardless of message strength.

The present analysis of impression involvement posits that people facing the prospect of publicly presenting their position about a message

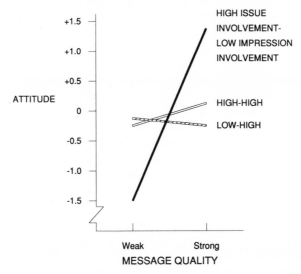

FIGURE 3.1. Results of the Leippe and Elkin (1987) study. Higher numbers indicate greater agreement with the message. From "When Motives Clash: Issue Involvement and Response Involvement as Determinants of Persuasion" by M. R. Leippe and R. A. Elkin, 1987, *Journal of Personality and Social Psychology, 52,* 269–278. Copyright 1987 by the American Psychological Association. Reprinted by permission.

issue become concerned with their public self-identity. In the absence of competing goals such as ego-protecting validation, they desire to present an attitude—a visible part of the self, however small—that is socially acceptable but not blatantly inconsistent with other aspects of the self. In the Leippe and Elkin (1987) study, since the professor/discussant's attitude was unknown, a middle-of-the-road attitude would serve this purpose. At least the discussant and participant would be in the "same ballpark."

The goal of presenting a public self-identity that the anticipated audience finds desirable should influence how impression-involved recipients process the message. We (Leippe & Elkin, 1987) argued that our impression-involved participants engaged in message analysis that was *biased toward moderation*. That is, their message-relevant thinking was selectively tuned to searching out evidence from the message and from their own knowledge base that was evaluatively balanced. Consistent with this interpretation, we found that, following the message, impression-involved participants listed thoughts that were more evaluatively mixed than those of other participants. This suggests that, although they are open to change, the dominant mental strategy of impression-involved participants favors bolstering and highlighting those aspects of the self supporting the allowable self-identity that is most publicly appealing in the present context. As in the case of commitment, an audience—this time, an anticipated one—serves to guide attention and thought to a certain side of the self and a certain angle on self-relevant information in the message.

The evaluative consistency of thought evinced under impression involvement in the Leippe and Elkin (1987) experiment is a curious one: Message recipients consistently conjure up reasons for a moderate reaction to polarized arguments. Note, however, that if the significant audience is known to be opinionated in a specific direction, impression-involved people should seek to construct an attitude closer to the audience's. Under these circumstances, thinking will reflect a bias to find reasons to support the audience's side (cf. Cialdini, Levi, Herman, & Evenbeck, 1973).

Impression involvement—concern with the self-presentational consequences of one's attitude on an otherwise uninvolving issue—thus appears to instigate the goal of constructing an attitude that presents a desirable public self-identity. It could be argued that the goal is achieved superficially and disingenuously, by publicly presenting the self-presentationally useful attitude while privately holding to a different viewpoint (perhaps one more sensitive to objective message strength). However, the notion that the goal is achieved through the way people process the message is supported by Tetlock's important research on accountability. Tetlock (1983; Tetlock & Kim, 1987; Tetlock, Skitka, & Boettger, 1989) has found repeatedly that social pressure to justify one's attitudes and beliefs to others compels people to think complexly about the issue, so as to develop integrated, evaluatively balanced stances.

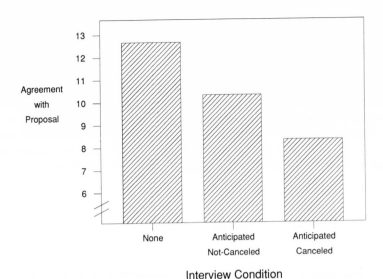

FIGURE 3.2. Results of the Manion and Leippe (1990) study, "strong message" conditions. From *Response Involvement and Biased Elaboration in Persuasion* by A. P. Manion and M. R. Leippe, 1990, paper presented at the meeting of the Midwestern Psychological Association, Chicago, IL.

A recent study (Manion & Leippe, 1990) confirms the genuineness of the audience-sensitive attitudes expressed by impression-involved subjects. A message on a rather unfamiliar topic (student input into tenure decisions) was presented to college students who either expected or did not expect to discuss the message with a professor who was *known to oppose* the message position. The impression-involved participants (those expecting the discussion) were less persuaded by a strong message than were those not expecting a discussion. Importantly, this inhibition of persuasive impact was evident even when impression-involved participants were informed immediately following the message that the interview would not take place. This result is displayed in Figure 3.2. It appears that public self-image concerns associated with the professor exerted a countermessage force on how participants processed the message.

When Self-Relevant Goals Compete

The foregoing discussion has generally treated the various involvement states in isolation, concentrating on the pure cases in which message-processing goals have only a single basis of relevance to the self. Often, of course, situational and personal circumstances will make salient two or more aspects of the self. Furthermore, the desired self-images associated with one aspect may not be consistent with the desired self-image asso-ciated with the other. What happens then? In the Leippe and Elkin (1987) study, such "clashing motives" were created in one experimental condi-tion. One group of students was both issue-involved and impression-in-volved: They both anticipated a discussion and believed that the message issue could affect them in the near future. The attitudinal result seemed to be a compromise—a blend in which message analysis reflected both the need to have an attitude that best fit the values and beliefs of the private self and the need to present a favorable public identity. These participants were more influenced by message strength than were participants who

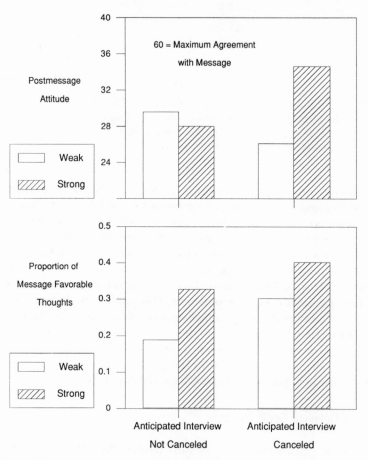

FIGURE 3.3. Results of the Leippe (1990) study. From *Sticking to Your Guns: Impression Involvement and Attitudinal Reactions to a Counterattitudinal Message* by M. R. Leippe, 1990, unpublished manuscript, Adelphi University.

were only impression-involved, but they were far less influenced by message strength than were participants who were only issue-involved (see Figure 3.1).

A more complex outcome of competing goals was evident in a study I recently completed (Leippe, 1990). By means of a pretest, college students committed themselves to an extreme antimessage stand before hearing the message, and some of these students were led to expect a post-message interview by a professor. Furthermore, the message was issue-involving: It concerned campus parking, a troublesome problem at the university. The major persuasion results appear in Figure 3.3. The post-message attitudinal responses of those recipients expecting an interview, and thus impression-involved, suggested that the goal of presenting a public self-image of consistency and prostudent sentiment "won." These participants were quire resistant to persuasion, whether the message was weak or strong. Instead of adopting a moderate attitude that would not be too distant from any stance the professor took, they chose a public image of "sticking to their guns." However, it is interesting that an analysis of the thoughts that participants listed about the message revealed greater positive responsiveness to the strong message than their expressed attitudes would suggest. Moreover, an additional group of participants, for whom the interview was cancelled just after the message, were more persuaded by a strong message than by a weak one. The goal of satisfying the needs of the private self for constructing an attitude consistent with values-related message information seems to have had at least some impact after all—impact that was revealed only after participants were "released" from impression involvement by interview cancellation.

This study raises two crucial points. First, it makes clear that more than one self-relevant goal may simultaneously influence cognitive and affective reactions to persuasive information. More than one desired self-image may be activated and shape thought in a persuasion setting. Second, it also seems that some "facework" was involved in the resistance of impression-involved message recipients. When "deinvolved" by cancellation of the interview, they expressed less disagreement with a strong message. It may be that, as a means of dealing with competing needs, these individuals expressed one stance (resistance) while privately accepting information supportive of another stance (a moderate attitude that was not totally oblivious to the message).

The inconsistency or facework however, may have been more apparent than real. Both responses, that is, may have been genuine. After all, both attitude and thought responses were made privately in the study. Moreover, the idea of multiple selves—of self-identities that differ depending on whether people are looking inward or outward, or what the external situation prompts them to think about themselves—is consistent with the social-psychological idea that attitudes are not so much points as they are ranges (what Sherif & Hovland, 1961, referred to as latitudes of acceptance). It also concurs with the view that the point within the range that people express is partly a function of what aspect of the attitude (specific beliefs, emotions, memories of past behavior, etc.) is activated by the situation (Zanna & Rempel, 1988). The resisting attitudes of those for whom the interview was not cancelled may have been the most extremely resisting version of a range that included more moderate positions. Participants expressed the most salient self at the moment. Importantly, had they proceeded to an actual interview with the professor, they probably would have continued to express the extreme form of their attitude, which would have made it a stronger and more influential aspect of self in the future. Recent research by Gilbert and Osborne (1989) demonstrates that a faulty judgment resulting from biased processing may influence subsequent related judgments even after the initial faulty judgment is detected and corrected. Similarly, if a recipient of a persuasive message contemplates a rather nonrepresentative attitude, this mental act may gradually make that attitude more representative.

IMPLICATIONS FOR THE WOULD-BE PERSUADER

Let us sum up. I have argued that people effortfully process persuasive communications to the extent that the communications are self-relevant. A message, however, can be self-relevant for different reasons and may demand different responses in order to serve the aspect of self made salient by the persuasion context. States of attitude involvement, or attitude self-relevance, can be categorized according to whether the private or public self is made salient and whether self-esteem and integrity associated with the activated self are best maintained by validating an existing attitude or constructing a new one. When one (or more) of these four involvement states is engaged, the persuasive message is processed with the goal of establishing or sustaining a desired self-image. Since cognition tends to be evaluatively consistent, continued contemplation of the message will yield increasing change or resistance in the service of that self-image, making the impact on the larger self more pronounced and more durable.

What are the implications of this analysis? Can the findings of largely laboratory-based studies be applied more broadly to the persuasion that must be accomplished to improve mental health, eliminate prejudice, or move mountains? Here are some ways (admittedly speculative) in which I think they can. In keeping with the "social–clinical interface" theme of this volume, most of my examples will involve therapy.

Ego Involvement and "Disengaging the Self"

Counterattitudinal messages aimed at attitudes that are strongly linked to the individual's most central and self-defining values and beliefs arouse a strong motive to protect the private self-image by resisting the message. Therapists since Freud have been well aware of the problem of resistance, noting that in many cases it is the biggest therapeutic hurdle (Wachtel, 1982). Thus, let us consider a female client who is unable to establish a lasting, intimate relationship with a man. It appears that she endorses an extremist and rigid, yet self-defining, brand of feminism that prevents her from sharing in the kinds of mutual dependencies and compromises necessary in intimacy. Because she is ego-involved in her feminism, trying to help her improve her relationships by persuading her to moderate that broad philosophy will be unsuccessful. In the same vein, messages aimed at more specific attitudes and feelings about dependency in relationships will also fail if they touch too closely on feminist themes.

A more effective strategy may be to disengage, at least initially, the self from the specific attitudes in need of change. The counselor might deliberately couch suggestions and arguments in ways that distance them from the core self-defining beliefs. Only when these arguments are accepted and have been responded to with considerable "cognitive work" would the change agent move arguments toward more fundamental attitude issues surrounding the feminist self.

A related strategy would be for the counselor, through knowledge of the client, to construct a "self-distance scale" in which behaviors and attitudes in need of change are ordered from least to most related to the dominant themes in the client's private self-image. Therapeutic persuasion efforts would begin with the less self-defining attitudes and gradually move to more self-defining ones—relying on positive thoughts about the message to grow through evaluative consistency, and thus to "soften" resistance at each succeeding step.

The paradoxical strategy studied by Swann, Pelham, and Chidester (1988) is another one that may break down ego involvement. These researchers discerned that people who are highly certain of their attitudes—as ego-involved people usually are—refuse to agree with statements that reflect attitudes even slightly different from the ones they hold. Let me illustrate by expanding on the experimental example employed by Swann et al. Consider a woman who is highly certain of her conservative views about gender roles. If she is asked what she likes about "sensitive men," she may reply bluntly that it is that "they know I won't date them." But if she is ego-involved in a specific stance, she may also resist statements or questions suggesting an attitude that is on the same side as hers but more extreme. She may counterargue that proattitudinal point and, by doing so,

55

move her private self-image ever so slightly in the other direction—the one the change agent desires. Thus, if the woman is asked, "Why do you sympathize with the feelings of some men that women are better kept barefoot and pregnant?" she may reject the implication, find herself sounding almost liberal in the process, and begin a shift that the change agent can now work with.

We can look at this effect in terms of self-identity. The validation motive of preserving private self-identity is activated by a message that threatens that identity from the other side. By counterarguing to preserve that self-identity, the client has planted the seeds of receptivity to a new self-identity consistent with the counterarguments.

The therapist strategy of "joining" in family therapy reflects an implicit recognition of the self-image rationale of the paradoxical strategy. One recommended way for the therapist to "join"—become enmeshed in and accepted by the troubled family system—is to initially "confirm" positive qualities of family members and their explanations for their negative behaviors (Minuchin & Fishman, 1981). The therapist bestows value on members' valued self-images, rather than assaulting their behavior as an indictment of those values. This allows the therapist to gain acceptance into both the family system and the individual self-systems of family members. Once "joined," the therapist, in effect, is a part of each member's private self-image, at least regarding the topics and family problems at issue. Thus members are more likely to be motivated to incorporate the therapist's later, more constructively critical statements into a self-image that the therapist has reinforced and that they seek to maintain.

Finally, a self-relevance analysis suggests that ego-involved resistance can be penetrated by casting the advocated message position as actually supporting the target's most cherished private self-image. This approach concurs with functional theories, which maintain that attitudes serve needs and that the best way to persuade someone to adopt a different attitude is to show the person how the new attitude better serves the need (Herek, 1986; Katz, 1960; Snyder & DeBono, 1985, 1987; Smith, Bruner, & White, 1956). Consider a workaholic man whose constant preoccupation with work is an outward reflection of his need to see himself as on the fast lane to career success—a need that may further reflect unconscious insecurities. His attitude toward work is that the more he does, the faster he will reach unchallengeable success. Instead of trying to persuade him that all work and no play makes Jack a dull and overly anxious boy who is a stranger to his children, the change agent might argue that success will come faster if he takes time to relax. Note also that if Jack's attitude toward work changes, this might be a start toward changing more fundamental self-images, and might ultimately bring deep insecurities to light.

Commitment: Untying and Tying Images to the Self

What about public self-concerns associated with commitment? Because the sense of commitment to an attitude and the resulting efforts to validate that attitude may occur unconsciously, it makes sense for change agents to inform their targets about "foolish consistencies." But the message must speak to the self, as it were, arguing that to give up the commitment concurs with self-defining values and creates a public image of intelligence, sensitivity, flexibility, and so forth.

Therapists, like social psychologists, have long known about the power of commitment and choice, often using them in various ways such as by having clients choose their own therapy or make verbal promises to execute certain therapeutic acts. A self-image analysis of persuasion suggests that they could go further. Commitment to one attitude will cause subsequent information and experience to be thought about in a manner consistent with that attitude. Now if further messages tie the committed attitude to other attitudes, beliefs, or aspects of self, this polarizing thought may create change in those other self-relevant aspects. In an attempt to maintain a public self-image of integrity and consistency on one issue, a person may gradually be changing related private self-images—with a little help from the therapist's messages.

Impression Involvement and Deliberately Created Evaluation Apprehension

There often are good reasons to avoid being judgmental in a therapy or counseling setting. But the subtle effects on message processing of anticipated public scrutiny of attitudes suggest that sometimes a little apprehension about the therapist's or some other significant other's judgment will help change attitudes and behavior in a positive direction. Imagine that, under appropriate circumstances, the client is instructed to "think about today's session and this advice I am going to give you, because I would like you to present your ideas about it next week to Dr. Jones, whom I've asked to be a consultant." Perhaps the client's thinking will be influenced by how Dr. Jones will judge him or her, and as a result the client will reach some self-convincing therapeutic conclusions himself or herself. To an extent, impression involvement effects may help drive beneficial reactions to the techniques of rational–emotive therapy (Ellis, 1962). Alternatively, if a marriage counselor asks one partner to see whether he or she can impress the spouse for 3 days, and the partner tries to do so, he or she may analyze the problem in a way that brings about change. Note (see the earlier discussion) that even if the clients in both cases disingenuously present a public self-image, the thinking and emotion that goes into "the act" may have real effects on the self.

Issue Involvement: Desirable but Not Bias-Free

To the extent that a therapist or other influence agent can make the target issue-involved, the possibility of desirable change is increased—provided that the message has perceivable merit. Issue involvement is associated with the most objective processing (Petty & Cacioppo, 1986) and is characterized by comparing and contrasting the message arguments and the values, beliefs, and knowledge associated with the private self. Change agents can encourage issue involvement by stressing the immediate and important implications of their messages and by giving the impression of credibility and genuineness.

Of course, relating the message to the private self does not guarantee a desirable change. There has to be some aspect of the private self—some value, some core belief—with which the message resonates. There must be something in which to plant the seeds of change. Another problem is that even open-minded people with the goal of constructing the "right attitude" often cannot help being biased by the self-identities they hold dear. Lord, Ross, and Lepper's (1979) well-known study of biased assimilation is a good case in point. After carefully reading the same information suggesting an "undecided" verdict on the deterrent capability of capital punishment, people for and against the death penalty actually moved further apart: They became more extreme advocates or opponents. Filled with self-values-related beliefs about the issue, they selectively interpreted the information as consistent with their original viewpoint.

What can be done? Exercises that encourage clients to "consider the opposite" have been shown to "de-bias" interpretation and promote change (Lord, Lepper, & Preston, 1984). Making people accountable to credible others who know the truth may likewise yield more objective processing—but, as we have seen, processing can also be biased toward moderation under these conditions (see Tetlock et al., 1989).

CONCLUSION

The closing "moral of the story" is that all roads to effective persuasion about issues and things that matter to people seem to lead through the self. Hence, messages must be equipped with the proper "wheels" to make it through. Perhaps the easiest way through is to hitch a ride on a public or private self-image that is pointed in the desired direction.

ACKNOWLEDGMENTS

I would like to thank Rebecca Curtis and Abe Tesser for their insightful suggestions after reading an earlier draft of this chapter. Thanks also are due Andrew Manion for preparing the figures.

REFERENCES

Baumeister, R. F. (1982). A self-presentational view of social phenomena. *Psychological Bulletin, 91*, 3–26.

Baumeister, R. F., Hutton, D. G., & Tice, D. M. (1989). Cognitive processes during deliberate self-presentation: How self-presenters alter and misinterpret the behavior of their interaction partners. *Journal of Experimental Social Psychology, 25*, 59–78.

Baumeister, R. F., & Tice, D. M. (1984). Role of self-presentation and choice in cognitive dissonance under forced compliance: Necessary or sufficient causes? *Journal of Personality and Social Psychology, 46*, 5–13.

Baumeister, R. F., & Tice, D. M. (1986). Four selves, two motives, and a substitute process regulation model. In R. F. Baumeister (Ed.), *Public self and private self* (pp. 63–74). New York: Springer-Verlag.

Bem, D. (1972). Self-perception theory. In L. Berkowitz (Ed.), *Advances in experimental social psychology* (Vol. 6, pp. 1–62). New York: Academic Press.

Brehm, S. S., & Smith, T. W. (1986). Social psychological approaches to psychotherapy and behavior change. In S. L. Garfield & A. E. Bergin (Eds.), *Handbook of psychotherapy and behavior change* (3rd ed., pp. 69–115). New York: Wiley.

Brickman, P., Redfield, J., Harrison, A. A., & Crandell, R. (1972). Drive and predisposition as factors in the attitudinal effects of mere exposure. *Journal of Experimental Social Psychology, 8*, 31–44.

Cacioppo, J. T., & Petty, R. E. (1979). Effects of message repetition and position on cognitive responses, recall, and persuasion. *Journal of Personality and Social Psychology, 37*, 97–109.

Carver, C. S., & Scheier, M. F. (1990). Origins and functions of negative affect: A control-process view. *Psychological Review, 97*, 19–35.

Chaiken, S. (1980). Heuristic versus systematic information processing and the use of source versus message cues in persuasion. *Journal of Personality and Social Psychology, 39*, 752–766.

Cialdini, R. B. (1987). Compliance principles of compliance professionals: Psychologists of necessity. In M. P. Zanna, J. M. Olson, & C. P. Herman (Eds.), *Social influence: The Ontario Symposium* (Vol. 5, pp. 165–184). Hillsdale, NJ: Erlbaum.

Cialdini, R. B., Levi, A., Herman, C. P., & Evenbeck, S. (1973). Attitudinal politics: The strategy of moderation. *Journal of Personality and Social Psychology, 25*, 100–108.

Cialdini, R. B., & Petty, R. E. (1981). Anticipatory opinion effects. In R. E. Petty, T. M. Ostrom, & T. C. Brock (Eds.), *Cognitive responses in persuasion* (pp. 217–235). Hillsdale, NJ: Erlbaum.

Cooper, J., & Fazio, R. H. (1984). A new look at dissonance theory. In L. Berkowitz (Ed.), *Advances in experimental social psychology* (Vol. 17, pp. 229–266). New York: Academic Press.

Devine, P. G., Sedikides, C., & Fuhrman, R. W. (1989). Goals in social information processing: The case of anticipated interaction. *Journal of Personality and Social Psychology, 56,* 680–690.

Elkin, R. A., & Leippe, M. R. (1988). When motives clash: Issue involvement and response involvement as determinants of persuasion. *Journal of Personality and Social Psychology, 52,* 269–278.

Ellis, A. (1962). *Reason and emotion in psychotherapy.* New York: Lyle Stuart.

Falbo, T., & Peplau, L. A. (1980). Power strategies in intimate relationships. *Journal of Personality and Social Psychology, 38,* 618–628.

Fazio, R. H. (1979). Motives for social comparison: The construction–validation distinction. *Journal of Personality and Social Psychology, 37,* 1683–1698.

Fazio, R. H. (1986). How do attitudes guide behavior? In R. M. Sorrentino & E. T. Higgins (Eds.), *Handbook of motivation and cognition: Foundations of social behavior* (Vol. 1, pp. 204–243). New York: Guilford Press.

Fiske, S. T., & Taylor, S. E. (1984). *Social cognition.* Reading, MA: Addison-Wesley.

Freedman, J. L., & Fraser, S. C. (1966). Compliance without pressure: The foot-in-the-door technique. *Journal of Experimental Social Psychology, 4,* 195–203.

Gilbert, D. T., & Osborne, R. E. (1989). Thinking backward: Some curable and incurable consequences of cognitive busyness. *Journal of Personality and Social Psychology, 57,* 940–949.

Greenwald, A. G. (1968). Cognitive learning, cognitive response to persuasion, and attitude change. In A. G. Greenwald, T. C. Brock, & T. M. Ostrom (Eds.), *Psychological foundations of attitudes* (pp. 147–170). New York: Academic Press.

Greenwald, A. G. (1982). Ego-task analysis: An integration of research on ego-involvement and self-awareness. In A. H. Hastorf & A. M. Isen (Eds.), *Cognitive social psychology* (pp. 109–147). New York: Elsevier/North-Holland.

Greenwald, A. G., & Breckler, S. J. (1985). To whom is the self presented? In B. R. Schlenker (Ed.), *The self and social life* (pp. 126–145). New York: McGraw-Hill.

Grush, J. E. (1976). Attitude formation and mere exposure phenomena: A non-artifactual explanation of empirical findings. *Journal of Personality and Social Psychology, 33,* 281–290.

Hass, R. G. (1981). Effects of source characteristics on cognitive responses and persuasion. In R. E. Petty, T. M. Ostrom, & T. C. Brock (Eds.), *Cognitive responses in persuasion* (pp. 141–172). Hillsdale, NJ: Erlbaum.

Herek, G. M. (1986). The instrumentality of attitudes: Toward a neofunctional theory. *Journal of Social Issues, 42,* 99–114.

Higgins, E. T., & McCann, C. D. (1984). Social encoding and subsequent attitudes, impressions, and memory: "Context-driven" and motivational aspects of processing. *Journal of Personality and Social Psychology, 47,* 26–39.

Hoch, S. J. (1984). Availability and interference in predictive judgment. *Journal of Experimental Psychology: Learning, Memory, and Cognition, 10,* 649–662.

Hollon, S. D., & Garber, J. (1990). Cognitive therapy for depression: A social cognitive perspective. *Personality and Social Psychology Bulletin, 16,* 42–57.

Hovland, C. I., Janis, I. L., & Kelley, H. H. (1953). *Communication and persuasion.* New Haven, CT: Yale University Press

Johnson, B. T., & Eagly, A. H. (1989). Effects of involvement on persuasion: A meta-analysis. *Psychological Bulletin, 104,* 290–314.

Katz, D. (1960). The functional approach to the study of attitudes. *Public Opinion Quarterly, 24,* 163–204.

Kendall, P. C. (1987). Cognitive processes and procedures in behavioral therapy. In G. T. Wilson, C. M. Franks, P. C. Kendall, & J. P. Foreyt, *Review of behavior therapy: Theory and practice* (Vol. 11, pp. 114–153). New York: Guilford Press.

Kruglanski, A. W. (1988). Knowledge as a social psychological construct. In D. Bar-Tal & A. W. Kruglanski (Eds.), *The social psychology of knowledge* (pp. 109–141). New York: Cambridge University Press.

Kruglanski, A. W., & Mayseless, O. (1987). Motivational effects in the social comparison of opinions. *Journal of Personality and Social Psychology, 53,* 834–842.

Leippe, M. R. (1979). *Message exposure duration and attitude change: An information processing analysis of persuasion.* Unpublished doctoral dissertation, Ohio State University.

Leippe, M. R. (1990). *Sticking to your guns: Impression involvement and attitudinal reactions to a counterattitudinal message.* Unpublished manuscript, Adelphi University.

Leippe, M. R., & Elkin, R. A. (1988). *Dissonance reduction and accountability: Effects of assessment and self-presentational concern on mode of inconsistency resolution.* Unpublished manuscript, Adelphi University.

Leippe, M. R., & Ferrari, J. R. (1985). *Polarization versus reversal of persuasion: Effects of processing set and message exposure duration.* Paper presented at the meeting of the Eastern Psychological Association, Boston, MA.

Lord, C. G., Lepper, M. R., & Preston, E. (1984). Considering the opposite: A corrective strategy for social judgment. *Journal of Personality and Social Psychology, 47,* 1231–1243.

Lord, C. G., Ross, L., & Lepper, M. R. (1979). Biased assimilation and attitude polarization: The effects of prior theories on subsequently considered evidence. *Journal of Personality and Social Psychology, 37,* 2098–2109.

Manion, A. P., & Leippe, M. R. (1990). *Response involvement and biased elaboration in persuasion.* Paper presented at the meeting of the Midwestern Psychological Association, Chicago, IL.

Markus, H. (1977). Self-schemata and processing information about the self. *Journal of Personality and Social Psychology, 35,* 63–78.

Mayseless, O., & Kruglanski, A. W. (1987). What makes you so sure? Effects of epistemic motivations on judgmental confidence. *Organizational Behavior and Human Decision Processes, 39,* 162–183.

McCullough, J. L., & Ostrom, T. M. (1974). Repetition of highly similar messages and attitude change. *Journal of Applied Psychology, 54,* 395–397.

McGuire, W. J. (1964). Inducing resistance to persuasion: Some contemporary approaches. In L. Berkowitz (Ed.), *Advances in experimental social psychology* (Vol. 1, pp. 191–229). New York: Academic Press.

Minuchin, S., & Fishman, H. C. (1981). *Family therapy techniques.* Cambridge, MA: Harvard University Press.

Ostrom, T. M., & Brock, T. C. (1968). A cognitive model of attitudinal involvement. In R. P. Ableson, E. Aronson, W. J. McGuire, T. M. Newcomb, M. J. Rosenberg, & P. H. Tannenbaum (Eds.), *Theories of cognitive consistency: A sourcebook* (pp. 373–389). Chicago: Rand McNally.

Pallak, M. S., Mueller, M., Dollar, K., & Pallak, J. (1972). Effects of commitment on responsiveness to an extreme consonant communication. *Journal of Personality and Social Psychology, 23*, 429–436.

Petty, R. E., & Cacioppo, J. T. (1984). The effects of issue involvement on responses to argument quantity and quality: Central and peripheral routes to persuasion. *Journal of Personality and Social Psychology, 46*, 69–81.

Petty, R. E., & Cacioppo, J. T. (1986). The elaboration likelihood model of persuasion. In L. Berkowitz (Ed.), *Advances in experimental social psychology* (Vol. 19, pp. 123–205). New York: Academic Press.

Petty, R. E., Cacioppo, J. T., & Goldman, R. (1981). Personal involvement as a determinant of argument based persuasion. *Journal of Personality and Social Psychology, 41*, 847–855.

Petty, R. E., Cacioppo, J. T., & Heesacker, M. (1981). Effects of rhetorical questions on persuasion: A cognitive response analysis. *Journal of Personality and Social Psychology, 40*, 432–440.

Petty, R. E., Ostrom, T. M., & Brock, T. C. (Eds.). (1981). *Cognitive responses in persuasion*. Hillsdale, NJ: Erlbaum.

Rosnow, R. L., & Suls, J. M. (1970). Reactive effects of pretesting in attitude research. *Journal of Personality and Social Psychology, 15*, 338–343.

Rule, B. G., & Bisanz, G. L. (1987). Goals and strategies of persuasion: A cognitive schema for understanding social events. In M. P. Zanna, J. M. Olson, & C. P. Herman (Eds.), *Social influence: The Ontario Symposium* (Vol. 5, pp. 185–206). Hillsdale, NJ: Erlbaum.

Scheier, M. F., & Carver, C. (1980). Private and public self-attention, resistance to change, and dissonance reduction. *Journal of Personality and Social Psychology, 39*, 390–405.

Schlenker, B. R. (1982). Translating actions into attitudes: An identity-analytic approach to the explanation of social conduct. In L. Berkowitz (Ed.), *Advances in experimental social psychology* (Vol. 15, pp. 193–247). New York: Academic Press.

Schlenker, B. R. (1986). Self-identification: Toward an integration of the private and public self. In R. F. Baumeister (Ed.), *Public self and private self* (pp. 21–62). New York: Springer-Verlag.

Sherif, C. W., Kelly, M., Rogers, H. L., Sarup, G., & Tittler, B. I. (1973). Personal involvement, social judgment, and action. *Journal of Personality and Social Psychology, 27*, 311–328.

Sherif, M., & Cantril, H. (1947). *The psychology of ego-involvement*. New York: Wiley.

Sherif, M., & Hovland, C. I. (1961). *Social judgment: Assimilation and contrast effects in communication and attitude change*. New Haven, CT: Yale University Press.

Sivacek, J., & Crano, W. D. (1982). Vested interest as a moderator of attitude–behavior consistency. *Journal of Personality and Social Psychology, 43*, 210–221.

Smith, M., Bruner, J., & White, R. (1956). *Opinions and personality*. New York: Wiley.

Snyder, M., & DeBono, K. G. (1985). Appeals to image and claims about quality: Understanding the psychology of advertising. *Journal of Personality and Social Psychology, 49*, 586–597.

Snyder, M., & DeBono, K. G. (1987). A functional approach to attitudes and persuasion. In M. P. Zanna, J. M. Olson, & C. P. Herman (Eds.), *Social influence: The Ontario Symposium* (Vol. 5, pp. 107–128). Hillsdale, NJ: Erlbaum.

Swann, W. B., Jr., Pelham, B. W., & Chidester, T. R. (1988). Change through paradox: Using self-verification to alter beliefs. *Journal of Personality and Social Psychology, 54*, 268–273.

Taylor, S. E., & Fiske, S. T. (1978). Salience, attention, and attribution: Top of the head phenomena. In L. Berkowitz (Ed.), *Advances in experimental social psychology* (Vol. 11, pp. 249–288). New York: Academic Press.

Tedeschi, J. T., Schlenker, B. R., & Bonoma, T. V. (1971). Cognitive dissonance: Private ratiocination or public spectacle? *American Psychologist, 26*, 685–695.

Tesser, A. (1978). Self-generated attitude change. In L. Berkowitz (Ed.), *Advances in experimental social psychology* (Vol. 11, pp. 289–338). New York: Academic Press.

Tesser, A., & Moore, J. (1986). On the convergence of public and private aspects of self. In R. F. Baumeister (Ed.), *Public self and private self* (pp. 99–116). New York: Springer-Verlag.

Tetlock, P. E. (1983). Accountability and complexity of thought. *Journal of Personality and Social Psychology, 45*, 74–83.

Tetlock, P. E., & Kim, J. I. (1987). Accountability and judgment processes in a personality prediction task. *Journal of Personality and Social Psychology, 52*, 700–709.

Tetlock, P. E., Skitka, L., & Boettger, R. (1989). Social and cognitive strategies for coping with accountability: Conformity, complexity, and bolstering. *Journal of Personality and Social Psychology, 57*, 632–640.

Wachtel, P. L. (1982). *Resistance: Psychodynamic and behavioral approaches.* New York: Plenum.

Webster, D. M., & Kruglanski, A. W. (1990). *Group members' reactions to an opinion deviant under high or low need for closure.* Paper presented at the meeting of the American Psychological Society, Dallas, TX.

Wood, W. (1982). Retrieval of attitude relevant information from memory: Effects on susceptibility to persuasion and on intrinsic motivation. *Journal of Personality and Social Psychology, 42*, 798–810.

Zanna, M. P. (in press). Message receptivity: A new look at the old problem of open- vs. closed-mindedness. In A. Mitchell (Ed.), *Advertising exposure, memory, and choice.* Hillsdale, NJ: Erlbaum.

Zanna, M. P., & Rempel, J. K. (1988). Attitudes: A new look at an old concept. In D. Bar-Tal & A. W. Kruglanski (Eds.), *The social psychology of knowledge* (pp. 315–334). New York: Cambridge University Press.

Zimbardo, P. G. (1960). Involvement and communication discrepancy as determinants of opinion conformity. *Journal of Abnormal and Social Psychology, 60*, 86–94.

CHAPTER FOUR

The Potency and Fragility of Self-Evaluation in Reducing the Social Loafing Effect

KATE SZYMANSKI

In recent years, there has been a renewal of interest in the self and in self-evaluation processes. For example, Deci and Ryan (1985) developed a theory of intrinsic motivation and self-determination, a central tenet of which is that people possess an innate organismic need for competence that energizes a variety of behaviors. Greenwald and Breckler (1985) proposed an ego-task analysis, which specifies three facets of the self that are relevant for evaluation concerns: the public self, the private self, and the collective self. At the heart of this typology is the notion that behavior is motivated, in part, by concern for evaluation by these sources. Bandura (1986) included an account of the process of self-evaluation that includes self-observation, judgmental processes, and self-reactions. The self-evaluation process affects judgments of self-efficacy, which in turn affect a whole range of behaviors.

Each of these accounts of self-evaluation effects provides a theoretical framework that is relevant to the current research findings within the social loafing paradigm.

THE SOCIAL LOAFING EFFECT AND ITS
MEDIATOR—EVALUATION

"Social loafing" has been described as the phenomenon in which participants who work together generate less effort than do participants who work alone (Latané, Williams, & Harkins, 1979). This reduction in effort has been found to occur on tasks that require both physical effort (clapping—Harkins, Latané, & Williams, 1980; pumping air—Kerr & Bruun, 1981; shouting—Latané et al., 1979) and cognitive effort (brainstorming and vigilance—Harkins & Petty, 1982; solving mazes—Jackson & Williams, 1985; evaluating essays—Petty, Harkins, Williams, & Latané, 1977; and reacting to proposals—Brickner, Harkins, & Ostrom, 1986).

Although Latané et al.'s (1979) description implies that social loafing is simply a consequence of participants' "working together," Harkins (1987) has suggested that this reduction in effort is a consequence of a particular feature of the experiments in which this effect has been found. In all of the loafing experiments, when participants worked together, their outputs were combined. Thus, individual outputs were "lost in the crowd," and participants could receive neither credit nor blame for their performances. Harkins (1987) has argued that the lack of evaluation potential was what led to loafing in these experiments.

Consistent with this notion are the findings of Williams, Harkins, and Latané (1981) that when participants were led to believe that their individual outputs were identifiable, the loafing effect was eliminated, whether they worked individually or together. Williams et al. (1981) argued that these results suggest that identifiability is an important mediator of the loafing effect.

Subsequent research (Harkins & Jackson, 1985), however, has shown that identifiability of individual outputs alone is not sufficient to eliminate loafing: Participants must also feel that their outputs can be *compared* with those of others. Without this potential for evaluation, participants whose outputs were individually identifiable put out as little effort as those whose outputs were combined. These data suggest that, in the loafing paradigm, people are motivated by the potential for evaluation.

Requirements for Evaluation

Consistent with this analysis, Szymanski and Harkins (1987) argued that for evaluation to be possible, two pieces of information are necessary: some measure of task output, and a standard against which this output can be compared. The need for a standard can be satisfied in a number of ways. If a participant has had extensive experience with a given task, it is possible that he or she has some notion of how his or her current level of performance compares with the earlier levels. In this case, the standard would be the participant's own earlier performances. However, in most if not all loafing research, it is unlikely that this type of standard is available, because the tasks are unfamiliar to the participants. In the absence of a personal standard, the need for a standard can be satisfied by either an objective or a social criterion. For example, if participants were asked to monitor a visual display and to report the number of signals they saw, the objective standard for this task would be the number of signals that were actually presented. On the same visual task, a social standard would be the average number of signals detected by previous participants. On some types of tasks, there is no objective criterion for performance; thus only a social standard can be used. For example, on a brainstorming task, when participants are asked to generate as many uses as possible for an object, a social standard would be the average number of uses generated by previous participants. There can be no objective criterion on this task, since there is no "correct" solution; one simply produces as much as possible.

Sources of Evaluation in Social Loafing

In the social loafing paradigm, there are three potential sources of evaluation: the experimenter, the coactor (or coactors), and the participant. In previous research on social loafing, the role of the experimenter as evaluator has been emphasized. For example, Harkins et al. (1980) wrote:

> The results [social loafing] are easily explained by a minimizing strategy, where participants are motivated to work only as hard as necessary to gain credit for a good performance or to avoid blame for a bad one. When the experimenter was unable to monitor individual outputs directly, performers sloughed off. (p. 464)

When manipulation checks have been used, only the participants' perceptions of the experimenter's ability to evaluate individual outputs have been assessed (e.g., Harkins & Jackson, 1985; Harkins & Petty, 1982; Jackson & Williams, 1985). This assumption about the central role of the experimenter's evaluation in the loafing effect may have been made, at least in part, because the tasks typically used in this research were seen as "noncompetitive, boring, tiring" (Harkins et al., 1980, p. 463) and as "unlikely to be personally involving for students, providing intrinsic importance, personal meaning, or significant consequences for one's life" (Brickner et al., 1986, p. 764). It seems reasonable to think that external surveillance would be required to motivate performance on such tasks. However, Szymanski and Harkins (1987) have pointed out that combined outputs not only make it impossible for the experimenter to evaluate individual performance, but also leave the coparticipants and the participants themselves unable to do so. For example, when participants shouted (Latané et al., 1979), no evaluation was possible, because the masking noise eliminated the possibility that participants could hear or be heard. After the session, if the participants had access to the scores, it was possible for them to compare (evaluate) individual performances, but they were as unable as the experimenter to decompose group outputs. Thus, when outputs were combined, participants may have felt that they could not evaluate their own outputs, and that these outputs could not be evaluated by their fellow participants either. Thus, people may loaf not only because the experimenter cannot evaluate them, but also because they cannot be evaluated by the coactors and/or by themselves. This last possibility is particularly intriguing, because, as mentioned earlier, the tasks used in the loafing research have been described as dull and tiring. Is the potential for self-evaluation sufficient to motivate performance on such tasks?

Motivational Aspects of Self-Evaluation

Szymanski and Harkins (1987) tested the possibility that the potential for self-evaluation alone can motivate performance by orthogonally manipulating the potential for evaluation by the experimenter and the self. Pairs of participants were asked to generate as many uses as possible for a knife (the same task that was used by Harkins & Jackson, 1985). These uses were either collected separately by the experimenter or pooled. Crossed with this manipulation of experimenter evaluation was the opportunity for self-evaluation. Pilot work indicated that participants felt that they knew how many uses they had generated at the end of this brainstorming task (task output). This finding suggested that to manipulate the opportunity for evaluation, one need only provide or withhold some sort of standard. This was accomplished by leading participants to believe either that the average number of uses generated in the previous experiment (the standard condition) would be provided after their performances, or that it would be withheld (the no-standard condition). Analysis of the manipulation checks revealed that providing this information was sufficient to lead participants in the standard condition to report that they could self-evaluate to a reliably greater extent than could participants in the no-standard condition.

Analysis of participants' performances revealed that the opportunity for self-evaluation was sufficient to lead to performance equivalent to that achieved in the experimenter evaluation conditions. In these experiments, we simply provided participants with the opportunity to self-evaluate without attempting to motivate them to do so. As noted before, previous descriptions of the tasks used in loafing research (e.g., Harkins et al., 1980; Brickner et al., 1986) would suggest that taking part in these tasks may be sheer drudgery. Nevertheless, our finding suggests that, even on boring tasks, the opportunity for self-evaluation is also sufficient to eliminate the loafing effect.

The Opportunity for Self-Knowledge and Self-Validation

This opportunity for self-evaluation, even in this motivationally barren setting, may actually have provided the participants with two incentives. First, they could have learned something about how well they could perform the particular task (*where* they stood in comparison to some objective criterion of performance). This incentive corresponds to what Goethals and Darley (1987) have termed "self-knowledge," defined as "a generalized desire, need, wish or want [for people] to *know* how good they are at various ability-linked tasks" (p. 24). Second, participants could compare their scores to the performance of the average previous participant, and take pleasure from the fact that they *surpassed* it. In Goethals and Darley's (1987) terminology, this incentive corresponds to "self-validation," defined as "a desire to think well of their abilities—that is, to think that their abilities are high" (p. 24). As long as a social criterion serves as the standard, both incentives are available. Thus, in our (Szymanski & Harkins, 1987) research, participants could have been motivated by the opportunity for self-knowledge, and/or by the opportunity for self-validation.

Subsequent research (Harkins & Szymanski, 1988) that used a vigilance task with an objective standard confirmed the role of self-evaluation as a powerful source in motivating performance. When participants were provided only with the opportunity for self-knowledge (the opportunity to compare one's performance to an objective standard), the loafing effect was also eliminated. These findings are consistent with the assumptions of social comparison theory (Festinger, 1954; Goethals & Darley, 1987). As suggested by Festinger's original theory and its revised version formulated by Goethals and Darley, the opportunity for self-knowledge alone should be sufficient to motivate performance. In Festinger's (1954) theory, the role of self-knowledge is central. In fact, the original version (Festinger, 1954) suggested that one will turn to social comparison only when objective standards are not available. Goethals and Darley (1987), in their revision of Festinger's (1954) theory, incorporated self-validation as another source of motivation, by stating that individuals do not want simply to inform themselves about how they stand relative to others; they want to learn that they are *better* than these others. Of course, there was some suggestion of this in the original theory in Festinger's notion of the unidirectional upward drive for abilities, but in the revised version Goethals and Darley emphasized self-validation and self-knowledge equally. Harkins and Szymanski (1988) demonstrated that the motivational effect of self-evaluation persists even when the possibility of self-validation is eliminated.

IMPLICATIONS OF THE SELF-EVALUATION EFFECT

The findings outlined here contribute to an understanding of self-evaluation processes as described by current theories of self-evaluation (e.g., Bandura's [1986] theory of self-efficacy; Greenwald and Breckler's [1985] ego-task analysis). The overall pattern of results presented in this chapter confirms the notion that self-evaluation requires two pieces of information: task output and a standard. The notion that standards of comparison underlie the evaluation process is consistent with the approaches taken in several recent formulations of the self-evaluation process (Bandura, 1986; Higgins, Strauman, & Klein, 1986; Masters & Keil, 1987), although there are differences in the particular standards that are incorporated in the approaches.

Of these approaches, only Masters and Keil (1987) include what I have termed "objective standards." Masters and Keil describe them as "external reference standards," by which they mean standards that are used "to index information that may be used in a comparison that is summary in nature and does not invoke specific instances of or information about social or personal events" (p. 15). Examples would be a moral percept, a self-selected goal, an expectancy for a performance, or a minimum standard of performance. Based on our findings (Harkins & Szymanski, 1988), the inclusion of such standards is certainly warranted, although additional research will be required to determine the limits of this effect.

Each of these typologies includes social standards, but there are differences in the degree of specificity that is represented. For example, Higgins et al. (1986) describe three different social standards: "social category" (the average performances or attributes of some social category or group); "meaningful other" (the performances or attributes of another individual who is meaningful to the evaluator); and "social context" (the performances or attributes of people to whom the evaluator is currently exposed). Bandura (1986) includes only two social standards, "normative comparison" and "social comparison," which appear to correspond to Higgins et al.'s (1986) social category and social context, respectively; Masters and Keil (1987) satisfy themselves with a generic social standard as described above.

In our previous research (Szymanski & Harkins, 1987), participants in the standard condition were informed that they would be told the average number of uses generated in a previous version of the experiment. This social standard corresponds to Bandura's (1986) normative comparison and Higgins et al.'s (1986) social category reference point. In the later research (Harkins & Szymanski, 1988), it was found that the opportunity to compare one's outputs to one's partner's was sufficient to motivate performance. This standard corresponds to Higgins et al.'s (1986) social context and Bandura's (1986) social comparison. The findings of the motivational efficacy of such standards are consistent with the predictions of these approaches.

Each of the typologies also suggests that a person's own previous performances can serve as a standard. Bandura (1986) terms these standards "personal comparisons," Higgins et al. (1986) label them "autobiographical reference points," and Masters and Keil (1987) describe them as "personal-subjective comparisons," but each means by this a standard of comparison that results from a participant's previous experiences with the task. In our research, we have used tasks with which the participants are unlikely to have had any prior experience from which to develop personal standards, so that it appears unlikely that these standards could have played a role in our research; however, given sufficient experience with a task, it is likely that such standards could also motivate performance.

Thus, our research is consistent with the notion that these various types of standards motivate performance, but are they equally effective in doing so? It would seem possible that some types of standards could have more motivational potency than others. For example, although Festinger (1954) suggested that people turn to social comparison only when objective sources of comparison are unavailable, it seems plausible that the prospect of social comparison could be more potent than the opportunity for objective comparison. After all, in the former case, concerns about both self-validation and self-knowledge are aroused; in the latter case, concern should focus on self-knowledge alone. In this respect, personal standards seem more like objective standards, because personal standards also do not involve direct comparison with another person.

To turn to different types of social standards, the knowledge that one's performance can be compared against that of another person who is physically present may be more motivating than the prospect of the more remote comparison of one's performance against the average performance of previous participants. By incorporating these various types of standards into *one* design, we will be able to compare the potency of these various standards. This will allow us to determine whether finer-grained analyses are necessary, at least from the point of view of motivating performance.

By providing the necessities for self-evaluation (task output and a standard of some type), we have created the opportunity for self-evaluation. However, simply providing the opportunity to self-evaluate may not guarantee the motivation to do so. Obviously, some level of motivation must exist, and these experiments only begin to hint at what is necessary to arouse and to maintain it. Systematically examining the potency of various types of standards may provide some clues about when and how much participants are motivated by the prospect of self-evaluation. Of course, these possibilities represent only a few of the ways to proceed in an attempt to determine the limits of the self-evaluation effect.

Our line of research also provides data that are relevant to more general processes that underlie self-evaluation. For example, Festinger's theory of social comparison proposed that there exists a "drive" for people to evaluate their opinions and abilities. Although the notion of a "drive" may be dated, the notion that people learn that it is useful to have a fairly accurate idea of their talents and skills remains quite current (e.g., Goethals & Darley, 1987). Our research provides data that are entirely consistent with this assumption (i.e., that people are motivated by the potential of self-knowledge alone). As another example, Greenwald and Breckler (1985) formulated the notion of three motivational facets of self—public, private, and collective—and their relevant evaluation concerns. The public self is sensitive to the evaluation of others. In describing private self, Greenwald and Breckler argued: "The prevalent assumption heretofore has been that self-presentations are targeted at audiences of others. We have reviewed evidence that there is also an important inner audience, oneself" (p. 141). The collective self is the "we" facet of the self and is oriented toward collective achievement—achieving goals and fulfilling one's role in a reference group.

In our research, the operation of the public self can be seen in the finding that the potential for evaluation of individual performance by the experimenter is sufficient to motivate performance (e.g., Szymanski & Harkins, 1987). Findings from the same set of experiments described earlier have also been consistent with Greenwald and Breckler's (1985) notion of motivational efficacy of the private self. After all, in the condition where one has the opportunity for self-evaluation, the only person who will know how a given participant performed is that person himself or herself. We have also obtained data that demonstrate the operation of the third motivational facet, the collective self.

GROUP EVALUATION AS A FORM OF SELF-EVALUATION

Up to this point, the analysis of the social loafing effect has focused on evaluation of the individual. That is, it has been suggested that people in a group slough off because their *individual* outputs cannot be evaluated by the experimenter or the self. However, in addition to output at the individual level, there is also the group's output. This output can be compared with a standard, thus permitting evaluation at the group level. In the previous loafing research, participants did not have an opportunity for this group evaluation, because once again one or both of the required pieces of information—performance output and a standard—were missing.

Several recent formulations have suggested that the potential for group evaluation could motivate performance. In addition to Greenwald and Breckler's (1985) idea of the collective self, Goethals and Darley (1987) also have incorporated the notion of group comparison in their revised version of social comparison theory.

In our recent research (Harkins & Szymanski, 1989), the possibility that providing participants with the opportunity for group evaluation may improve performance has been tested. Participants were tested in groups of three and were told either that their individual outputs were identifiable or that they were pooled. Crossed with this manipulation was another one: Half of the participants were given a social standard, and the other half were not provided with this information.

Analysis of the manipulation checks revealed that pooled-output participants who were provided with a standard reported that they felt they could evaluate their group's performance to a greater extent than did pooled-output participants who were not provided with one. Analysis of participants' performances revealed that when given a standard, participants whose outputs were pooled performed as well as those who took part as individuals. These findings demonstrate that the opportunity for group evaluation is sufficient to motivate performance. They are consistent with Goethals and Darley's (1987) extension of social comparison theory to the group level, mentioned earlier. In this extension, Goethals and Darley incorporated Tajfel and Turner's (1986) social identity theory. Tajfel and Turner suggested that people strive to maintain a positive self-concept, which can be achieved by attaining a positive social identity. One means of gaining such a positive identity is to discover that one's group compares favorably with other groups. If, on the other hand, one's group fares badly in such comparisons, the individual will attempt to improve the group, or, failing that, will leave it. Goethals and Darley (1987) saw this concern about positive self-concept as corresponding to the self-validation aspect of their revised theory, but at the group rather than the individual level. They also proposed to add to their theory a group-level concern with self-knowledge. That is, in addition to a concern about how one's *group* stacks up against other groups, one may simply be concerned about gaining information about how well one's group does at various tasks, which should allow the group to function more effectively.

The setting provided by the social loafing paradigm seems ideal for testing Goethals and Darley's notions, because in the loafing condition the possibility of evaluation of individual performances is minimized. Providing or withholding access to group-level output and a standard thus permits the motivational properties of group evaluation to be examined.

In their elaboration of social comparison theory (Festinger, 1954), Levine and Moreland (1986) have developed a typology of outcome comparisons that incorporates three dimensions: type of comparison, social context, and temporal contest. In addition to the self–other comparison that has been the traditional focus of interest in this area, Levine and Moreland added self–self and group–group comparisons. These types of comparisons can take place within the group (intragroup) or across groups (intergroup), the social contexts proposed by Levine and Moreland; they can also occur in the same time period (intratemporal) or across time periods (intertemporal), the temporal context dimension of the model. To apply this perspective to the current research, our pooled-output/standard condition would fall in the group–group/intergroup/intertemporal cell of Levine and Moreland's typology, because participants were afforded the opportunity to compare their group's performance to the average performance of previous, different groups.

Each of these approaches incorporates the notion that the potential for group evaluation can motivate performance, but under what conditions? Breckler and Greenwald (1986) suggested that the collective self's ego task is "achieving the goals of and fulfilling one's role in a reference group" (p. 148), which may include religious organizations, clubs, athletic teams, and family. Apparently, then, performing a task in service of such a group engages this aspect of self. Levine and Moreland (1986) suggested that group–group comparisons are likely when "group membership is salient because of group competition, group dissimilarity, or status differentials between groups (Brewer, 1979), when group members seek to enhance their social identity through intergroup comparisons (Tajfel, 1978)" (p. 289). Along similar lines, Goethals and Darley (1987) suggested that "comparison is not always sought out, but will take place whenever another group is salient, available, or similar" (p. 33).

An initial examination of these approaches to group evaluation would not necessarily lead one to expect reliable effects in the loafing paradigm. Our "groups" were composed of strangers who only expected to be together for the duration of the experiment. These groups were not the coworkers, religious organizations, clubs, athletic teams, or families to which Breckler and Greenwald (1986) referred. The features that Levine and Moreland (1986) and Goethals and Darley (1987) described as making group–group comparison likely also do not seem to have been strongly operative in our settings. However, there were aspects of the settings in the loafing research that could motivate group performance. For example, it is likely that participants who made up the groups saw themselves as being highly similar to one another (the same age, likely to share most values); they generated a group product; and it is possible that they saw the task as having some minimal value. The data show that even these minimal groups are sufficient to arouse comparison motives.

The research described here emphasizes the importance of evaluation potential in reducing the social loafing effect. However, we do not propose that effects stemming from manipulations of evaluation account for all, or even most, motivation losses in groups. Any number of other variables may affect performance in group settings (e.g., dispensability of members' effort; Kerr & Bruun, 1983). Even when our attention is limited to the loafing paradigm, it is clear that other factors motivate performance, regardless of the potential for evaluation. For example, personal involvement (Brickner et al., 1986), partners' effort (Jackson & Harkins, 1985), task challenge and task uniqueness (Harkins & Petty, 1982), and group cohesion (Williams, 1981) have all been shown to eliminate the loafing effect, even though the potential for evaluation by each of the potential sources is minimized. In future research, it will be necessary to determine how these other factors interact with the potential for evaluation to motivate performance in these settings.

CONCLUSIONS

In this chapter, I have focused on the role that evaluation plays in eliminating the loafing effect. Borrowing Greenwald and Breckler's (1985) typology of ego-task analysis, I have identified three evaluative audiences—public, private, and collective—all of which motivate performance. A line of research has been presented that provides data relevant to each of these accounts of evaluation effect.

Given that most tasks used in the social loafing paradigm are seen as uninvolving, this chapter has centered on the motivational efficacy of the potential for self-evaluation. These current findings demonstrated that the opportunity for self-evaluation at the level of both the individual and the group reduces the loafing effect. This research not only contributes to the better understanding of the loafing paradigm, but also provides us with more understanding of the motivational properties of the potential for self-evaluation. The data are consistent with the accounts of self-evaluation effects generated by current theories of self-evaluation processes (e.g., Bandura, 1986; Goethals & Darley, 1987; Greenwald & Breckler, 1985; Levine & Moreland, 1986; Masters & Keil, 1987). The next step will be to determine the limits of the self-evaluation effect—in other words, to discover how powerful the "self" really is.

REFERENCES

Bandura, A. (1986). *Social foundations of thought and action: A social cognitive theory.* Englewood Cliffs, NJ: Prentice-Hall.

Breckler, S., & Greenwald, A. (1986). Motivational facets of the self. In R. M. Sorrentino & E. T. Higgins (Eds.), *Handbook of motivation and cognition: Foundations of social behavior* (Vol. 1, pp. 145–164). New York: Guilford Press.

Brewer, M. (1979). In-group bias in the minimal intergroup situation: A cognitive–motivational analysis. *Psychological Bulletin, 86,* 307–324.

Brickner, M., Harkins, S., & Ostrom, T. (1986). Personal involvement: Thought provoking implications for social loafing. *Journal of Personality and Social Psychology, 51*, 763–769.

Deci, E., & Ryan, R. (1985). *Intrinsic motivation and self-determination in human behavior.* New York: Plenum.

Festinger, L. (1954). A theory of social comparison processes. *Human Relations, 7*, 117–140.

Goethals, G., & Darley, J. (1987). Social comparison theory: Self-evaluation and group life. In B. Mullin & G. Goethals (Eds.), *Theories of group behavior* (pp. 21–47). New York: Springer-Verlag.

Greenwald, A., & Breckler, S. (1985). To whom is the self presented? In B. Schlenker (Ed.), *The self and social life.* (pp. 126–145), New York: McGraw-Hill.

Harkins, S. (1987). Social loafing and social facilitation. *Journal of Experimental Social Psychology, 23*, 1–18.

Harkins, S., & Jackson, J. (1985). The role of evaluation in eliminating social loafing. *Personality and Social Psychology Bulletin, 11*, 457–465.

Harkins, S., Latané, B., & Williams, K. (1980). Social loafing: Allocating effort or taking it easy? *Journal of Experimental Social Psychology, 16*, 457–465.

Harkins, S., & Petty, R. (1982). Effects of task difficulty and task uniqueness on social loafing. *Journal of Personality and Social Psychology, 43*, 1214–1229.

Harkins, S., & Szymanski, K. (1988). Social loafing and self-evaluation with an objective standard. *Journal of Experimental Social Psychology, 24*, 354–365.

Harkins, S., & Szymanski, K. (1989). Social loafing and group evaluation. *Journal of Personality and Social Psychology, 56*, 934–941.

Higgins, E. T., Strauman, T., & Klein, R. (1986). Standards and the process of self-evaluation: Multiple affects from multiple stages. In R. M. Sorrentino & E. T. Higgins (Eds.), *Handbook of motivation and cognition: Foundations of social behavior* (Vol. 1, pp. 23–63). New York: Guilford Press.

Jackson, J., & Harkins, S. (1985). Equity in effort: An explanation of the social loafing effect. *Journal of Personality and Social Psychology, 49*, 1119–1206.

Jackson, J., & Williams, K. (1985). Social loafing on difficult tasks: Working collectively can improve performance. *Journal of Personality and Social Psychology, 49*, 937–942.

Kerr, N., & Bruun, S. (1981). Ringelman revisited: Alternative explanations for the social loafing effect. *Personality and Social Psychology Bulletin, 7*, 224–231.

Kerr, N., & Bruun, S. (1983). Dispensability of member effort and group motivation losses: Free-rider effects. *Journal of Personality and Social Psychology, 44*, 78–94.

Latané, B., Williams, K., & Harkins, S. (1979). Many hands make light the work: The causes and consequences of social loafing. *Journal of Personality and Social Psychology, 37*, 823–832.

Levine, J., & Moreland, R. (1986). Outcome comparisons in group contexts: Consequences for the self and others. In R. Schwarzer (Ed.), *Self-related cognitions in anxiety and motivation* (pp. 285–303). Hillsdale, NJ: Erlbaum.

Masters, J., & Keil, L. (1987). Generic comparison processes in human judgment and behavior. In J. Masters & W. Smith (Eds.), *Social comparison, social justice, and relative deprivation* (pp. 11–54). Hillsdale, NJ: Erlbaum.

Petty, R., Harkins, S., Williams, K., & Latané, B. (1977). The effects of group size on cognitive effort and evaluation. *Personality and Social Psychology Bulletin, 3*, 579–582.

Szymanski, K., & Harkins, S. (1987). Social loafing and self-evaluation with a social standard. *Journal of Personality and Social Psychology, 53*, 891–897.

Tajfel, H. (1978). Social categorization, social identity, and social comparison. In H. Tajfel (Ed.), *Differentiation between social groups: Studies in the social psychology of intergroup relations* (pp. 61–76). London: Academic Press.

Tajfel, H., & Turner, J. (1986). The social identity theory of intergroup behavior. In S. Worchel & W. Austin (Eds.), *Psychology of intergroup relations* (pp. 33–48). Chicago: Nelson-Hall.

Williams, K. (1981, May). *The effects of group cohesiveness on social loafing*. Paper presented at the meeting of the Midwestern Psychological Association, Detroit, MI.

Williams, K., Harkins, S., & Latané, B. (1981). Identifiability as a deterrent to social loafing: Two cheering experiments. *Journal of Personality and Social Psychology, 40*, 303–311.

CHAPTER FIVE

Social Identities: Thoughts on Structure and Change

KAY DEAUX

In the novel *Billy Bathgate*, E. L. Doctorow (1989) places his young hero in some complicated and often contradictory situations. Beginning as a young street kid, Billy Bathgate idolizes and then becomes an apprentice to Dutch Schultz, the leading gangster of the era. From ragamuffin to young peacock, Billy Bathgate is transformed in appearance. His locale changes as well, as the raucous world of the Bronx is traded for gentility in upper New York State, and Bible studies are substituted for gambling lessons. Perplexed by these rapid changes, Billy muses on the meaning of self-definition: "None of these things made sense except as I was contingent to a situation" (p. 183). Contemplating this state of continued fluctuation in identity, Billy formalizes his observations as the "license-plate theory of identification" (p. 183).

Billy Bathgate is clearly a social psychologist in the making, using situations to account for the major portion of variance. And although I argue in this chapter that there are important stabilities in the identities we claim as well, this recognition of multiplicity and of change is central to my approach.

THE CONCEPT OF IDENTITY

"Identity" is an intellectually seductive concept, capable of drawing on a number of diverse literatures, from the structural concerns of sociology on the one hand to psychoanalytic probes of individual personality on the other. Yet because the intellectual roots are so diffuse, and the connotations quite varied (Gleason, 1983), I should clarify the assumptions that I make when I use this term. This will place my work in the line of some traditions while distinguishing it from others.

My analysis of identity includes three specific aspects: first, an emphasis on social identity, as defined by membership in recognizable social groups; second, a notion of multiplicity; and third, a premise of social construction.

1. As defined by the late Henri Tajfel, social identity is "that part of an individual's self-concept which derives from his knowledge of his membership of a social group (or groups)" (1981, p. 255). Thus, in defining ourselves as women, professors, or New Yorkers, we speak not only of personal characteristics but of attributes potentially shared with a large number of other people. In Tajfel's framework, this process of self-categorization is a way to foster self-esteem. Individuals gain esteem through their group membership, in large part by comparing themselves to other groups. This recognition that self-esteem derives from group membership is an important supplement to the more individualistic tradition of self-esteem research, which focuses primarily on intrapsychic experience. And, as the recent work of Crocker and her colleagues has shown, self-esteem associated with collective identities is conceptually and empirically distinct from personal self-esteem (Crocker & Luhtanen, 1990; Luhtanen & Crocker, 1988).

2. Second, I assume that individuals have a multiplicity of identities. George Herbert Mead was an early proponent of this position. "We divide ourselves up in all sorts of different selves with reference to our acquaintances," he said, and he went on to add that "a multiple personality is in a certain sense normal" (1934, p. 142). More recently, the work of Sheldon Stryker and his colleagues assumes a variety of social identities, each tied to different relationships and different situations, much as Billy Bathgate proposes (Stryker, 1968, 1987; Stryker & Serpe, 1982).

3. The assumption that social identities are constructed through experience rather than accepted as givens can also be linked to the pioneering work of Mead. Mead (1934) led social scientists to appreciate the interplay between self and society, according priority to context in the development of a sense of self. Mead argued that meaning always emerges from social interaction, and thus that categories of meaning are socially constructed. Stryker continues to develop this viewpoint, arguing for appreciation of the interplay between structural provisions and individual choices: "The proper question is under what circumstances will . . . behaviour be more or less heavily constrained, more or less open to creative constructions" (1987, p. 93). Arriving at a similar position from the perspective of personality psychologists, Rosenberg and Gara state that "social identities are . . . identities elaborated by the individual within seemingly broad social constraints" (1985, p. 88).

In sum, when I speak of identity, I assume that people have several distinct senses of themselves, that these identities are linked in some degree to group memberships, and that people give individual meaning to these categories as a result of their own subjective experiences. Accepting these assumptions suggests a number of important questions for theory and research, including issues of dimensionality, structure, content, and stability.

DIMENSIONS AND CATEGORIES OF IDENTITY

The general concept of social identity used here includes a variety of exemplars, including social roles (e.g., parent), demographic categories (e.g., woman), and membership in organizations (e.g., Republican). For the most part, these categories are treated interchangeably in discussions of social identity. Yet it seems reasonable to assume that these various identities differ in psychologically meaningful ways. Some social categories such as gender and age are visible to observers, for example, while other categories are not so readily identified. Some identities, such as spousehood or occupation, may be freely chosen, while others, such as ethnicity or deafness, are not subject to personal choice. Variations may also exist in the degree to which a social category implies shared membership and common characteristics—features essential to Tajfel's theoretical formulation.

Relatively little attention has been paid to these dimensions of difference and their consequences for identity-relevant behavior. Believing that these distinctions are important, a colleague and I have begun to explore the domain (Deaux & Ethier, 1990). In our initial study, we asked people to rate a set of social categories on a variety of psychological dimensions, such as importance, stability, specificity of goals, and visibility. Our data are still preliminary, but they serve to illustrate the possible distinctions. Social categories are plotted on two dimensions in Figure 5.1: "desirable–undesirable" and "voluntary–involuntary." When these two dimensions are used, four distinct clusters of identities emerge.

These differences should be important. Identities that are voluntarily chosen, for example, may require more effort to maintain. Identities perceived to be voluntary should also provide different attributional alternatives when explaining identity-relevant behavior. Similarly, the desirability or undesirability of an identity surely influences the degree to which that identity will be proclaimed or hidden—will serve as a source of self-esteem or be cause for shame. Recognizing and formalizing these conceptual distinctions should lead to greater understanding of the processes by which identities are claimed and maintained.

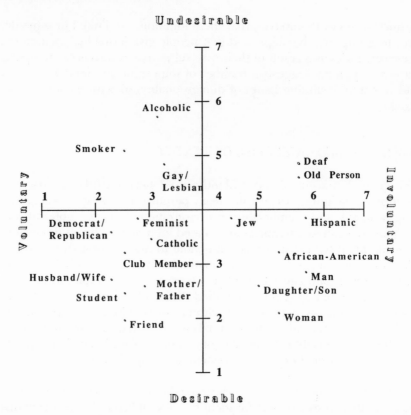

FIGURE 5.1. Ratings of selected social categories on dimensions of desirable–undesirable and voluntary–involuntary. From [Dimensions of Social Identity] by K. Deaux and K. Ethier, 1990, unpublished raw data.

STRUCTURE AND HIERARCHY

If one assumes that people have a number of important social identities, then obvious questions are raised about the structural relationships among identities. Some writers have addressed this question, but the issues are far from resolved.

Stryker (1987) proposes that identities are hierarchically ordered according to their salience, defined in terms of the individual's level of commitment to the underlying roles. He also suggests that certain categories such as age, gender, and ethnicity serve as master statuses, influencing the definition of other identities. Turner (1987) suggests that self-categorization can be represented in terms of three levels of abstraction: (1) a superordinate level of human being; (2) an intermediate level of social categories, such as woman, black, and student; and (3) a subordinate level of "personal self-categorizations" based on differentiations within one's ingroup. Within each of these levels, Turner suggests there can be finer grades of categorization: For example, at the intermediate level one could claim membership in both national and supranational ingroups.

Both Stryker's and Turner's models of the identity hierarchy are theory-driven. In contrast, Rosenberg and his colleagues have developed a data-driven approach, in which the structure of individual identities emerges from the empirical base (DeBoeck & Rosenberg, 1988; Rosenberg, 1988, 1989; Rosenberg & Gara, 1985). Eliciting both identities and the features associated with those identities from the individuals themselves, Rosenberg uses statistical techniques (specifically, hierarchical classification) to discover individual identity structures. His findings (and our own preliminary work) suggest substantial variation in the structural patterns of identities: Whereas some individuals show a clear hierarchy, the identity patterns of other individuals are best represented at the same level of inclusiveness. Thus one person might have a "master identity" as a black, and all other identities would be subordinate to that guiding identity. Another person, in contrast, might give equal importance to identities such as professor, Latina, and mother, with none superordinate to any other. These empirical findings must inform our theoretical analyses of identity structure.

DESCRIPTIVE WORK ON IDENTITY

Adopting a bottom-up approach to the analysis of social categories, my colleagues and I are gathering descriptive data on the nature of people's identities. Our general approach is straightforward: We ask people to identify those categories or labels that have meaning for them, and to tell us about the attributes that characterize each identity. (It is worth noting that people find this task quite easy to do and seem to enjoy doing it.)

Two different subject populations have been sampled. The first sample consisted of 12 women and 12 men, ranging in age from 24 to 64 (Deaux, 1988). They were selected to represent a range of occupation, ethnicity, and marital status. These 24 adults were interviewed on two occasions, separated by an interval of 5 months. The second sample, chosen to explore specific issues of ethnic identity and threats to that identity, consisted of 45 Hispanic students attending one of two Ivy League universities, who were interviewed on three separate occasions over the course of their first academic year (Ethier & Deaux, 1990a, 1990b). The group was homogeneous in age and divided approximately 60%–40% between male and female; it included students of both Mexican and Puerto Rican descent.

TABLE 5.1. Identities Mentioned Most Frequently in 24-Adult Study

Identity	Percent
Occupation	88
Spouse/lover	71
Friend	58
Daughter/son	54
Gender	46
Parent	46
Religion	17
Political party	8
Ethnicity	8

Respondents in both studies claimed approximately 7 identities each (6.5 in the first study and 7.8 in the Hispanic student study), with a range of 3 to 12. Testifying to the importance of assessing identities "from the inside out" (Ryff, 1984), we observed both "Type I" and "Type II" errors. In other words, there were instances when people claimed an identity that they did not objectively possess, such as that of spouse when they were not yet married, or failed to claim an identity, such as Hispanic, when an observer (or college official) would categorize them as such. Tables 5.1 and 5.2 provide lists of the identities that people in the two studies most frequently claimed.

TABLE 5.1. Identities Mentioned Most Frequently in Hispanic Student Study

Identity	Percent
Hispanic	87
Student	84
Friend	80
Daughter/son	78
Sister/brother	49
Religion	44
Political party	36
Gender	27
Leader/role model	22

Note. The data are from Ethier and Deaux (1990a).

Not all self-relevant characteristics need to be conceptualized as identities. People may characterize themselves in terms of personality traits without necessarily claiming an identity, as in the statement "I am a kind person." Such traits may be a key feature of one particular identity, or they may be overarching characteristics common to a number of different identities. From the particular theoretical perspective taken here, the concern is not with these generally abstract traits, but rather with more concrete categories of membership.

A major tenet of the present formulation is that a person's identities cannot be assumed in advance or stipulated from the outside. Rather, they are subjectively determined and must be assessed accordingly. In studying the parent identity, for example, Karen Dion (1989) finds that approximately 80% of women but only 50% of men who have children—an objective status—list parent as one of their salient psychological identities. Similarly, Lau (1989) reports varying degrees of correspondence between objective categorization and subjective identity, from 15%–20% in the case of political affiliations to 80% for U.S. African-Americans.

The reverse is also possible: People may claim identities that they seem objectively not to have. In the adult sample we interviewed, at least two women claimed an identity as a mother when the objective evidence was not supportive. One woman claimed both mother and spouse as among her most important identities, though at the time of the interview she was neither a mother nor a spouse. She was, however, engaged, and one can surmise that the "possible self" had a subjective reality in terms of her self-definition. These cases underline the importance of a methodology that allows some ideographic analysis.

Beyond the question of how identities are defined is the question of the meaning associated with an identity. Addressing this issue, Rosenberg and Gara (1985) define an identity as "an amalgam of features—personal characteristics, feelings, values, intentions, and images—experienced by the individual" (p. 90). This position assumes that identities often represent widely accepted social categories, but that the meaning associated with acceptance of that categorical membership is constructed by the individual.

Empirical analysis of people's identities makes the issue of individual variation clear. Even when a stated identity is the same, two people may differ widely in the meaning that they associate with that category. As an example, several women named the identity of mother as an important one. Yet consider how different the meanings of this identity can be. One woman characterized her identity as a mother with the words "loving, understanding, sympathetic, reliable, sincere, and conscientious"; another woman, for whom the identity was equally important, described her mother-self as "strict, bossy, organized, clean, and worried." The validity of these descriptions is unknown, but the differences in the subjective definitions are quite striking.

Similarly, Hispanic students varied their characterizations of a Hispanic identity. One student described her Puerto Rican identity as "proud, loyal, happy, lucky, cared for, social, religious, and standing out in both good and bad ways." In contrast, a Mexican-American student described her Hispanic identity as "proud and representative," but also as "confused, mixed, questioning, a token, and excluded."

How stable are these reported identities? It is important to determine whether the reports are casual responses that are influenced by a current situation or whether they represent more stable depictions of self. Results from both studies attest to the basic stability of these social identities. In the study of 24 adults, most of the respondents showed relatively little change in their claimed identities over the 5-month interval between interviews (average common-element correlation $= +.70$; cf. McNemar, 1969). Not only were the identities themselves reasonably stable, but the attributes used to describe these identities on the two occasions remained quite similar as well ($r = +.58$). Similarly, in the sample of Hispanic students, there was consistency across the two-semester span ($r = +.70$ in the 6-month interval between Time 1 and Time 3).

SALIENCE OF IDENTITIES

Equipped with a set of stable identities, individuals have some latitude as to what identity will come to the forefront. At any given time, in any given interaction, one identity may be more prominent than others, guiding behavior and influencing the sequence of events (Deaux & Major, 1987). What conditions make identities salient? In considering the specific case of gender, we (Deaux & Major, 1987) proposed a framework in which one could account for the presence of sex differences on some occasions and their absence in others. Relevant to the present discussion was the consideration of gender identity as one of a number of possible identities, and an analysis of factors that could make that specific identity salient in any given situation.

Numerous factors influence the likelihood that an identity will be salient. From the internal or stable individual perspective, people differ in the importance and salience of various aspects of themselves. Notions of hierarchy, whether generated from a top-down or bottom-up approach, attempt to depict these variations in importance.

Why is any one identity more prominent, and what identities are most likely to take top billing? Stryker (1987; Stryker & Serpe, 1982) suggests that one's commitment to an identity, and hence its prominence in the identity hierarchy, is related to the number of interactions one has that are defined in terms of that identity. McGuire and his colleagues suggest that the salience of an identity is influenced by stable household patterns. School children who come from households in which their sex is in a minority, for example, are more likely to define themselves in terms of gender than are children whose sex is in the majority (McGuire, McGuire, & Winton, 1979).

In the case of the student sample, Hispanic identity was related to the strength of the students' cultural background (Ethier & Deaux, 1990a). An index of cultural background consisted of variables such as language spoken in the home, percentage of Hispanics in the community, percentage of high school friends who were Hispanics, country of origin, and the like. The index was then correlated with strength of the Hispanic identity, assessed both by rated importance and by the Identity subscale of Luhtanen and Crocker's (1988) Collective Self-Esteem Scale. Cultural background did not differ for the men and women in the sample, yet the relation of this background to identity importance was significant only for men ($r = +.38$).

This pattern persisted over time. Six months later, the relationship still continued to be strong for men ($r = +.69$) and nonsignificant for women ($r = +.17$). On the one hand, this pattern of correlations verifies the seemingly obvious connection between one's Hispanic background and an endorsed Hispanic identity. On the other hand, the variation shows that the strength of this background does not necessarily predict identity salience. With regard to the women, it should be noted that although their Hispanic identity was not related to cultural background, Hispanic identity was significantly stronger for them than for the men. Furthermore, although the women's Hispanic identity was not linked to general cultural background, it was strongly related to the specific identity of daughter, suggesting somewhat different constructions of identity for women and men. The selection factors involved in college entrance for Hispanic women versus men must also be considered in interpreting these differences.

In addition to these internal influences, numerous situational and contextual influences come into play, pulling out some identities and making others irrelevant. If an identity is tied to a particular setting or role relationship, for example, it will tend to be invoked when that context is salient. The individual entering a classroom brings out the professor or student identity; the individual moving into an operating room takes on the identity of surgeon, nurse, or patient. These identities are brought out because of strong situational demands.

Demographic characteristics of a setting vis-à-vis the individual can prime a particular identity. The influence of minority status, shown by McGuire and his colleagues in terms of long-term influence, has more momentary effects as well. School children are more likely to refer to their ethnicity, height or eye color when these attributes are distinctive in their classroom (McGuire, McGuire, Child, & Fujioka, 1978). College students in experimenter-assembled groups show the same pattern with regard to sex (Cota & Dion, 1986). At a more general level, Turner (1987) has suggested that there is a functional relationship between categorization and context; that is, the salience of a given category will depend on its fit to the environmental reality.

More subtle influences can also bring a particular identity to the fore, as the extensive work on priming has shown. Actions of other people in the setting, environmental cues, casual comments by onlookers—any of these can be the trigger for bringing a particular identity into the working self-concept, ready to influence subsequent behavior.

It is also important to consider the motivational forces exerted by the individual—the motivated strategies, the goal-directed behaviors, the intentions and purposes that are an equally importance source of identity shifts. Individuals often approach situations with particular goals in mind and then consciously choose which identity or aspect of self to depict.

To the extent that various identities overlap in their features, then the issue of salience is less important. However, if identities are markedly different in their features, meanings, and behavioral implications, then shifts in salience should be accompanied by sharply different behavioral choices. These consequences need to be explored further.

IDENTITY AND CHANGE

Despite this flexibility in their use, identities are relatively stable self-constructions. As such, many identity-relevant activities consist of strategies to maintain important identities. Social-psychological work on self-verification, for example, stresses the active engagement of the individual in presenting a persona and selecting a context in which self-defined identity can be maintained (Swann, 1983, 1984). A sociological perspective reminds us that identities are defined in the context of social relationships, and thus habitual role relationships are likely to persist unchanged. At a still broader level, one can look to the ecological context as providing a system of support for particular identities. These forces for stability provide a means of organizing experience, insuring predictability, and stabilizing self-esteem.

Yet despite these forces for stability, it is equally apparent that there are changes in an individual's identity structure over the life course. Some of the changes seem to be almost inevitable consequences of the life sequence. People typically get married and begin careers in their 20s, for example, and become parents and grandparents at later points. Even here, however, when taking a subjective perspective, one must recognize that not all individuals set the same pace through the life course. There are many "off-time" examples, such as the early occurrence of life-threatening illness or first-time parenthood for a man in his 50s. These examples attest to the variation in both claimed identities and invested meaning.

Beyond the reasonably predictable sequential changes in identity that have been explored by life span developmentalists, other forces—both internal and external—pressure for alteration of an existent identity structure. Significant others can die, for example, making one's identity as spouse, parent, or son/daughter no longer viable. Employment settings can provide new identities (e.g., that of an assistant professor or a newly elected partner) or can take away identities, as in the case of unemployment and job termination (Breakwell, 1986). Even an event as impersonal as a state lottery can create a new identity, if one is suddenly thrust into the million-dollar winners' group.

One case from our study of adult identities can be used to illustrate identity change. This case is particularly interesting, because some of the identities mentioned in the first interview were in a sense "possible selves" rather than actual selves. In the words of Markus and Nurius (1986), possible selves serve "as cognitive bridges between the present and future, specifying how individuals may change from how they are now to what they will become" (p. 961). I would argue that these possible selves, while not consistent with objective criteria, are nonetheless meaningful identities.

The reported identities of this 27-year-old secretary are shown in Table 5.3. At the time of the first interview, this woman was engaged and had clearly developed identities as mother and spouse, preparatory to assuming those objective roles. Between our two interviews, the engagement was broken, and the "possible selves" no longer seemed likely.

TABLE 5.3. Case Study of Identity Change

Identities named at Time 1	Identities named at Time 2
Mother[a]	Woman[a]
Teacher[a]	Daughter[a]
Lover[a]	Aunt[a]
Spouse	Sister
Supervisor	Friend
Psychologist	Tutor
Child	Girlfriend
	Lover
	Secretary

[a]Indicates identity was named as one of three most important.

Replacing those identities were such familial positions as daughter, sister, and aunt, along with the broader identity as a woman.

Changes such as these do not occur without stress. Indeed, we can hypothesize that the process of reconstruction is inherently stressful, requiring changes in both internal meaning and external relationships. Consistent with a hypothesis that changes in important identities are associated with stress, we found a correlation of −.49 between the stability of identities from the first to the second interview and scores on the Perceived Stress Scale (Cohen, Kamarck, & Mermelstein, 1983). More change was associated with more stress.

Many things can challenge an identity structure, creating a need for what I would call, with a nod to Erving Goffman, "identity work." Long-term changes in identities occur in at least three different forms. First, the change can take place in the characteristics associated with an identity. In general, it is probably easier for people to change the meanings associated with an identity than to change the category itself. Certainly this is true in the case of ascribed identities or biologically determined identities. One may change what it means to be black or female or short, for example, whereas the category is basically inalterable.

One of the Hispanic students furnished a vivid and wrenching example of changes in meaning, as well as esteem, as he attempted to cope with the threats to his Hispanic identity that he perceived at college. In the first interview, after only a few weeks on campus, this young man described being Hispanic as "happy, proud, and strong," yet tempered by "questioning, unsureness, and a sense of being isolated." Three months later, the attributes associated with being Hispanic continued to be primarily positive, though with an increasing awareness of being "different" (one of the adjectives used); he also talked about a dual role and the use of inner strength to overcome adversity. By the end of his first year, this picture was much bleaker: Attributes associated with being Hispanic included "alienated, confusion, upsetting, doubt, and disgust."

Change in the meaning of an identity is one form of change. A second form of identity change is a shift in importance—or, to use Stryker's (1987) terms, a shift in the salience hierarchy. The Hispanic student just described is one example of this. While devaluing the category of Hispanic, he also claimed it to be much less important at the end of the year, possibly as a means of protecting his overall self-esteem (cf. Crocker & Major, 1989). Many other examples of change in importance could be cited. One student whose parents separated in midyear attached increased importance to being a son and a brother at the end of the year. Another student of mixed parentage—one Hispanic parent, one black parent—initially claimed both identities but rated black as far more important than Hispanic. By the middle of the year, however, he had raised the importance of Hispanic substantially—and by the end of the year he no longer claimed black as one of his identities. One might speculate that this identity shift was a self-protective strategy—choosing the identity that was more acceptable in the primarily white Ivy League environment.

This deletion of a black identity (whether temporary or permanent) represents a third form of identity change—one in which either an existent identity is dropped or a new identity is added. In some cases, an identity may gradually decrease in importance until in some sense it atrophies and ceases to be a meaningful part of the identity structure. In other cases, a person will actively choose to discard an identity, particularly a negatively valued one. Overweight people may shed pounds and their identity as fat in the process; the person in an unsatisfactory marriage may discard the spouse identity. Thus individuals often make conscious choices and design specific strategies for reconfiguring their identity structure.

In other cases, identities are lost through external forces and events. Sometimes these can be anticipated. Retirement, for example, generally causes a loss of occupational identity, for which one can plan and restructure. Often, the loss of positive identities is not so clearly anticipated. The employee who is fired and told to clear out the desk immediately experiences a sharp and sudden loss of identity (Breakwell, 1986). The death of parents makes the identity of son or daughter somewhat empty, and the death of a spouse forces alterations in one's identity as wife or husband.

People also consciously choose to add identities to their repertoire. Getting married or deciding to have a child, for example, represents a conscious choice to add an important identity. So, typically, does the decision to enter college (cf. Hormuth, 1990). Initially, these identities may be represented as possible selves. The mental representation then can serve as a motivator, directing the individual to take actions that will realize that potential.

Added identities may also take their shape from previous related identities. One man we interviewed, for example, listed boyfriend as an identity on the first occasion and, having married in the interval, listed husband at the second interview. In such cases of identity work, the individual may take aspects of the earlier identity and incorporate them into the new identity (what Parkes, 1975, would call "encapsulation"). In the case of the boyfriend turned husband, we were able to correlate the pattern of attributes used to describe the two identities. The obtained correlation was only +.31, suggesting some but not substantial overlap between the two roles. (However, it is also worth noting in this case that the original girlfriend did not become the wife, perhaps accounting for a lower degree of overlap than might be expected.) In contrast, the woman described in Table 5.3 who initially claimed mother as an identity and later claimed an identity as aunt showed a correlation of +.66 between these two identities, suggesting that the attributes of mother had been substantially included in the newly claimed identity of aunt. Here, to go back to Billy Bathgate, the "license plate" may be shifted but the "car" remains the same.

CONSTRUCTING SOCIAL IDENTITIES

The construction of a social identity involves at least three interrelated processes: (1) self-definition in terms of group membership; (2) the acquisition of relevant information about group characteristics; and (3) public proclamation of belonging to the group. First and most obvious is defining oneself as an "X." As a possible self becomes a claimed identity, individuals presumably see themselves not only as attorneys or parents, for example, but as sharing some characteristics with other attorneys or parents. Thus the group takes on personal meaning. As Baker (1989) has reported, more positive feelings about one's social identity tend to be associated with greater identification with ingroup members.

Identity construction is also facilitated by the acquisition of relevant information. Cultural stereotypes are one source of information; direct experience with people in the category is another. This information both influences the initial selection of an identity and gives meaning to the identity once selected. Yet identity construction involves much more specific information search processes as well. In making the transition to motherhood, for example, a woman actively seeks information from books, physicians, and friends prior to the birth of the child (Deutsch, Ruble, Fleming, Brooks-Gunn, & Stangor, 1988).

A third mechanism involved in the construction of a social identity can be termed "self-proclamation." Self-proclamation refers to those actions that an individual takes to announce to others that he or she is a member of a particular group or the holder of a particular role. As Gollwitzer and his colleagues (Gollwitzer, 1986; Wicklund & Gollwitzer, 1982) have argued in discussing symbolic self-completion, the recognition by an audience of the identity may be particularly important, although some degree of self-persuasion is probably involved as well. (A distinction is made here between "self-verification" [Swann, 1983], which typically refers to actions directed toward confirming an existent identity, and self-proclamation, which is concerned with the initial acquisition of an identity. The similarity and areas of possible overlap are recognized, however.)

Several tactics of self-proclamation are possible. A person may display symbols of a particular group membership, such as college sweatshirts, distinctive hairstyles, or lapel pins (cf. Hormuth, 1990; Wicklund & Gollwitzer, 1982). To the extent that an identity is not otherwise visible, symbolic proclamation should be more likely. (Transsexuals contemplating surgery constitute a particularly clear example of this, insofar as they are generally required to cross-dress and act as members of the other sex for some period of time before surgery; cf. Morris, 1974.) Performing activities associated with group membership, such as subscribing to topical magazines or marching in parades, is another means of self-proclamation (and may in some cases facilitate the acquisition of relevant skills as well). Perhaps in recognition of these activities, persons who are members of groups judge that social identity to be more visible than do those who are not members: Thus, for example, the Catholic, the Democrat, and the club member believe that these social identities have greater visibility than others think they do (again, I am reporting some preliminary data from our investigations; Ethier & Deaux, 1990b).

These activities of self-proclamation are carried out to establish one's credentials as a member of a group. To the extent that this membership is in doubt, self-proclamation activities should be more intense. Ingroup favoritism has also been shown to be stronger when membership status is ambiguous (Brown & Wade, 1987) and when there are doubts about the legitimacy of one's claim to a particular social identity (Breakwell, 1979).

CONCLUDING THOUGHTS

Many questions about Billy Bathgate's "license plates" remain to be answered. The structure and change in identities—those categories that we live by—require a social-psychological analysis to supplement earlier sociological and developmental accounts. Much of the basic research on self can help us understand the processes by which identities are added, deleted, or maintained in the face of threat. At the same time, general processes of self, often studied in abstraction without context or interrelationships, will gain explanatory power by being connected to those senses of identity that are embedded in the social context.

ACKNOWLEDGMENTS

Research reported in this chapter has been conducted in collaboration with Kathleen Ethier, Jamila Pittalwala, and Margaret Miele. Conversations with them, with Yael Bat-Chava, and with members of the Identity Research Group have been important in my thinking about these issues.

REFERENCES

Baker, D. (1989). Social identity in the transition to motherhood. In S. Skevington & D. Baker (Eds.), *The social identity of women* (pp. 84–105). London: Sage.
Breakwell, G. (1979). Illegitimate group membership and intergroup differentiation. *British Journal of Social and Clinical Psychology, 18*, 141–149.

Breakwell, G. (1986). *Coping with threatened identities*. London: Methuen.

Brown, R., & Wade, G. (1987). Superordinate goals and intergroup behavior: The effect of role ambiguity and status on intergroup attitudes and task performance. *European Journal of Social Psychology, 17*, 131–142.

Cohen, S., Kamarck, T., & Mermelstein, R. (1983). A global measure of perceived stress. *Journal of Health and Social Behavior, 24*, 385–396.

Cota, A. A., & Dion, K. L. (1986). Salience of gender and sex composition of ad hoc groups: An experimental test of distinctiveness theory. *Journal of Personality and Social Psychology, 50*, 770–776.

Crocker, J., & Luhtanen, R. (1990). Collective self-esteem and ingroup bias. *Journal of Personality and Social Psychology, 58*, 60–67.

Crocker, J., & Major, B. (1989). Social stigma and self-esteem: The self-protective properties of stigma. *Psychological Review, 96*, 608–630.

Deaux, K. (1988, August). *Incipient identity*. Carolyn Wood Sherif lecture presented at the annual meeting of the American Psychological Association, Atlanta.

Deaux, K., & Ethier, K. (1990). [Dimensions of social identity]. Unpublished raw data.

Deaux, K., & Major, B. (1987). Putting gender into context: An interactive model of gender-related behavior. *Psychological Review, 94*, 369–389.

DeBoeck, P., & Rosenberg, S. (1988). Hierarchical classes: Model and data analysis. *Psychometrika, 53*, 361–381.

Deutsch, F. M., Ruble, D. N., Fleming, A., Brooks-Gunn, J., & Stangor, C. S. (1988). Information-seeking and maternal self-definition during the transition to motherhood. *Journal of Personality and Social Psychology, 55*, 420–431.

Dion, K. (1989, May). [*Gender differences in parental roles*]. Paper presented at Nags Head Conference on Sex and Gender, Nags Head, NC.

Doctorow, E. L. (1989). *Billy Bathgate*. New York: Random House.

Ethier, K., & Deaux, K. (1990a). Hispanics in Ivy: Assessing identity and perceived threat. *Sex Roles, 22*, 427–440.

Ethier, K. A., & Deaux, K. (1990b, August). *Maintaining the stability of a social identity during a life transition*. Poster presented at the annual meeting of the American Psychological Association, Boston.

Gleason, P. (1983). Identifying identity: A semantic history. *Journal of American History, 69*, 910–931.

Gollwitzer, P. M. (1986). Striving for specific identities: The social reality of self-symbolizing. In R. F. Baumeister (Ed.), *Public self and private self* (pp. 143–159). New York: Springer-Verlag.

Hormuth, S. E. (1990). *The ecology of the self: Relocation and self-concept change*. Cambridge, England: Cambridge University Press.

Lau, R. R. (1989). Individual and contextual influences on group identification. *Social Psychology Quarterly, 52*, 220–231.

Luhtanen, R., & Crocker, J. (1988). *Collective Self-Esteem Scale: Self-evaluation of one's social identity*. Unpublished manuscript, State University of New York at Buffalo.

Markus, H., & Nurius, P. (1986). Possible selves. *American Psychologist, 41*, 954–969.

McGuire, W. J., McGuire, C. V., Child, P., & Fujioka, T. (1978). Salience of ethnicity in the spontaneous self-concept as a function of one's ethnic distinctiveness in the social environment. *Journal of Personality and Social Psychology, 36*, 511–520.

McGuire, W. J., McGuire, C. V., & Winton, W. (1979). Effects of household sex composition on the salience of one's gender in the spontaneous self-concept. *Journal of Experimental Social Psychology, 15*, 77–90.

McNemar, Q. (1969). *Psychological statistics* (4th ed.). New York: Wiley.

Mead, G. H. (1934). *Mind, self, and society: From the standpoint of a social behaviorist* (C. W. Morris, Ed.). Chicago: University of Chicago Press, 1962.

Morris, J. (1974). *Conundrum*. New York: Harcourt Brace Jovanovich.

Parkes, C. M. (1975). What becomes of redundant world models? A contribution to the study of adaptation to change. *British Journal of Medical Psychology, 48*, 131–137.

Rosenberg, S. (1988). Self and others: Studies in social personality and autobiography. In L. Berkowitz (Ed.), *Advances in experimental social psychology* (Vol. 21, pp. 57–95). New York: Academic Press.

Rosenberg, S. (1989, March). *Social self and the schizophrenic process: Theory and research*. Paper presented at the Second Kansas Series in Clinical Psychology, Lawrence, KS.

Rosenberg, S., & Gara, M. A. (1985). The multiplicity of personal identity. *Review of Personality and Social Psychology, 6*, 87–113.

Ryff, C. D. (1984). Personality development from the inside: The subjective experience of change in adulthood and aging. In P. B. Baltes & O. G. Brim, Jr. (Eds.), *Life span development and behavior* (Vol. 6). New York: Academic Press.

Stryker, S. (1968). Identity salience and role performance. *Journal of Marriage and the Family, 30*, 558–564.

Stryker, S. (1987). Identity theory: Developments and extensions. In K. Yardley & T. Honess (Eds.), *Self and identity: Psychological perspectives* (pp. 89–103). Chichester, England: Wiley.

Stryker, S., & Serpe, R. T. (1982). Commitment, identity salience, and role behavior: Theory and research example. In W. Ickes & E. Knowles (Eds.), *Personality, roles and social behavior* (pp. 199–218). New York: Springer-Verlag.

Swann, W. B., Jr. (1983). Self-verification: Bringing social reality into harmony with the self. In J. Suls & A. Greenwald (Eds.), *Psychological perspectives on the self* (Vol. 2, pp. 33–66). Hillsdale, NJ: Erlbaum.

Swann, W. B., Jr. (1984). Quest for accuracy in person perception: A matter of pragmatics. *Psychological Review, 91*, 457–477.

Tajfel, H. (1981). *Human groups and social categories*. Cambridge, England: Cambridge University Press.

Turner, J. C. (1987). *Rediscovering the social group: A self-categorization theory*. Oxford: Basil Blackwell.

Wicklund, R. A., & Gollwitzer, P. M. (1982). *Symbolic self-completion*. Hillsdale, NJ: Erlbaum.

CHAPTER SIX

An Ecological Perspective on the Self-Concept

STEFAN E. HORMUTH

Over the last several years I conducted a program of research in which I studied processes of change in the relationship between self and the environment. This includes a theoretical framework, which I call a "social–ecological" one, as well as its empirical realization. I chose relocation as a research paradigm to study changes in the person–environment relationship.

DEFINITION AND THEORETICAL DEVELOPMENT OF THE SELF

The self can be understood as a moderator between person and society, because a person's understanding of self is acquired and develops in social experiences. This basic idea has guided almost all theory and empirical research on self-concept and identity in modern psychology and sociology, beginning in 1890 with William James's chapter on the "self"; continuing with Cooley's (1902) "looking-glass self"; on to Mead's (1934) *Mind, Self, and Society*; and finally to the integration of identity, role, and self-concept in Stryker and Statham's (1985) chapter in the most recent edition of the *Handbook of Social Psychology*. On this common ground, psychologists are more concerned with the relationship between "mind" and "self" (i.e., cognitive representation and self), whereas sociologists are more concerned with the relation between "self" and "society" (i.e., the self-concept and social structure). Therefore, the self is a theoretical concept that uniquely links psychology and sociology.

Sociologists, like social psychologists, emphasize the social nature of one's understanding of self. The person is seen as a product of the interaction between individual and society—an idea that can be traced back to the Scottish moral philosophers of the 18th century. Mead (1934) presented the most completely developed theory about the relationship between self and society. Here, the "self" is an object that acquires meaning through social interaction, but at the same time is also subject to this social interaction. Therefore, the self is—in the words of Morris Rosenberg (1981)—both "social product" and "social force." The self as a process and the self-concept as its empirically accessible product are therefore connected to the individual social situation as well as to the greater social structure. The social situation is the context in which identities are created and maintained in social exchange.

Over the past two decades, psychologists have again become interested in the self-concept. On one hand, within the framework of social cognition, they treat the self-concept as a specific cognitive structure; on the other hand, they investigate the function of the self-concept (e.g., in the activation of specific contents of this cognitive structure).

THE SOCIAL–ECOLOGICAL APPROACH

My own approach, which I consider a "social–ecological" approach to self-concept research, also rests on the basis that is common to most theories of the self-concept and identity.

The social and physical constituents of the self can be described as an ecological system. These constituents include *other persons* as direct sources of social experience; *things*, which mediate and perpetuate social experiences; and *environments*, which are the settings for social behavior. These external components are reflected in self-related cognitions. The self forms this system and is its reflection: It is its object and subject at the same time. Development and change take place in this ecological system.

The first function of others for one's concept of oneself is to reflect and react to one's own behavior. Continuous development and change of the self necessitate experiences with a variety of different social–behavioral possibilities. But social experiences are also generalized and symbolized in various forms: in rules and expectations, but also in related objects and things.

The physical environment, which consists of things and environments, also has social character. Aspects of the physical environment can have different functions for the self-concept. For one, either geographical settings or instruments can allow the realization of certain identities: A skier needs a mountain, a tennis player a racket. Things and environments can also initiate self-concept-relevant cognitions (e.g., memories, or projections of future goals). Examples would be the scenes of one's childhood or a picture of oneself, even in a mirror. Third, the environment and things can be used to present oneself to others, through, for instance, the style of one's house or the objects displayed therein. Finally, the physical environment can carry in it rules of social conduct, such as in a court of law or a church. Thereby, its function in this respect for the self-concept can be compared to role prescriptions.

None of these aspects has been neglected in psychological or sociological theory or research. However, they have been examined separately in social psychology, in sociology, in environmental psychology, and even in developmental perspectives. If one puts these different approaches together, however, the appropriateness of the ecological metaphor becomes obvious. The self functions in interdependence with its social–ecological system, consisting of others, things, and environments. Thereby, it connects social reality and social cognitions.

The program of research that I describe in this chapter centered on changes in this system, and therefore on changing person–environment relationships. Before going on to a theoretical discussion of the conditions for stability and change, I provide an overview of the research program and the methods selected.

OVERVIEW OF THE RESEARCH PROGRAM

The research program addressed the effects of changes in self–environment relations on social behaviors and experiences, and the perception of the environment in its function for the self-concept. I chose relocation as a quasi-experimental paradigm to study such changes in the relation between a person and his or her environment. A relocation presents opportunities for change, and also presents a person with the necessity of maintaining the self-concept in the face of challenges.

This theoretical framework required direct empirical access to the social situation where, in exchanges with others, social experiences were being created. This direct access to the social situation was made possible through the method of "experience sampling," which involved obtaining random samples of everyday behavior in natural environments (Hormuth, 1986). Research participants received beepers that were preprogrammed to remind the subjects to fill out a questionnaire; the beepers went off at random eight times a day for 1 week. The questionnaire assessed the actual social situation and addressed specifically the last social interaction before the beep sound; it asked about the actual and desired self and other disclosure during a social encounter.

A series of seven studies investigated changes in self-concept-relevant behaviors and perceptions before, during, and after a relocation. The

TABLE 6.1. Research Methods and Designs

	Study						
	S1	S2	S3	S4	S5	S6	S7
Method							
Telephone survey	×	×					
Mail survey				×	×	×	×
Experience sampling			×				×
Autophotography			×			×	×
Questionnaires	×	×		×	×	×	×
Design							
Cross-sectional	×						
Longitudinal					×		×
Quasi-experimental		×	×			×	
n	500	300	110	70	85	50	100

studies employed longitudinal, cross-sectional designs. More than 1,200 research participants were recruited from the general population and from among students. Methods used included telephone and mail surveys, as well as random samples of everyday behavior over a time span of several months (see Table 6.1). Figure 6.1 illustrates the designs of the seven studies.

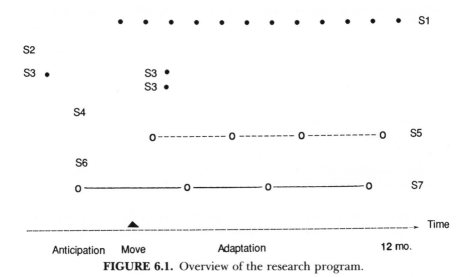

FIGURE 6.1. Overview of the research program.

The first study (S1; Hormuth, 1984), employing a cross-sectional design, collected data via telephone on social behaviors of persons whose relocation had occurred within the last year. Another telephone-survey study (S2), employing a sample of the general population, assessed the relationships among life changes, social behaviors, and satisfaction with self. Two other studies (S4, S6) addressed the anticipation of change. Yet another study, employing a quasi-experimental design (S3), compared a group of persons who had moved from a different city, another group who had moved within the city, and a third group who had lived at the same residence for at least 2 years. This study employed experience-sampling methodology to obtain random samples of everyday behavior. It also made use of "autophotography"—the use of Polaroid cameras to take photographs of self-concept-relevant aspects of the environment. In the latter studies, we studied subjects' social experiences and social perceptions during the first few weeks in a new location.

The first longitudinal design (S5) was a mail survey. Based on these experiences, a larger longitudinal study (S7) of students new in town began with data collection in the anticipation phase before the students moved to Heidelberg and then followed those students with beepers and cameras until they became increasingly familiar with their new environment in the second semester. During the anticipation phase, satisfaction with self and specific expectations for the new person–environment situation were assessed. After moving to the new environment, the students participated in three "waves" of data collection, distributed over about 9 months. During each wave, for 1 week each, the students reported eight times daily on their social experiences and activities. For the first and third waves, participants received cameras to take pictures of self-relevant aspects of their environment.

CONDITIONS FOR STABILITY AND CHANGE: COMMITMENT

What are the conditions for stability and change in the ecology of the self? In the sphere of social relationships, the interdependence between the stability of the self-concept and the stability of the social–ecological system can be understood in terms of the concept of commitment to an identity. The sociologist Becker (1960) has pointed out in his "Notes on the Concept of Commitment" that a person's commitment to a relationship is stabilized through a system of "side bets" (i.e., dependencies or side commitments). For instance, giving up a marriage affects one's relationships to in-laws, to one's children, and to common friends. Thus, a social commitment stabilizes a system of social relationships, which in turn stabilizes the person's self-concept.

Stryker (1980), in his identity theory, also links social structure to individual behavior through the self-concept. Identity theory differentiates between sociological and psychological components of commitment: "Interactive commitment" is the number of relationships affected if an identity is given up, and "affective commitment" refers to the emotional costs involved.

However, Becker's and Stryker's concepts of commitment neglect psychological components. On a psychological level of analysis, too, the beginning or end of a social commitment has implications for stability and change of the self-concept. The beginning or end of a central social relationship is usually tied to an evaluation of self, both by oneself and by a significant other. The offer to enter a social relationship that involves commitment is preceded by an evaluation of that person's past, so as to be able to project this past into the future of the relationship. Therefore, the possibility of engaging in such a social relationship is a reinforcement of the self-concept as it is. On the other hand, a person's self-concept is questioned through an evaluation that leads to the end of a commitment. Satisfaction or dissatisfaction with self is the consequence. Therefore, the concept of satisfaction with self carries implications for the effects of stability in a person's social structure and the concomitant psychological evaluation.

OPERATIONALIZATIONS OF COMMITMENT

To do justice to this psychological as well as sociological conceptualization of commitment, the research program employed multiple operationalizations that were related to each other in empirical validations.

In one approach, a colleague and I developed a scale to assess satisfaction with self (Hormuth & Lalli, 1988). This scale takes the ecological theoretical approach into account by considering the self-concept as both product and force—as both subject and object in a social–ecological system that involves different aspects of the social and physical environment. The subscales cover different self-concept-relevant life spheres: family, spouse/partner relationships, social relationships, work, and the immediate environment (such as one's home). The scale has been proven to have high construct and concurrent validity; its external validity has been demonstrated in relation to life events and actual social behavior.

Of particular interest is the relation of satisfaction with self to changes in the social structure. To assess these changes, we developed a method to assess the implications of changes in social relationships for a person's social structure. Subjects were asked to indicate first the kinds of social relationships that had changed within the last 3 months:

Parents O   O Spouse/partner
Children O   O Close relatives
In-laws O   O Distant relatives
Colleagues O   O Boss/supervisor
Employees/supervisees O   O Customers, etc.
Close friends O   O Acquaintances
Neighbors O   O Other friends

(Note: For specific populations—e.g., students—the list could be altered.)

In the next step, they had to indicate whether a change in relationship to one person affected other relationships as well, by drawing an arrow to those. Using this simple method, we could determine whether a change in social relationship was isolated or affected the social structure of that person in some way.

Figure 6.2 shows an interaction effect in a 2 × 2 analysis of variance, with nature of the change and number of others affected as independent variables, and satisfaction with self as the dependent variable (S2; Hormuth & Lalli, 1988). As can be seen from the figure, dissatisfaction with self was highest if a separation from a person affected the social structure as well. This effect was replicated in a second study. These results support one of the basic theoretical assumptions about the relationship between social structure and self-concept—namely, that the self-concept is linked to the social structure through interactive commitment.

In our first study (S1; Hormuth, 1984), a cross-sectional telephone survey of 500 persons who had moved sometime within the last 14 months,

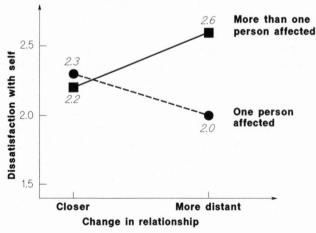

FIGURE 6.2. Satisfaction with self by type and centrality of change in commitment. Interaction: $F\ (1,\ 70) = 7.55$, $p \le .01$.

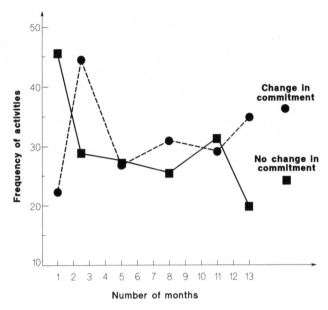

FIGURE 6.3. Distribution of "solitary–social" activities over time by commitment analysis.

interviewees were asked directly: "Sometimes moving from one place to another has something to do with the end of a social relationship—for instance, a separation or the loss of a job. In other cases, a new commitment is started—for example, a new place of work or a new personal relationship. Was either of these true in your case?" The effects of change in commitment, thus operationalized as a variable, showed that the course of social adaptation in a new location (as indexed by the distribution of "solitary–social" activities over time; see Figure 6.3) varied depending on this variable. "Solitary–social" activities are those where, though the individual is alone, a social world is created through a medium, such as books, letters, or long-distance phone calls. It became clear in this study that commitment was indeed a concept worthy of further investigation because it influenced the course of adaptation to a new person–environment relationship.

SUMMARY OF THE THEORY

The basic elements of the theoretical framework of the ecology of the self can now be summarized: The self-concept is developed and exists in interaction with its social and physical environment, and thus forms a social–ecological system, reflected in self-related cognitions. Certain factors of the cognitive and social organizational structure serve to stabilize this ecological system. Among them are central social relationships, or commitments.

The questioning of the self-concept can only lead to its change if the ecological system allows for change. This may be made easier through external changes in the environment that the person can utilize. Using environmental opportunities facilitates an active process of self-concept change, in which the individual can be an agent of his or her own change. The mechanism that provides stability for the cognitive structure and the self-concept within its social and physical environment consists of *implicative relationships* between elements of the cognitive representations of self and elements of the social–ecological system. A single cognition or element, by being linked to other elements, gains meaning because it implies at the same time other predictions or constructs. Through the linking of new experiences to existing ones, new experiences gain meaning. Through the linking of new social relationships to existing ones, social commitments are created, and the self-concept is stabilized in its social structure.

THE ROLE OF THINGS IN SELF-CONCEPT CHANGE

I offer here a three-stage model of the role of things in self-concept change. These stages are (1) the *acquisition* of new knowledge about the self; (2) the *stabilization* of that knowledge as part of the self-concept; and (3) the *maintenance* of these elements of the self-concept, even in the face of challenges.

1. New knowledge about the self is acquired through action (cf. Vallacher & Wegner, 1985). One important function of things is instrumental: the facilitation of action. For instance, a stereo can be used to produce the type of music that allows an adolescent to experience himself or herself, as described by Csikszentmihalyi and Rochberg-Halton (1981). This experience can also link an adolescent to his or her peers through social implications. Or a tennis racket can be a tool allowing an activity that will both provide a test of one's physical capabilities through social comparison and give access to a specific social group. The self-concept relevance of these activities comes from their being embedded in a social context. It is the link of the activity to its social context that provides self-relevant meaning, not the physical object by itself.

2. In the second stage, once new information about oneself is acquired, it has to be stabilized. "Stabilization" here means establishing implicative links to other elements of the self-concept. For instance, one way of doing this is to establish a social reality. Social reality, as shown by Wicklund and Gollwitzer (1982), can be established through the display of

symbols for an element of the self-concept. Objects can thereby function in a self-presentational manner by announcing an attribute of the person to others. In this way, a public commitment has been established. Giving it up would now incur some type of cost to the individual. The role of objects in this process is self-presentational and provides links between the new element of self and its social and temporal context. The social function of objects at this stage implies that they have to have a meaning that can be shared and understood by others.

3. In the third stage, after an element of the self-concept has been acquired and established, it has to *maintain* its stability even in the face of challenges. Stability is created through links to other elements of the self-concept. Therefore, objects are especially relevant insofar as they signify the relationship to the social, spatial, and temporal context of a person's self-concept. Objects that are reminders of persons, places, or events serve such a function. However, at this stage, their meaning does not necessarily have to be communicable to others—it can be idiosyncratic—but it must be clearly understood by the person himself or herself.

PICTURES OF THE ECOLOGY OF THE SELF: AUTOPHOTOGRAPHY

To understand the function of the physical environment and of things for the process of changing personal–environment relationships, my colleagues and I obtained subjects' perceptions of self-relevant aspects of the environment. "Autophotography," a method initially employed by Ziller (see Ziller & Lewis, 1981), was further developed for the purposes of the present research. Subjects were asked to take seven photographs of persons, things, and environments that they considered to be part of or expressive of their self-concept. The participants provided brief comments concerning the content of each picture on the back of the picture.

Our use of the method diverged from Ziller's in that we developed a completely different way of rating the pictures, based on the theoretical assumptions of the ecological model of the self. In a first step, the *content* was rated: persons, things, or environments. The next step assessed the *function* of the content of the photographs for stability and change in the self-concept. Dimensions were derived from previous research and were based on my own theoretical analysis of the function and meaning of the ecology of the self for a person's self-concept.

The following findings from a longitudinal study of students' first year at a university (our seventh study, or S7; Hormuth, 1990) illustrate the changing meaning of the environment in the process of acquiring a new ecological system for the self. The findings closely follow the three-stage

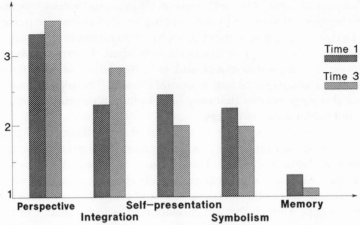

FIGURE 6.4. Change in photo content and functions between Time 1 and Time 3. Multivariate analysis: F (6, 69) = 29.9, $p \leq .01$; all differences were statistically significant.

model of the role of things in self-concept change as described above. The study spanned a time period of 9–10 months after students moved into the university city; it employed experience sampling as well as autophotography. The longitudinal design included four measurement points. The first was before the actual move, in the anticipation phase; at this stage, we made use of questionnaires mailed to the students' old home addresses, assessing satisfaction with self and specific expectations for changes in the new environment. After the students actually moved to the new environment, experience sampling was employed three times (hereafter referred to as Times 1, 2, and 3) for 1 week each; autophotography was employed twice, once in the new students' first and once in the second semester (Time 1 and Time 3, respectively).

The results of autophotography showed that while no change could be noted for the relative *content* of objects, persons, and environments over time, the self-relevant *meaning* changed considerably between the Time 1 and Time 3 measurement points (see Figure 6.4). Several categories of meaning were assessed. The first category was the *perspective* taken—that is, a close-up versus a very distant approach to the object depicted—which served as an indicator of psychological closeness or involvement (Wofsey, Rierdan, & Wapner, 1979). Among our subjects at Time 1 in the new environment, a more distant perspective was taken, whereas several months later (Time 3) the pictures showed a closer perspective.

Second, the *integration* of the object in the context of the picture was rated. Was the object presented in an isolated way, or was it integrated into a context? This could indicate the perceptual structuring of a new environment and the degree of integration of self-concept-relevant items in the new environment through the links that had been established to other objects. As the results show, items were less isolated and more integrated in their context when the environment became more familiar.

The next dimension assessed was that of *self-presentational* aspects of the objects in the photos: Did the objects give a clear message about what kind of a person the subject was? I have stated earlier that this function should be more dominant in the early stages of self-concept change. Indeed, the self-presentational value of the pictures' content decreased over time; greater self-assurance may diminish the need for self-presentation in a new environment. (However, no change over time was found in the *instrumental* value of the pictures' content, which was generally low. It is likely that while an object still has only instrumental value, it may not be considered to be self-concept-relevant and thus may not be included in such pictures as these.)

Some objects have value for the *memories* they revive. They are links to the past and thus can be used to create stability for one's self. Their role for self-concept change lies in the presentation of continuity with the past and the possibility to project this into the future. For the subjects in this study, the memory value of pictured items decreased slightly but significantly over time, although it was overall the least important category. This suggests that the transition to university is one that implies, more than others, a break with the past and a new beginning.

A decrease was also found in the *symbolic* value of the pictures' content. "Symbolism" as used here refers to the extent to which the meaning of objects is socially shared and generally understood. It is considered relevant in my model for the stabilization of the self-concept by establishing links between self and others. Symbolism was made use of more often in the first few weeks in the new environment; over time, the idiosyncratic, personal meaning of the pictures increased.

Overall, it seems that the pictures subjects took immediately after arriving in their new environment made more use of the meaning categories that indicated the kinds of persons they were and had been before: self-presentation, symbolism, and memory. These functions of things for the self-concept are, as defined here, mainly functions that make use of generally shared information to present a clear picture of oneself. Over time, these functions of things in the new physical environment decreased, and the subjects felt more strongly that they were part of that environment. The presentation of self to others now became less important, and elements of the environment, as they were incorporated into the self-concept, acquired more idiosyncratic meaning.

To summarize these results, the study indicated that indeed in the beginning persons showed a more distant perspective and items were less integrated into a context. More use of socially shared symbols, more self-presentation, and more memories showed this to be a state of orientation, as well as of reliance on one's past. After 8 months, the environment was perceived more closely and things were more integrated into it; self-presentation and memories became less important, and the symbols used became more personal. These findings closely represent what would be expected in the second stage (stabilization) and the third stage (maintenance) of the three-stage model presented above.

VARIABILITY OF BEHAVIOR

Another set of data from this study (S7) described the variability of social behaviors. The within-subject variability of individual answers from the experience-sampling data of the study constituted this set of data (see Figure 6.5).

In the new environment of our research participants, behavior first took place in an increasing number of different settings, but with a smaller variety of other persons present. Over time, the settings relevant for the behavior were established, while the variety of activities taking place in those settings increased. Social interactions were perceived as more important and as more meaningful, and more personal information was exchanged in interactions.

PREDICTORS OF THE COURSE OF ADAPTATION

After this descriptive analysis of the course of adaptation to new person–environment relationships, I now consider the predictors of differential

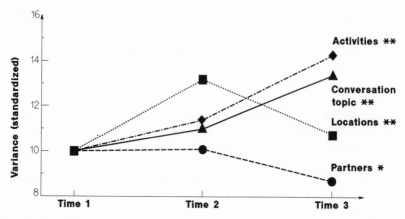

FIGURE 6.5. Situational variance in social behavior over time. $^*p \leq .05$; $^{**}p \leq .01$.

courses of adaptation. Which are the better predictors: the self-concept-relevant variables that I have identified (satisfaction with self and commitment), or rather the specific and concrete expectations with which one enters a new environment?

The model assumes that change is the consequence of questioning of or dissatisfaction with the self-concept, concomitant to a change in the person–environment relationship. If, on the other side, a person is satisfied with his or her self-concept and is being reinforced, existing elements of the self should be strenghtened. Presumably, also, the process of active self-concept change consists of initial exposure to a large number of possible experiences, followed by a later concentration on some few experiences. These are finally linked to other elements of the ecology of the self, and thereby provide new structure and stability to the system.

The empirical results, presented in detail elsewhere (Hormuth, 1990), show that indeed the variables of commitment and satisfaction with self—in some studies (S6 and S7), collected as predictors in the old environment—contributed significantly to the social behaviors, experiences, and perceptions of persons in a new environment, and even explained a significant portion of the variance of the development up to a year after the move. The destabilization of the social structure and dissatisfaction with self did not, however, immediately lead to active attempts to change. Rather, these persons tried to have fewer new social experiences in the beginning and withdrew initially from the new environment. The percentage of variance in social behavior in a new environment, as determined by satisfaction with self, was clearly higher than the percentage of variance explained by the contribution of specific expectations.

CONCLUSION

This program of research found support for some of the assumptions about the function of a social ecology of the self in the process of self-concept change. At the same time, the need to develop and sharpen this approach further has become clear.

In today's psychology and sociology, the self-concept and identity have once again become central topics of theorizing and research—rightly so, I think. The self-concept is the cognitive representation of the social experiences of a person, and influences in turn the social perceptions and behaviors within a given social and physical environment. As a concept of social-psychological theory and research, the self-concept is especially suited to bridge the gap between the social cognitions and the social reality of a person. If cognitions are seen as social, they have to be connected to social structure and social action. To provide this link between social reality and social cognition is one of the tasks of a social–ecological approach in social psychology.

REFERENCES

Becker, H. S. (1960). Notes on the concept of commitment. *American Journal of Sociology, 66,* 32–40.

Cooley, C. H. (1902). *Human nature and the social order.* New York: Scribner.

Csikszentmihalyi, M., & Rochberg-Halton, E. (1981). *The meaning of things: Domestic symbols and the self.* Cambridge, England: Cambridge University Press.

Hormuth, S. E. (1984). Transitions in commitments to roles and self-concept change: Relocation as a paradigm. In V. L. Allen & E. van de Vliert (Eds.), *Role transitions: Explorations and explanations* (pp. 109–124). New York: Plenum.

Hormuth, S. E. (1986). The sampling of experiences *in situ. Journal of Personality, 54,* 262–293.

Hormuth, S. E. (1990). *The ecology of the self: Relocation and self-concept change.* Cambridge, England: Cambridge University Press.

Hormuth, S. E., & Lalli, M. (1988). Eine Skala zur Erfassung der bereichsspezifischen Selbstzufriedenheit [A scale to assess life-sphere specific satisfaction with self]. *Diagnostica, 34,* 148–166.

James, W. (1890). *The principles of psychology* (2 vols.). New York: Dover, 1950.

Mead, G. H. (1934). *Mind, self, and society: From the standpoint of a social behaviorist* (C. W. Morris, Ed.). Chicago: University of Chicago Press, 1962.

Rosenberg, M. (1981). The self-concept: Social product and social force. In M. Rosenberg & R. H. Turner (Eds.), *Social psychology: Sociological perspectives* (pp. 591–624). New York: Basic Books.

Stryker, S. (1980). *Symbolic interaction: A social structural version.* Menlo Park, CA: Benjamin/Cummings.

Stryker, S., & Statham, A. (1985). Symbolic interaction and role theory. In G. Lindzey & E. Aronson (Eds.), *Handbook of social psychology* (3rd ed., Vol. 1, pp. 311–378). New York: Random House.

Vallacher, R. R., & Wegner, D. M. (1985). *A theory of action identification.* Hillsdale, NJ: Erlbaum.

Wicklund, R. A., & Gollwitzer, P. M. (1982). *Symbolic self-completion.* Hillsdale, NJ: Erlbaum.

Wofsey, E., Rierdan, J., & Wapner, S. (1979). Planning to move: Effects on representing the currently inhabited environment. *Environment and Behavior, 11,* 3–32.

Ziller, R. C., & Lewis, D. (1981). Orientations: Self, social, and environmental percepts through auto-photography. *Personality and Social Psychology Bulletin, 7,* 338–343.

PART THREE

Integrative Approaches from Clinical Psychology and Psychoanalysis

The first two chapters in this section focus upon the self as a processor of experiences. Epstein presents a theory of the self with separate rational and experiential processing systems, and Curtis and Zaslow explore how one gains knowledge about one's "self," both rationally and experientially. Both of these chapters acknowledge the unconscious, subjective affective experiences attended to by the psychoanalysts, but also address the conscious, objective data of cognitive scientists.

The next two chapters explore cultural influences upon the self from a psychoanalytic vantage point. In doing so, they question some of the assumptions about the self held by Western psychologists and analysts. These chapters represent a significant departure from the tendency of many psychoanalysts to ignore situational and cultural variables.

Roland contrasts the "familial" organization of the self of Asians with the "individualized" organization of the self of Westerners. More specifically, Roland speaks of the "familial–communal self" of the Indians and the "familial–group self" of the Japanese. Other conceptions of the self pointed out by Roland are the "spiritual self" and the "expanding self" (the latter takes into account sociocultural forces). His exploration questions psychoanalytic assumptions about separation and autonomy, and delineates some areas in which Western psychoanalytic styles will be misunderstood and probably nontherapeutic.

Westen argues that cultural unconscious and affective aspects of the self need to be integrated with data from experimental investigations. He sees experimental research as misleading because of its reliance upon self-report and reaction time data, and clinical theory as of limited use because of the frequent failure to operationalize constructs. Clinical data from clients with narcissistic personality disorders and victims of sexual abuse are provided to demonstrate the need for research tapping the unconscious and emotional aspects of self. The emphases on individuation, personal control, and self-schemas in contemporary psychology and psychoanalysis are viewed as manifestations of a particular historical epoch characterized by rapid cultural changes and threats to coherent views of the world.

CHAPTER SEVEN

Cognitive–Experiential Self-Theory: An Integrative Theory of Personality

SEYMOUR EPSTEIN

INTRODUCTION

Cognitive–experiential self-theory (CEST; Epstein, 1980, 1983, 1990) is a broad, integrative theory of personality that is compatible with major aspects of a wide variety of other theories, including psychoanalytic theory, particularly ego psychology, object relations theory, and psychoanalytic self-theory; Adler's individual psychology; Jung's analytical psychology; the phenomenological self-theories of Carl Rogers and others; existential theories; learning theories; George Kelly's personal construct theory; and modern cognitive approaches. A potential weakness in an eclectic theory is that it will achieve its breath at the cost of coherence. There is the concern that it will provide a diet that, instead of being a rich source of nourishment, is a source of indigestion. I therefore hasten to add that I did not set out to develop an eclectic theory. I did not winnow from the major theories what I regarded to be their most significant insights and then consider how to combine them into a coherent whole. I simply developed a theory of personality, and I was surprised when others from widely divergent backgrounds pointed out that my thinking was compatible with theirs.

Despite its apparent simplicity, CEST is capable of explaining almost everything that psychoanalysis does and much that it does not, and it is able to do so in a more parsimonious and scientifically defensible manner. It not only provides a framework for understanding everyday rational and irrational behavior, but it elucidates broader human concerns and enterprises, such as religion, spirituality, advertisement, and politics, about which most personality theories have little to say.

CEST is deceptive in its simplicity. Major aspects of it are so consistent with common sense that it is in some danger of being dismissed as simplistic. Many think that because behavior is complicated and often irrational, only theories that employ exotic concepts, such as archetypes, libidos, ids, and superegos, can adequately plumb its depths. Others react so negatively to such an esoteric approach that they eschew anything suggestive of a dynamic unconscious, and choose instead to adopt surface explanations of behavior. There is a middle road, the one taken by CEST. According to CEST, the most important mental functioning is not what occurs in consciousness, nor is it in the stirrings that occur in deep, inaccessible regions of the mind. Rather, it is the reactions that occur at a preconscious level of awareness—a level at which people automatically interpret reality. It is a level that influences our feelings, behavior, and conscious thinking.

Figure 7.1 presents three major perspectives on levels of consciousness. First, let us consider the Freudian model. Most of the iceberg, which is far below the surface and therefore not visible, corresponds to the unconscious mind. What is visible, corresponding to the conscious mind, is but the tip of the iceberg. Just beneath the surface is the preconscious mind, which Freud did not regard as very important, and about which he had little to say. Its only function for him was as a gateway between the other two levels. It is here that censorship takes place, which the conscious mind uses to protect itself from awareness of distressing thoughts, images, and impulses in the unconscious mind. However, the preconscious mind is assumed to have no rules of inference of its own, but simply to function as extension of the conscious mind. The conscious and unconscious minds, on the other hand, operate by their own separate rules of inference. The unconscious mind operates by the "primary process," which is the logic of the dream: associationistic, symbolic, and knowing nothing of cause and effect or of constraints imposed by time and place. The conscious mind operates by the "secondary process," which follows conventionally established rules of logic and cause and effect.

In the iceberg representing traditional mainstream psychology in Figure 7.1, emphasis is on consciousness as the main source of behavior: "What you see is what you get." Anyone wanting to know something about a person should simply ask the person or give him or her a standardized questionnaire to fill out. Although a subconscious is recognized, it is vastly different from the dynamic unconscious of psychoanalysis, which strives for expression and is held down by forces of repression. It is a subdued subconscious that simply contains information of which the individual is momentarily unaware.

CEST does not deny the importance of the conscious or unconscious mind (although it conceptualizes the deep unconscious somewhat differently from Freud), but it considers the preconscious level of awareness as

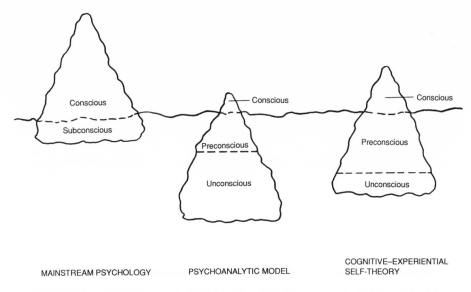

MAINSTREAM PSYCHOLOGY   PSYCHOANALYTIC MODEL   COGNITIVE–EXPERIENTIAL SELF-THEORY

FIGURE 7.1. "Iceberg" representations of levels of consciousness in three theoretical approaches.

considerably more important than Freud did. It is at this level that cognition automatically interprets and organizes experience, directs behavior, and influences conscious thought. Accordingly, in the representation of CEST in Figure 7.1, the largest portion of the iceberg is assigned to the preconscious. Because of its location between the conscious and deeper unconscious processing of information, it is also the center that has the potential for integrating the entire mind.

As I point out shortly, Freud was even more right than he realized when he said that behavior is unconsciously determined. His only problem, from the perspective of CEST, is that he had the wrong unconscious. According to CEST, most behavior is automatically regulated by an "experiential conceptual system" that operates primarily at the preconscious level of awareness, and that functions according to its own rules of inference. These rules are different from those operating in the systems that function primarily at the conscious and the deeper unconscious levels.

COMPARISON OF BASIC ASSUMPTIONS IN CEST AND PSYCHOANALYSIS

Before I provide a more detailed description of CEST, it will be helpful to compare some of its major features with those of traditional psychoanalytic theory, the most influential personality theory that has emphasized unconscious processes.

Freud's great contribution was that he developed the first comprehensive theory of personality. Not surprisingly—because it was meant to be a beginning, not an end—it contains some serious flaws. Before Freud's time, mental illness was attributed either to inhabitation by evil spirits or to organic malfunctioning. It was widely assumed then, as it often is now, that people's behavior could be understood as rational attempts to contribute to their welfare. Yet it was apparent to any keen observer of human affairs not only that people act in strange ways, but that they often act in ways detrimental to their own welfare, as in the case of a woman who repeatedly falls in love with men who abuse her or of a man who repeatedly undertakes ventures that are doomed to failure. The ancient Greeks had an explanation for such self-destructive behavior: They attributed it to the Fates, three stern goddesses who were thought to control people's destinies.

Freud's genius was that he provided a theory that could account for humankind's irrational behavior without assuming imaginary physiological or supernatural causes. He provided a scientifically feasible explanation of an extremely important aspect of human behavior. The need for a theory of the unconscious was so great that Freud's theory became highly influential, despite its serious logical and empirical limitations. Any explanation was better than none, and Freud had an explanation that was scientifically more defensible than any of the alternatives that were available. The question remains whether, at this time, there is a better way to conceptualize unconscious processes and to otherwise improve on Freud's theory without sacrificing its tremendous scope. I believe that CEST offers such an alternative.

Table 7.1 presents a comparison of Freudian theory and CEST on a number of key issues. According to Freudian theory, there are two reasons why material is unconscious. One is that the material has arrived there at a preverbal period in the individual's development. Because the individual at this point has no words with which to conceptualize the experiences, they can not be consciously represented and remain in the unconscious. The more common reason given for material becoming unconscious is that it is repressed. Taboo material that is unacceptable to the conscious mind is said to be kept from awareness by an opposing repressive force. The result is unconscious conflict that is a direct source of tension and therefore of symptoms in its own right; worse yet, it is an indirect source of symptoms, because the repressed impulses are assumed to gain indirect expression in the form of symptoms, dreams, and maladaptive behavior. Thus, the Freudian theory of the unconscious is based on a "steam boiler" analogy (see Figure 7.2). Repressed impulses and thoughts create tension as

TABLE 7.1. Comparison of Freudian Theory and CEST

Freudian theory	CEST
Emphasis on repressed unconscious.	Emphasis on preconscious.
Pleasure principle as only source of motivation.	Four basic motives: pleasure principle, model of world, relatedness, self-esteem.
Unconscious conflict the basic source of all pathology.	Maladaptive beliefs, sensitivities, and compulsions the major sources of pathology.
Things are unconscious mainly because of repression; everything would be conscious if no resistance.	Things are unconscious mainly because that is their most natural and efficient state.
Repression the result of taboo impulses.	Repression the result of conceptual incongruity.
Healing through making the unconscious conscious.	Healing through differentiation and integration; establishing harmony within and between the systems and with external reality.

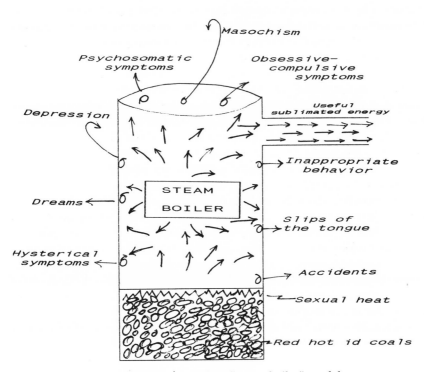

FIGURE 7.2. Freudian "steam boiler" model.

they strive for expression, and the tension must be expressed in one form or another or the whole system will blow up.

In summary, unconscious conflict between forces striving for expression and repressing forces is at the heart of psychoanalytic theory. All neurosis is assumed to be caused by such conflict. Because the problem is unconscious conflict, the solution is presumed to be to make the unconscious conscious. Psychoanalytic therapy is therefore based on a quest for insight. What was unconscious has to be made conscious; ego must replace what was id. Freud had great faith in the power of the conscious mind when it is not warped by unconscious influence. It is for this reason that he saw little of value in religion and regarded it as an institutionalized form of psychosis—one that could well be dispensed with to the advantage of humankind.

CEST does not deny that problems can be caused by unconscious conflict. It accepts much of what Freud had to say about the repressed unconscious, but relegates it to a much smaller aspect of unconscious functioning than does psychoanalytic theory. From the perspective of CEST, repression is simply a learned avoidance response. There is no steam boiler generating pressure that must be expressed in one form or another. There is simply an area of experience that is problematic because it is dissociated, and therefore cannot be assimilated into the broader conceptual system of the individual. It is also a source of sensitivity, avoidance, and unconscious generalization.

In his first and more influential theory, Freud assumed that there is one basic source of motivation, the pleasure principle. Later he became aware that people under certain conditions have a need to re-experience distressing events—a need that takes precedence over the pleasure principle. He never adequately solved the issue of what this other principle was, but in *Beyond the Pleasure Principle* (Freud, 1920), he launched into some wild speculation to account for what he labeled as a "repetition compulsion." He attributed the repetition compulsion to the operation of a death instinct, which he said often prevails over a life instinct. CEST offers a more satisfactory explanation. According to CEST, there are four basic sources of motivation: the pleasure principle; the need to assimilate the data of reality and therefore to maintain the stability of the assimilating system; the need to maintain relatedness; and the need to enhance self-esteem. These motives—particularly the need to maintain the stability of a person's experiential conceptual system, as will be seen shortly—readily account for the repetition compulsion.

According to CEST, most thought occurs below the threshold of awareness—not because it is taboo, as Freud maintained, but because that is its natural state. Most behavior is determined by cognitions that automatically organize reality and direct behavior, and for which consciousness would be an unnecessary burden. One is reminded of the centipede who forgot how to walk when asked to describe the order in which it moved its many feet. According to Freud, everything would be conscious if there were no force of resistance. According to CEST, consciousness is a special state, and it would be inefficient to be conscious of all of one's interpretive and decision-making processes.

Whereas some cognitions are subconscious (i.e., not conscious) in the sense that they occur automatically and require no conscious deliberation, other cognitions are unconscious because there is resistance to their becoming conscious. The resistance occurs not only because material is taboo, as in the case of unacceptable aggressive or sexual thoughts, but, more generally, because it is unassimilable in the rational system. Material can also be unassimilable in the experiential system, in which case it will be dissociated and will not be available to the rest of the experiential system. In any event, whereas the emphasis in psychoanalytic theory is on taboo cognitions as the source of repression, in CEST it is on unassimilable cognitions, of which taboo ones are a subset.

Pathology, from the viewpoint of CEST, does not derive necessarily from unconscious conflict, as it assumed in psychoanalysis; more often, it derives from maladaptive preconscious cognitions. If a person is unaware of these cognitions, it simply adds a level of complication in remedying them. However, making the individual conscious of them, which is the emphasis in psychoanalysis, is usually not sufficient, and often does no more than transform a repressed neurotic into an insightful one. Healing, according to CEST, results mainly from corrective emotional experiences, both actual and fantasized, that facilitate differentiation and integration at an automatic, preconscious level. Insight can be helpful in this process but it is not always necessary, meaning that people can get better without knowing why.

THE BASIC THEORY

The Nature of Personal Theories of Reality

According to CEST, everyone develops an implicit theory of reality that contains subdivisions of a self-theory, a world theory, and propositions connecting the two. A personal theory of reality is a hierarchically organized set of "schemas" and networks of schemas. The most basic schemas are referred to as "postulates." Among the most important postulates are four derived from the basic functions of a personal theory of reality, which are discussed shortly. The four basic postulates include (1) the degree to which the world is viewed as benign versus malevolent; (2) the degree to which the world is viewed as meaningful (including predictable, controllable, and just) versus chaotic; (3) the degree to which others are viewed as a source of support and happiness rather than as a source of insecurity and un-happiness; and (4) the degree to which the self is viewed as worthy (including capable, good, and lovable) rather than the opposite.

Because the basic postulates represent the highest constructs in the hierarchy of a personal theory of reality, invalidation of any one of them has a destabilizing effect on the entire personality structure. As one descends the hierarchy, schemas become narrower in scope and more closely associated with direct experience. The very lowest-order schemas are situation-specific cognitions, which are not very informative about a person's personality in the absence of knowledge about their connections to higher-order constructs. Relatedly, lower-order constructs can readily change without affecting the higher-order structure. Thus, the upper structure can maintain stability while the lower-level constructs can allow for a high degree of flexibility, which is one of the important advantages of a hierarchical structure of a personal theory of reality.

There are two kinds of basic beliefs, or schemas; descriptive and motivational. Descriptive schemas are beliefs about what the self and the world are like, as in the four basic postulates described above. Motivational schemas are beliefs about what one has to do to obtain what one desires and avoid what one dislikes. Motivational beliefs, like other schemas in the experiential system, are derived primarily from emotionally significant experiences, and are thus emotionally charged (i.e., they are "hot," not "cold," cognitions about how to act in the world). Consider the case of a child with a rejecting mother. Such a child is likely to develop descriptive beliefs that the world is malevolent and untrustworthy, and motivational beliefs that the only way to get by in the world is to look after one's own needs, trust no one, and avoid deep attachments. (Unless stated otherwise, it should be understood that I am referring to preconscious beliefs in the experiential system, which may be quite different from a person's conscious beliefs.) Motivational schemas, like descriptive schemas, exist at various levels of generality and complexity, and subsume constructs such as values, goals, and plans.

Personal theories of reality, in common with scientific theories, serve the purpose of organizing the data of experience and directing behavior. In the case of scientific theories, the data that are organized are the subject matter of the science, and the behavior that is directed is the scientist's pursuit of knowledge. In the case of personal theories of reality, the data that are organized are the experiences of everyday living, and the behavior that is directed is how the individual goes about living his or her daily life.

An important difference between the two is that the scientist is motivated only to understand the phenomena he or she wishes to study, but the person in everyday life is motivated to live in an emotionally satisfying way. It is important to recognize that a personal theory of reality is emotionally driven.

The Four Basic Functions of a Personal Theory of Reality

Personal theories of reality have four basic functions: to assimilate the data of reality (which subsumes the need to maintain the conceptual system that does the assimilating); to maintain a favorable pleasure–pain balance; to maintain relatedness to others; and to maintain a favorable level of self-esteem. It is noteworthy that different personality theories emphasize one or another of these functions, but only CEST attributes a central role to all four. In fact, one of the more important contributions of CEST is the explanatory power that is derived from the interplay of these four functions.

According to learning theory and psychoanalysis, the most important motive in human behavior is to maximize pleasure and minimize pain. This is referred to as the "pleasure principle" in psychoanalysis and is regarded as the source of reinforcement, and therefore of learning, in learning theory. According to phenomenological self-theories (e.g., Lecky, 1945; Snygg & Combs, 1949; Rogers, 1951) and Kelly's (1955) theory of constructive alternativism, the most basic human motive is to assimilate the data of reality into a coherent conceptual system and, relatedly, to maintain the conceptual system that does the assimilating. For Bowlby (1973) and for object relations theorists, such as Mahler, Fairbairn, and Kernberg, there is no need more influential than the need to maintain relatedness to others (Cashdan, 1988). For social psychologist Allport (1927) and psychoanalyst Kohut (1971), the need for self-esteem is of major importance.

According to CEST, the four motives above are all of central importance, and any one of them can dominate the others, depending on the individual and circumstances. It is assumed that all four motives normally play an equally important role in directing behavior. That is, behavior is viewed as a compromise among the four basic motives. It follows that they provide a series of checks and balances on one another's influence, thereby keeping behavior within adaptive limits. Once one is aware of this, it is possible to explain a wide variety of human behavior that otherwise appears to be anomalous. For example, recent research has demonstrated that most normal people are not accurate in their self-appraisals, but exhibit a self-serving bias (see review in Taylor & Brown, 1988). This has led some to suggest that reality awareness has been overrated as an important criterion of mental health. From the perspective of CEST, all that these findings demonstrate is that normal people not only have a need to realistically assimilate the data of reality; they have an equally important need to enhance self-esteem. If we put the two together, we get a compromise, leading to the prediction that normal people should exhibit a tendency to overestimate their vitures, but only within limits. If a consideration of reality were unimportant, then, given a need to enhance the self, everyone would develop delusions of grandeur.

An imbalance among the four basic functions is a common source of maladaptive behavior. Such an imbalance can be produced by a serious threat to any one of the functions. Thus, a severe threat to self-esteem can produce overcompensation to the point that the need to enhance the self overwhelms the other functions, resulting in, for example, a delusion of grandeur. Repetitive self-destructive behavior, such as the behavior that Freud attempted to explain by his concepts of the repetition compulsion and the death instinct, can be explained by a need to maintain the coherence of the conceptual system that assimilates the data of reality. A person who has had severely negative experiences incorporates these experiences into a basic belief about the nature of the world. Any experiences that violate this view are a threat to the stability of the person's conceptual system. The person therefore is motivated to produce validating negative experiences. In other words, in cases of people suffering from a repetition compulsion, the need to maintain the stability of the conceptual system takes precedence over the need to maximize pleasure and minimize pain. According to CEST, different disorders are associated with dominance of different basic needs (Epstein, 1980).

The Four Basic Beliefs Associated with the Four Basic Functions

Associated with the four basic functions are four basic beliefs. In order for the experiential system to fulfill the four basic functions, it is necessary for it to assess their status. As already noted, there are four basic assessments, or belief dimensions, related to the four basic functions. Accordingly, everyone has an intuitive belief about (1) the degree to which the world is benign; (2) the degree to which life is meaningful (including predictable, controllable, and just); (3) the degree to which people are desirable to relate to; and (4) the degree to which the self is worthy (including capable, good, and lovable).

The Three Conceptual Systems

According to CEST, there are three conceptual systems; a rational conceptual system, an experiential conceptual system, and an associationistic conceptual system. The rational system operates predominantly at the conscious level, where it functions according to socially prescribed rules of inference. CEST has nothing new to say about this system. The experiential and associationistic systems have their own separate rules of operation. Since the experiential conceptual system is the system of greatest concern to CEST, it is described here in greatest detail. The associationistic system corresponds to a state of altered consciousness and is similar to Freud's unconscious system, which operates according to the rules of the primary process. However, in common with Jung's views, CEST also considers the associationistic system as a source of creativity; as a system for making inferences about the future as well as the past; and, in general, as a more sophisticated system than the Freudian unconscious. This is not the place for a detailed discussion of the associationistic system. Further discussion of the associationistic and rational systems, including their topographical representation, can be found in a previous article (Epstein, 1983). For now, let us turn to a more detailed discussion of the experiential system.

The Experiential Conceptual System

The experiential conceptual system is a more "natural" system than the rational conceptual system, in the sense that it is less responsive to cultural training, has a stronger biological component because of its close association with emotions, and has a longer evolutionary history. When therapists such as Horney (1945) and Rogers (1951) speak of a "natural" or "organic" self and contrast it with an "inauthentic" self, they are referring to beliefs that are derived directly from emotionally significant experience, as opposed to beliefs that are acquired from others. In other words, they are referring to representations in the experiential system as contrasted with those in the rational system. A common source of problems, they note, is a person's becoming alienated from his or her natural self because of his or her need to please others. It is apparently the existential fate of humans to have two selves that chafe against each other, one derived more from our animal past, and the other from our cultural and social conditioning.

If one dates the evolutionary development of the experiential system from the first appearance of human-like creatures (which is a highly conservative assumption, as lower-order creatures also operate by the same system), then it has evolved over at least 7 million years. Contrast this with 5,000 years in the development of the rational system as we know it today. The use of written symbols, signs, and numbers was introduced less than 5,000 years ago. The first alphabet and pure mathematics were introduced by the Greeks 2,500 years ago. The modern scientific method is no more than 500 years old. Thus, the evolutionary development of the rational system is but a drop in the bucket compared to that of the experiential system. Nature does not give up its hard-won gains easily. It is therefore unthinkable that the experiential system was simply abandoned once humans developed more abstract, conscious ways of apprehending reality. Given its long evolutionary history, it can be assumed that the experiential system is highly adaptive, for, if it were not, we would not be here today.

It remains to be seen how adaptive the rational system will turn out to be. It may turn out to be the greatest blunder in evolutionary history—one that may not only result in the demise of the species that uses it, but in the demise of all other species as well. At any rate, my point is that we should not assume that the rational system is necessarily the superior system. There is much inherent wisdom in the experiential system. Of course, there is no need to take sides between them; like it or not, we are stuck with both. They each have advantages and disadvantages, and the task we are faced with is how to employ both in a supplementary and harmonious manner.

Attributes of the Experiential System

Unlike the rational system, which guides behavior by direct assessment of stimuli, the direction of behavior by the experiential system is mediated by feelings, or "vibes." These include subtle feelings of which individuals are usually unaware, as well as full-blown emotions of which they usually are aware. The experiential system is assumed to operate in the following manner. When an individual is confronted with a situation that, depending on past experience, is appraised as significant for the person's welfare, the person experiences certain feelings or vibes. The vibes motivate behavior to enhance the feeling state if it is a pleasant one and to terminate it if it is an unpleasant one. The whole process occurs with great rapidity, so that to all appearances the behavior is an immediate reaction to the eliciting stimulus. The same process guides the behavior of higher-order infrahuman animals. In the case of humans, however, the vibes produce not only tendencies to act in certain ways, but also tendencies to think in certain ways. Thus, people are less in control of their conscious thinking than they like to believe.

Table 7.2 compares the rules of operation of the rational and experiential systems. The list has been derived from an analysis of people's thinking when they discuss highly charged emotional issues, in comparison to their thinking when they discuss impersonal issues. It has also been influenced by analysis of the nature of the appeals made in advertising and in politics; by research on constructive thinking (Epstein & Meier, 1989); and by experimental cognitive research (e.g., Kahneman & Miller, 1986; Kahneman & Tversky, 1982; Epstein, Lipson, & Huh, in review).

Several of the features in Table 7.2 contribute to a major adaptive characteristic of the experiential system, which is that it promotes rapid assessment and decisive action. Included among such features are the holistic and categorical appraisal of events, and the experience of the outcome of the appraisal process as self-evidently valid.

The experiential and rational systems each have advantages and disadvantages. The rational system is better suited for analysis and for consideration of long-term consequences. However, without the experiential system, the rational system is devoid of passion. Moreover, an analytic approach is not necessarily the best approach for solving all problems. For example, a holistic approach is less apt to lose the forest for the trees. Moreover, a rational, analytic approach is apt to overlook significant sources of data that may be attended to by a more intuitive, holistic

TABLE 7.2. Comparison of the Experiential and Rational Systems

Experiential system	Rational system
More holistic.	More analytic.
More emotional—Pleasure- and pain-oriented (what feels good).	More logical—reason-oriented (what is sensible).
More associationistic.	More cause-and-effect analysis.
More outcome-oriented.	More process-oriented.
Behavior mediated by "vibes" from past experiences.	Behavior mediated by conscious appraisal of events.
Encodes reality in concrete images and metaphors.	Encodes reality in abstract symbols (words and numbers).
Rapid processing—oriented toward immediate action.	Slower processing—oriented toward delayed action.
Relatively slow to change—changes with repetitive experience, direct or vicarious.	Changes relatively rapidly—can change with speed of thought.
Crudely differentiated; broad generalization gradient; categorical thinking.	More highly differentiated; dimensional thinking.
Crudely integrated—dissociative, organized into emotional complexes (cognitive–affective modules).	More highly integrated.
Experienced passively and preconsciously: We are seized by our emotions.	Experienced actively and consciously: As if we are in control of our thoughts.
Self-evidently valid: "Experiencing is believing."	Requires justification via logic and evidence.

approach. Thus, a rational approach may arrive at solutions that, although reasonable from an external frame of reference, are counterproductive because they fail to take into account the emotional consequences of a decision. Given that each system has advantages and disadvantages, the most adaptive solution is to employ both systems; this requires awareness of and respect for the operation of the experiential system.

Although the rational and experiential systems are independent, they are capable of communicating with and otherwise influencing each other. For example, the rational system can employ metaphor and imagery, which more commonly fall in the domain of the experiential system, and the experiential system can employ words, which fall more commonly in the domain of the rational system. Words, of course, can be used to paint word pictures and pictures can be used to present analytical material (e.g., pictures in anatomy textbooks).

As has already been noted, the experiential system influences the rational system by producing feelings, or vibes, that guide thought as well as action. On its part, the rational system, by becoming aware of the experiential system, can often override its influence, as indicated by resolutions of conflicts between the heart and the mind in favor of the mind. It is when the conflict is not recognized that the experiential system is most apt to dominate and influence the rational system unreasonably. The rational system can also influence the experiential system by directing the person to have certain experiences, either in reality or in fantasy.

EVIDENCE FOR THE EXISTENCE OF A SEPARATE EXPERIENTIAL CONCEPTUAL SYSTEM

Now that I have made a strong appeal for recognizing the importance of an experiential conceptual system, what is the evidence that there actually exists such a system that is independent from a rational conceptual system? Actually, a wide array of evidence points to the existence of two separate conceptual systems. It is important to note that the consideration here is of a distinction between two cognitive systems that operate in parallel, and not between a cognitive system and a presumably noncognitive emotional system, which I do not believe exists.

First, let us consider the so-called conflicts between the heart and the mind, unreflectively attributed by many to a conflict between emotion and reason. What would it actually mean if there were a conflict between emotion and reason? Such a conflict is meaningless unless emotions include a cognitive decision-making component that can operate in opposition to the cognitive decision-making component of the rational system, and in that case the conflict would be between two cognitive systems. When someone says, "I was in conflict between studying and going to the movies," was not the conflict actually between two different decision-making processes, and therefore between two different cognitive systems? The cognitive system that is associated with emotions exists in the experiential system, and the other in the rational system. They are both capable of adaptively interpreting and directing behavior, but they do it on a different basis. One attends to feeling states based on past memories and inferences from past memories, and the other attempts to "be reasonable" by keeping feeling states out of the decision-making process.

As previously noted, it should not be assumed that the "reasonable" solution is always the more adaptive. There is reason to suspect that people pay a high price in happiness and health, as well as in the more conventional criteria of success, if they sufficiently ignore either system (Epstein, 1990, in press; Epstein & Meier, 1989).

Irrational fears provide additional evidence of an experiential system that operates independently from a rational system. There are many people who despite knowing that it is far safer to travel by air than by automobile, elect to do the latter because being on the ground "feels" safer. This means that the experiential system, on the basis of past experience with heights and its own form of inference, computes that it is safer. The difference between insight and intellective knowledge in therapy provides another example of the difference between the two systems. Therapists know that it is often useless to provide clients with intellectual information about their difficulties. On the other hand, providing knowledge through emotionally significant experiences, such as a transference relationship, can profoundly influence behavior. Apparently, there is knowledge and knowledge, and experiential knowledge has different consequences from intellectual knowledge. Cigarette advertisements provide still further evidence of the existence of two systems. Why is it that tobacco companies are willing to pay great sums for advertisements that carry the message that their product can have dire consequences? They and their advertising agencies are intuitively aware that their message in the form of a picture easily overrides the factual written warning. The reason for the greater potency of the picture is that pictures are better suited than words for communicating with the experiential system. I doubt whether tobacco companies would be willing to pay for ads that were required to include a small picture of a burial scene, or of someone in a hospital bed with tubes coming out of his or her nose and distressed relatives at the bedside.

A particularly interesting example of the two systems is provided by an experiment reported by Piaget (1973). Young children were given the task of getting a tetherball into a box by twirling and releasing the string at the appropriate moment. With some practice they succeeded. However, when asked to explain how, they incorrectly said they released the ball when it was pointing at the target. When older children were given the same task, they correctly reported that they released the ball when it was at a right angle to the target. Piaget's point was that unless a child has an appropriate conscious schema for assimilating information, he or she is unable to report the nonverbal knowledge that he or she has acquired. For present purposes, the example well illustrates the existence of two different systems of knowing, one based on experience and the other on intellectual knowledge. The experiential system can apparently function highly effectively in many circumstances without conscious articulation.

Sappington and his coworkers (Sappington, 1981, 1989; Sappington, Rice, Burleson, & Gordon, 1981; Sappington, Richards, Spiers, & Fraser, 1983; Sappington & Russell, 1979; Sappington, Russell, Triplett, & Goodwin, 1980) propose a model that distinguishes between two kinds of beliefs, "intellectually based beliefs" and "emotionally based beliefs." They note that this division is highly similar to the one in CEST between the rational and experiential systems. They are impressed with the degree to which people are aware that they have emotionally based beliefs in conflict with their rational beliefs. In a series of experiments, they found that emotionally based beliefs tend to have a stronger influence on behavior than intellectually based beliefs. In one study (Sappington et al., 1981), they demonstrated that assessments of subjects' emotionally based beliefs about the use of aversive techniques with autistic children more accurately predicted their willingness to use the techniques than did assessments based on their intellectual beliefs about the effectiveness of the techniques. In another study (Sappington et al., 1980), they found that emotionally based beliefs predicted handling a snake more accurately than did the intellectually based belief of how dangerous it is to do so. In a "lottery" study (described in Sappington, 1989), subjects' expectancies about winning and their actual betting behavior were significantly influenced by an experimental manipulation that increased their emotionally based beliefs. Their intellectually based beliefs were unaffected by the manipulation. Moreover, their emotionally based beliefs, but not their intellectually based beliefs, were significantly related to their actual behavior.

A series of studies by Miller, Tversky, Kahneman, and others (e.g., Kahneman & Miller, 1986; Kahneman & Tversky, 1982; Johnson 1986; Miller & McFarland, 1986; Miller, Turnbull, & McFarland, 1990) provides further evidence consistent with the distinction in CEST between an experiential and a rational system, although these authors do not interpret their results from such a perspective. By having subjects respond to vignettes by indicating in which of two conditions people would be more upset, they explore the kinds of situations in which people tend to make what they refer to as "counterfactual" judgments. The research has revealed that subjects are more likely to make irrational decisions concerning bad outcomes following near rather than far misses, following acts of commission rather than acts of omission, following free rather than constrained choices, and following unusual rather than customary responses. The irrational responses are produced despite subjects' intellectual awareness that the likelihood of the negative outcome is the same for both conditions. As an example, subjects report that a person who is 30 minutes late with respect to scheduled flight time but misses his or her flight by 5 minutes because the flight was accidentally delayed will be more distressed than someone who misses his or her flight by the full 30 minutes because it left on time. When subjects are asked to respond rationally, they say the person should not be affected differently by the two conditions. Likewise, subjects report that a person who loses a sum of money by switching to a different stock will be more upset than a person who loses the same amount of money by failing to switch, even though they intellectually believe that one reaction is no more likely to result in a negative outcome than the other.

In a recent study (Epstein et al., in review), in which my colleagues and I used vignettes similar to those used by Miller, Tversky, and Kahneman, we replicated their results and found that by increasing the magnitude of negative outcomes, we were able to increase the degree to which people responded irrationally. In other words, by increasing the emotionality of the situations, we were able to drive the responses further in the direction of the experiential system. In responding to the vignettes, we had subjects indicate how most people would respond, how they themselves would respond, and what they thought was the most logical way to respond. Responses with respect to the behavior of others and themselves indicated that the subjects believed that, in situations such as the ones described, people (including themselves) do not respond rationally. Of particular interest, they were nevertheless well aware of what the most reasonable responses were, as indicated by their responses in the rational condition. Thus, people are aware that they have two sets of beliefs, rational and emotional, and that their emotional beliefs are often more important in determining their behavior.

The findings on irrational responses to vignettes are entirely consistent with what would be expected from the operation of an experiential system. As I have noted above, people report they would be more distressed following near misses than following remote misses, following acts of commission than acts of omission, following unusual responses than customary responses, and following choices when there were many as opposed to few options. It is noteworthy that all of these responses are usually adaptive in everyday behavior. In the normal world of everyday experience for both human and nonhuman animals, what is learned from a near miss can prevent a hit in the future. Making unusual responses is more apt to be dangerous than making tried and true responses. Acts of commission are a more likely source of conditioning and other forms of learning than acts of omission, which provide nothing specific to be conditioned. It is understandable, therefore, that in the world of nature, which is the world in which the experiential system evolved, it is generally more adaptive to be concerned with acts than with nonacts. By the same token, there is less to be learned from making a bad response when there is no choice than from making a bad response when there is a choice. The experiential system is geared for rapid processing of information and rapid responding, and its reactions are mediated by feelings. A system that responds in this manner will sometimes behave illogically when judged by the rules of the rational system, but under most circumstances that arise naturally in the environment, it is highly adaptive.

Resistance to Awareness of an Experiential Conceptual System

If the experiential system is as important as I have claimed, how is it possible that it has been overlooked for so long? There are several reasons for this. One is that the experiential system provides the background of mental activity, whereas conscious thinking is in the foreground. As Thomas Carlyle noted, if a fish had an inquiring mind, the last thing it would discover is water. People look out onto reality, and not reflexively back onto how they automatically construct it.

A second reason why people are able to avoid awareness of the experiential system is that, no matter what the actual cause of their behavior, they are usually able to give a rational explanation (i.e., they "rationalize").

People also resist awareness of their experiential system because awareness is burdensome. Worse yet, awareness of one's automatic thinking can be distressing because it can make one aware of one's role in producing one's emotions. For example, if people are angry at someone, they can feel righteously indignant. The other person is seen as a bad person and the self as good. If one were to become aware of one's preconscious thoughts, it would become evident that the other person's badness is contingent on ones own interpretation of what happened. There is the possibility that one could interpret the event differently and not be angry. There is even the possibility that one might learn that one uses emotions manipulatively, which would make it difficult to continue behaving that way. Many people would rather believe they are passive victims of their emotions than accept responsibility for them.

A fourth reason for resistance to acknowledging an experiential system that operates automatically without awareness is that there are already well-established theories that emphasize unconscious processes. Most psychologists are satisfied with their explanations of irrational behavior and thus see no reason to adopt a new system. As Kuhn (1970) has reminded us, old paradigms die hard.

A final reason is that people believe that what I attribute to an experiential and conceptual system is nothing new, because it can be accounted for by a distinction between emotions and cognitions. They fail to realize that emotion versus cognition is an unsatisfactory distinction, because emotion includes cognition. Those who contrast emotion with cognition generally equate cognition with conscious thought. They ignore the fact that a great deal of cognition occurs automatically without consciousness awareness or verbal representation. Piaget, one of the foremost cognitive psychologists, did not confine his study of cognition to conscious, reportable information; he also studied nonverbal cognition, as in the example of the children and the tetherball cited earlier, and in his more general views on sensory–motor intelligence.

Emotions and Moods

Emotions are of particular interest to CEST because they are the royal road to a person's preconscious beliefs. Thus, one of the most effective ways of learning about the basic beliefs in a person's theory of reality is to examine the person's emotions. Emotions can reveal preconscious cognitions in two ways. First, emotions serve as a barometer of the significance of beliefs in a personal theory of reality. The greater the emotional reaction a person has in a situation, the more it can be assumed that a significant belief in the person's theory of reality was implicated. For example, if someone becomes very distressed when his or her intelligence is impugned, it can be assumed that intelligence is very important in the person's preconscious self-system. Thus, if one wishes to determine the important schemas in a personal theory of reality, a particularly useful procedure is to observe the kinds of situations that cause the person to react emotionally. Of particular interest, in this respect, is the fact that emotional responses often belie conscious beliefs, so emotions provide a way of acquiring information about schemas in the experiential system that are distinguishable from those in the rational system.

The second way in which emotions can reveal underlying conditions is that particular cognitions are associated with particular emotions. For example, the most common preconscious cognitions underlying anger are that someone has behaved badly and deserves to be punished. The most common preconscious cognitions underlying sadness are that something of importance to one's happiness has been or will be lost and that nothing can be done about it. The most common preconscious cognitions underlying fear are that something dangerous will happen in the future and that escape is possible from it. Notice that in each case the cognitions include an interpretation of a situation and of a possible response (for a more extensive discussion of the relation of specific cognitions and emotions from the perspective of CEST, see Epstein, 1984). Because of the connection between specific emotions and preconscious cognitions, some of a person's most important preconscious cognitions can be inferred from knowledge about the person's disposition to experience certain emotions. Thus, people who are frequently angry tend to assume the role of judge and jury; they view themselves as good or right, and other people as bad or wrong and as deserving therefore to be punished.

The recognition that preconscious cognitions are the usual effective stimuli that instigate emotions also has important implications for the control of emotions, for it follows that if cognitions instigate emotions, then by altering cognitions it is possible to change emotions. The fact that this relationship has important implication for behavior change has not been lost on cognitive therapists, such as Beck (1976) and Ellis (1962).

What has been said about emotions is also true of moods, but on a grander scale. Emotions are cognitive–affective modules, somewhat like multiple personalities. The same is true of moods. They differ in that emotions are episodic reactions instigated by the interpretation of specific stimuli, whereas moods are more enduring and profound states that often occur in the absence of identifiable stimuli. Like the waves in relation to the tide, emotions are superimposed on moods. A person in a sad mood may experience an emotion of joy when given pleasant news, only to have the affect shortly return to the baseline of the more enduring mood. In time, of course, moods also shift, but they do not do so as readily as emotions.

Whereas emotions are instigated by preconscious appraisals of specific events, moods are instigated by preconscious appraisals that are broader in scope and that have more serious implications for a person's long-term welfare. The preconscious appraisals are apt to include interpretations of people's prospects, if they continue on their present course, of finding love or happiness or of achieving success in their lives. This is not meant to deny that moods can also be influenced by other factors, including biological ones. Nor is it meant to deny that the influence between cognitions and feeling states goes in both directions. A depressed person is apt to interpret a particular stimulus in a different manner from the way he or she would in a happier frame of mind. Thus, it is obvious that feeling states influence cognition as well as vice versa.

Sensitivities and Compulsions

According to CEST, the primary sources of schemas in personal theories of reality are emotionally significant experiences. To a large extent, the schemas are simply generalizations from experience. A person who has been raised in a rejecting, destructive family environment is likely to develop the beliefs that people are rejecting and the world is destructive. A person raised under more benign circumstances is likely to develop more optimistic and benign views about people and the world. It is, of course, adaptive to develop a belief system that accurately represents one's experiences. Most beliefs are reasonably flexible, in the sense that they change as a function of cumulative experience. Sensitivities and compulsions, however, are resistant to change. The person who has experienced a rejecting mother should ideally be able to change his or her generalized views about people's being rejecting upon encountering people who are not rejecting. Beliefs that are inflexible are, according to CEST, a major source of maladjustment. It follows that sensitivities and compulsions should be particularly important sources of maladjustment.

"Sensitivities" refer to exaggerated, rigid beliefs in the experiential system that certain kinds of situations or events are dangerous. An example of a sensitivity is a person's reacting to mice as if they are life-threatening beasts, and, as a result, being continuously alerted to the presence of mice and reacting to any possibility of their presence with intense fear. "Compulsions" refer to experientially derived generalizations that certain kinds of behavior are effective ways of reducing threat. Both are resistant to extinction or modification because they have been learned under conditions of high emotional arousal, and have, over time, become nuclei of cognitive and behavioral networks. Sensitivities correspond to preconscious descriptive beliefs, and compulsions to preconscious motivational beliefs.

Sensitivities and compulsions, as the terms are used in CEST, differ from their more traditional use in abnormal psychology in one very important respect. When used to describe abnormal behaviors, they refer to narrowly defined classes of stimuli and behavior. Thus, individuals are diagnosed as having a hand-washing compulsion or a compulsion to engage in certain other private rituals. In CEST the meaning of the terms is expanded to include more complex patterns of behavior that, although maladaptive, are not abnormal in the usual sense of the word, because they are relatively common, often simply defining the most salient characteristics of people.

The hallmark of a sensitivity is that whenever certain stimuli or situations arise, the individual becomes excessively distressed. Sensitivities can be identified by situations that "get to people," that "bug them," that their friends recognize they must avoid if they wish to maintain peace. The hallmarks of a compulsion are as follows: (1) The person acts in a rigid way across a variety of situations, such as always having to be dominant or always having to be ingratiating; (2) the person experiences distress whenever he or she is unable to behave in the manner dictated by the compulsion; and (3) the compulsion becomes exaggerated when the person is threated, particularly when the threat involves a relevant sensitivity. It is assumed that sensitivities were learned under conditions of extreme threat and that compulsions were learned as ways of coping with sensitivities. In order to understand the fundamental nature of sensitivities and compulsions, it will be helpful first to consider the nature of anxiety.

Anxiety became established as part of the inherited repertoire of higher-order species because of its adaptive significance. As an example, consider a rabbit that has been attacked by a hawk. From that point on, whenever a stimulus that is reminiscent of the original threatening stimulus appears, the anxiety alarm sounds and the rabbit automatically responds with whatever actions it previously made that were followed by a reduction in anxiety. Normally, the anxiety and the responses it evokes are adaptive, because they provide the rabbit with an automatic warning signal and with automatic responses for escaping from the danger. In time, if similar stimuli are experienced in the absence of real danger, the anxiety gradually subsides, which of course is also adaptive. The greater the initial anxiety, the broader the gradient of generalization, and the more resistant the responses to the anxiety-inducing stimulus are to extinction. The stimuli that threafter evoke anxiety as a result of being associated with the original stressor are sensitivities. The automatic responses that are produced to these stimuli as a way of reducing anxiety are compulsions.

From the viewpoint of CEST, sensitivities and compulsions, not unconscious conflict and repression, are the most fundamental sources of maladaptive behavior. Unconscious conflict and repression are simply complications that make the sources and sometimes the nature of the sensitivities and compulsions unavailable to awareness. Accordingly, in many cases, removing repression (i.e., making the unconscious conscious) is not enough to correct maladaptive behavior, because the initial sensitivities and compulsions remain. As I have noted earlier, all that may be accomplished by such a procedure is to transform a neurotic without insight into one with insight. As I have likewise already indicated, sensitivities correspond to descriptive schemas that identify sources of danger. Compulsions correspond to motivational schemas about how to avoid or escape from danger. The maladaptiveness of these schemas depends on how general (undifferentiated, rigid, inflexible) they are and how resistant they are to modification. The earlier such schemas are acquired, and the greater the intensity and repetition of the emotional experiences on which they are based, the more likely they are to become central postulates in a personal theory of reality and therefore to be broadly influential and self-maintaining.

The acquisition of sensitivities and compulsions can account for many of the phenomena that psychoanalysts attribute to unconscious conflict. There is thus the danger that behavior will be diagnosed and treated by psychoanalysts as if unconscious conflict is present, when in fact it is not. To state this is not to deny the importance of unconscious conflict, but to indicate that it is less general than psychoanalysts assume, and to draw attention to another kind of unconscious (or, more accurately, preconscious) thinking with which it is often confused.

IMPLICATIONS

CEST has important implications for psychological research, psychotherapy, education, politics, mental and physical well-being, and an understanding of religion and spirituality. It is obviously beyond the scope of this chapter to discuss any of these in depth. However, a brief comment on each is in order.

If there are two conceptual systems, then the usual practice of referring to "*the* conceptual system" is misguided. Research should study the characteristics of each of the systems and examine the implications of discrepancies between the systems. It is particularly important to determine the attributes of the experiential system that distinguish it from the rational system. As a beginning, the hypothesized attributes of the experiential system as presented in Table 7.1 could be tested. An important area for research is establishing the relative contribution of each system to behavior under different circumstances, as in the studies by Sappington and colleagues using instructions meant to engage the emotional and rational systems, and in the studies by Kahneman, Miller, and Tversky examining anomalies in thinking with specially constructed vignettes.

Social-psychological research can examine the efficacy of different kinds of messages for communicating with the two systems and of the influence of attitudes or beliefs within each of the systems on social behavior. It can be expected that emotional, visual, and experientially based messages will be found to be more effective in reaching the experiential system, and that beliefs in the experiential system will under many (but not all) circumstances exert a greater influence on social behavior than beliefs in the rational system. Personality research could examine individual differences in tendencies to rely on one of the systems more than the other. The tendancy to direct one's life predominantly by one system or the other is an extremely important variable that should affect the influence of other variables on the individual. An important issue for clinical psychology is the relationship to adjustment of extreme approaches that rely almost exclusively on either the experiential or the rational system, in contrast to a more balanced approach.

An important implication for psychotherapy is that if one wishes to understand an individual, according to CEST, it is necessary to become aware of the basic schemas in a person's preconscious theory of reality. This means knowing the person's most fundamental descriptive and motivational postulates, and, in particular, identifying the person's sensitivities and compulsions. From the viewpoint of CEST, significant changes in psychotherapy require changes in the experiential system. This can be accomplished in two ways: by reaching the experiential system through the rational system, and by reaching the experiential system more directly through actual experience or fantasy. The former can be accomplished by informing the rational system about the nature of the experiential system and how it can be changed by providing it with appropriate experiences and by disputing inappropriate construals and coping responses. The latter can be accomplished by providing corrective experiences in therapy and in homework assignments, and by employing imagination and visualization techniques. An important area for research in psychotherapy is determining the most efficient ways of producing experientially based changes. According to CEST, imagery techniques are particularly promising, because the experiential system reacts to imagination in the same way as it reacts to reality.

The major implication of CEST for education is that it is at least as important to train the experiential mind as the rational mind. Although what evidence there is suggests that the experiential system is more important than the rational system for success in living (Epstein, in press; Epstein & Meier, 1989), 12 years of public education are required of all citizens for training their rational systems and none for training their experiential systems. By drawing on experiences from their everyday lives as well as using standard situations, children could be taught to identify their rational and experiential reactions, and to take both into account in their decisions. It is particularly important in a democracy to train citizens to identify appeals by self-serving politicians to the experiential system for problems that are best solved by the rational system.

CEST has obvious implications for mental and physical well-being, because it considers the experiential system to be intimately associated with the experience of emotions, which are related to stress and physiological reactions. It has been demonstrated with the Constructive Thinking Inventory (CTI) that the constructiveness of people's automatic thinking is related to the amount of stress they experience in everyday life and to their mental and physical health (Epstein, 1990, in press; Epstein & Meier,

1989). According to CEST, humans are caught in an existential dilemma because they have two different systems for apprehending and coping with reality—an experiential and a rational system. As a result, they, alone in the animal kingdom, are alienated from their natural state and have the difficult task of finding an integrative approach, one that can establish harmony between the two systems. From this viewpoint, effective adjustment requires not merely the extirpation of areas of conflict or the extinction of sensitivities and compulsions, or the domination of the experiential system by the rational system, but the use of both systems to their fullest advantage in a harmonious manner.

Why does there appear to be a universal need for religion? Throughout recorded history societies have practiced religion. They have invented either multiple gods or a single God, and have done monumental deeds, both for human welfare and against it, in the service of these gods. Freud denigrated religious beliefs by referring to them as institutionalized delusions that are used as crutches by insufficiently developed societies. According to CEST, religion fulfills an important human need because it reaches the experiential mind in a way that science and reason have not, through its use of imagery, music, concrete symbolization, and social support. The experiential mind can comprehend a personified God in a way that it cannot an abstract principle. It is apparently so important for many people to apprehend their world in a manner appealing directly to their experiential system that they are willing to maintain beliefs that are clearly absurd from the perspective of the rational system. Moreover, throughout the course of history, they have been willing to defend these beliefs to the death and have been eager to force them on others. The power of religion has also been exhibited in its ability to effect miraculous cures from terminal illness. It remains for future research to establish ways in which the power of fantasy that has been exhibited in religious practice can be harnessed yet more effectively in scientific practice to contribute to human welfare.

ACKNOWLEDGMENTS

Preparation of this chapter and the research reported in it were supported by National Institute of Mental Health (NIMH) Research Grant No. MH01293 and NIMH Research Scientist Award No. K05 MH00363. I wish to acknowledge the contribution of Carolyn Holstein, who did the computing on most of the studies that were reported. I also wish to thank Albert Ellis and Alice Epstein for their constructive criticism. At the same time, I must acknowledge that I did not always take their advice, and that, although there was considerable agreement, it should not be assumed that they agreed with all the views expressed.

REFERENCES

Allport, G. W. (1927). *Pattern and growth in personality*. New York: Harcourt, Brace & World, 1961.

Beck, A. T. (1976). *Cognitive therapy and the emotional disorders*. New York: International Universities Press.

Bowlby, J. (1973). *Attachment and loss: Vol. 2. Separation, anxiety and anger*. New York: Basic Books.

Cashdan, S. (1988). *Object relations therapy: Using the relationship*. New York: Norton.

Ellis, A. (1962). *Reason and emotion in psychotherapy*. New York: Lyle Stuart.

Epstein, S. (1980). The self-concept: A review and the proposal of an integrated theory of personality. In E. Staub (Ed.), *Personality: Basic issues and current research* (pp. 82–132). Englewood Cliffs, NJ: Prentice-Hall.

Epstein, S. (1983). The unconscious, the preconscious and the self-concept. In J. Suls & A. Greenwald (Eds.), *Psychological perspectives on the self* (Vol. 2, pp. 219–247). Hillsdale, NJ: Erlbaum.

Epstein, S. (1984). Controversial issues in emotions theory. In P. Shaver (Ed.), *Annual review of research in personality and social psychology* (pp. 64–87). Beverly Hills, CA: Sage.

Epstein, S. (1990). Cognitive–experiential self-theory. In L. A. Pervin (Ed.), *Handbook of personality: Theory and research* (pp. 165–192). New York: Guilford Press.

Epstein, S. (in press). Constructive thinking and mental and physical well-being. In S. H. Filipp & L. Montada (Eds.), *Crises and loss experiences in the adult years*. Hillsdale, NJ: Erlbaum.

Epstein, S., Lipson, A., & Huh, E. (in review). *Irrational reactions to negative outcomes: Evidence for two conceptual systems*.

Epstein, S., & Meier, P. (1989). Constructive thinking: A broad coping variable with specific components. *Journal of Personality and Social Psychology, 57,* 332–349.

Freud, S. (1920). *Beyond the pleasure principle*. New York: Bantam, 1959.

Horney, K. (1945). *Our inner conflicts*. New York: Norton.

Johnson, J. T. (1986). The knowledge of what might have been: Affective and attributional consequences of near outcomes. *Personality and Social Psychology Bulletin, 12,* 51–62.

Kahneman, D., & Miller, D. T. (1986). Norm theory: Comparing reality to its alternatives, *Psychological Review, 93,* 136–153.

Kahneman, D., & Tversky, A. (1982). The simulation heuristic. In D. Kahneman, P. Slovic, & A. Tversky (Eds.), *Judgment under uncertainty: Heuristics and biases* (pp. 201–208). New York: Cambridge University Press.

Kelly, G. A. (1955). *The psychology of personal constructs* (2 vols.). New York: Norton.

Kohut, H. (1971). *The analysis of the self*. New York: International Universities Press.

Kuhn, T. S. (1970). *The structure of scientific revolutions* (2nd ed.). Chicago: University of Chicago Press.

Lecky, P. (1945). *Self-consistency: A theory of personality*. New York: Island Press.

Miller, D., & McFarland, C. (1986). Counterfactual thinking and victim compensation: A test of norm theory. *Personality and Social Psychology Bulletin, 12,* 513–519.

Miller, D., Turnbull, W., & McFarland, C. (1990). Counterfactual thinking and social perception: Thinking about what might have been. In M. P. Zanna (Ed.), *Advances in experimental social psychology* (Vol. 23, pp. 305–331). San Diego: Academic Press.

Piaget, J. (1973). The affective unconscious and the cognitive unconscious. *Journal of the American Psychoanalytic Association, 21,* 249–261.

Rogers, C. R. (1951). *Client-centered therapy.* Boston: Houghton Mifflin.

Sappington, A. A. (1981). Apollo and Bacchus in cognitive therapy: Emotionally based assessments. *The Southern Psychologist, 3,* 13–18.

Sappington, A. A. (1989). *The independent manipulation of intellectually and emotionally based beliefs.* Unpublished manuscript.

Sappington, A. A., Rice, J., Burleson, R., & Gordon, J. (1981). Emotionally based expectancies and willingness to use aversive therapy. *Basic and Applied Social Psychology, 2,* 227–234.

Sappington, A. A., Richards, S., Siers, M., & Fraser, M. B. (1983). *Relationship of intellectually and emotionally based perceptions of personal control to improvement in a pain clinic program.* Paper presented at the annual meeting of the Southeastern Psychological Association.

Sappington, A. A., & Russell, J. C. (1979). Self-efficacy and meaning: candidates for a uniform theory of behavior. *Personality and Social Psychology Bulletin, 2,* 327.

Sappington, A. A., Russell, J. C., Triplett, V., & Goodwin, J. (1980). Self-efficacy expectancies, response–outcome expectancies, emotionally based expectancies and their relationship to avoidance behavior. *Journal of Clinical Psychology, 37,* 737–744.

Snygg, D., & Combs, A. W. (1949). *Individual behavior.* New York: Harper & Row.

Taylor, S. E., & Brown, J. D. (1988). Illusion and well-being: A social psychological perspective on mental health. *Psychological Bulletin, 103,* 193–210.

CHAPTER EIGHT

Seeing with the Third Eye: Cognitive–Affective Regulation and the Acquisition of Self-Knowledge

REBECCA C. CURTIS
GARRY ZASLOW

Hamlyn, a philosopher, in his contribution to Theodore Mischel's 1977 volume entitled *The Self: Psychological and Philosophical Issues,* states that the Socratic dictum "Know thyself" certainly includes a moral dimension that contemporary psychology has largely failed to address. If self-knowledge involves more than knowing with the mind and "is nothing if it has no relation to one's life in general," as Hamlyn has argued (p. 174), then what is it?

This paper addresses two types of knowledge Epstein discusses elsewhere in this volume (see Chapter Seven) in greater detail: (1) rational knowledge and (2) affective or experiential knowledge. Other theorists have also postulated separate but similar representational systems. Paivio (1971, 1978, 1986), for example, a cognitive psychologist, has provided evidence for verbal and nonverbal informational processing systems. Bucci (1985, 1989) has found evidence for a logical, verbal system and an alogical, nonverbal representational system. She calls the connection between the two, which is the verbal labeling of nonverbal elements, "referential activity," borrowing from Paivio. Weinberger and McClelland (1990) have also described two conceptual systems—one conscious, that of self-reported explicit motives; the other unconscious or implicit, similar to Freud's id.

The thesis of the current chapter is that as people gain knowledge of their own affective systems, they become more aware of feelings of others, more knowledgeable about what hurts others, and more knowledgeable about how their own failings cause suffering in others. Although it is possible to have such knowledge and use it to hurt other people, it is argued in this chapter that when painful affects of the experiential system have no longer been warded off from the awareness of the rational system, the moral choices of people no longer favor "the self" over others. When this type of enlightened self-knowledge occurs, the distinctions between self and nonself become unimportant. Although the enlightened individual unlike the psychotic, can differentiate his or her own pain from that of others, the other's pain is felt as much as one's own. Thus, in the West, we advocate that people treat their neighbors as they would treat themselves. In the East, where the disappearance of the distinction between self and nonself is valued, people are taught instead, "Your neighbor *is* yourself."

Hamlyn (1977) has criticized experimental psychologists for examining only beliefs about the self and beliefs about the reactions of others— that is, what Epstein (see Chapter Seven) calls the rational conceptual system. The English word "knowledge" is itself a synthesis of words from two different roots—one meaning "to know with the mind," as in the German *wissen* or the French *savoir*; the other meaning "to know with the senses," as in the Latin *gnoscere* (*Compact Edition of the Oxford English Dictionary*, 1971, Vol. 1, p. 1550). Although the first type of knowledge has been more amenable to the domain of science, researchers are now beginning to explore the second type of knowledge (i.e., experiential or affective awareness).

Before we continue with this presentation, we wish to emphasize that our interest in this topic comes not from our expertise in the area, but from our own desire to become more knowledgeable in this domain. Readers will undoubtedly draw their own conclusions about how much of use we have to say on this topic, not only from our review of the literature and research, but also from how our presentation comes across. And, although we have only begun this journey, we have at least read reports from others about the road to follow.

Reviews of the functions and meaning of the self have been published recently by Greenwald and Pratkanis (1984) and by Baumeister (1986). The sense of "self" is frequently considered to be an awareness of unity and continuity (Cantor, Markus, Niedenthal, & Nurius, 1986), and sometimes also of differentiation (Baumeister, 1986). In the present chapter, the "self" is conceived of as a process in which the feelings, thoughts, and behaviors are recognized by the person as differentiated from those of another person (Curtis, 1991). According to this definition, not all individuals possess a sense of self, and in some cultures a self-system may include more than one individual (cf. Stoetzel, 1963; Westen, 1985). Awareness of an organization of feelings, thoughts, and behaviors into a continuous and coherent system is considered to be essential to the sense of self.

This chapter examines five types of self-knowledge: (1) recognition of the physical self; (2) awareness of the self; (3) the assessment of the self; (4) the emotional experience of the self; and (5) the disintegration of the self.

KNOWLEDGE OF THE PHYSICAL SELF: SELF-RECOGNITION

Self-knowledge begins with recognition of a physical self. Gallup (Gallup & Suarez, 1985, in press) has conducted many experiments on self-recognition, in which primates were first exposed to mirrors and then anesthetized while a red mark was placed on their faces. These studies indicate that upon awakening, only humans, chimpanzees, and orangutans appear to recognize that they are what is represented in a mirror and to use this information to explore the otherwise unseen red mark. Gallup has argued that self-recognition is the basis of self-awareness (Gallup, 1982, 1983), and that an organism that is aware of its own experience is able to model the experience of others (Gallup & Suarez, 1985). Gallup and Suarez (in press) state that "Knowledge of self provides a means of achieving an inferential knowledge of others." Interestingly, species that lack self-awareness fail to show evidence of empathy and deception.

Although various methodological problems exist with regard to the studies investigating the age when human infants recognize themselves in a mirror (Andersen, 1984; Gallup, 1979), the studies reveal that 70% of babies aged 18 to 24 months are able to do so (Lewis & Brooks-Gunn, 1979). Lewis and Brooks-Gunn, citing evidence that children as young as $2\frac{1}{2}$ years of age are able to show simple role-taking abilities (Fishbein, Lewis, & Keiffer, 1972; Masangkay et al., 1974), postulate that empathy "has its beginnings in the second year of life, emerging with the providing support for the child's emerging concept of self" (p. 261).

KNOWLEDGE OF THE AWARE SELF: "OBJECTIVE" SELF-AWARENESS

Research on "objective" self-awareness (Duval & Wicklund, 1972; Wicklund, 1975) demonstrated that the initial reaction to self-focused attention is self-evaluation; that self-focused attention generates attempts to escape when there are discrepancies between attainments and aspirations; and that discrepancy reduction occurs when there is no escape from self-focusing stimuli. Further research (Wicklund, 1978) showed that, although attributions in social situations are usually made toward whatever aspect of the situation is most salient, thus accounting for findings of increased attributions to the self under conditions of heightened self-

awareness, attributions to the self were not made when they were potentially ego-threatening (Federoff & Harvey, 1976). In an experiment by
Federoff and Harvey, the participants were given a brief training in the
administration of psychotherapy and then asked to attempt to treat a
patient who was phobic. Half of the participants met with success and half
with failure. Under conditions of high self-awareness (i.e., in front of a
camera), participants attributed more blame for the failure to the patient,
instead of to themselves, as had previously been the case in other experiments in which participants were made self-aware. Hull and Levy (1979)
also found that on a test of cognitive abilities, participants made self-aware
were more reluctant to characterize their performance outcome as failure.
Other research on self-awareness indicates that self-focus gives a person a
more accurate assessment of the causes and noncauses of arousal states
(Gibbons, cited in Wicklund, 1978); that affect becomes more extreme
when people are self-focused (Scheier & Carver, 1977); and that the effects
of affect can be more important than those of conformity to standards
under conditions of heightened self-focus (Scheier, 1976).

"Self-monitoring," as proposed by Snyder (1979), is a process in which
a system of rules established through self-knowledge governs the social
behavior of an individual. Self-monitoring processes are active only in
social situations. Individuals *high* in self-monitoring tend to adapt themselves to social situations by fitting their self-presentations to the
specifications of appropriateness for that particular situation. This sort of
individual strives to create an image of self that is flexible—one that can
easily mold itself to any situation. Individuals *low* in self-monitoring, on the
other hand, strive to maintain a relatively consistent self-image across
situations and value a similarity between "who they are" and "what they
do." They rely on dispositional accounts attributes within themselves.

People high in self-monitoring attend more to the relationship between intentions and actions than do people low in self-monitoring (Snyder, 1987). Those low in self-monitoring tend to possess a greater understanding of themselves and are able to draw upon that knowledge more
readily than those high in self-monitoring (Snyder & Cantor, 1980). However, there are times when it is appropriate for those with high self-
monitoring to exhibit attributes typical of low self-montoring. That is, they
will attribute more responsibility to the "self" (Schneiderman, Webb, Davis, & Thomas, cited in Snyder, 1987) and behave more in line with their
own attitudes in certain situations (e.g., Snyder & Kendzierski, 1982).

Thus, self-monitoring is a moderating variable, if we may call it that,
between self-knowledge and social interaction. It serves as a guide for the
individual, through which information about people and situations is actively translated into social behavior. The individual high in self-monitoring acquires self-knowledge by means of social interaction and has a

flexibility for situations lacked by individuals low in self-monitoring, whose self-knowledge is acquired more from the understanding of their attitudes, dispositions, and salient and relevant inner states (Snyder, 1979).

KNOWLEDGE OF ONE'S STRENGTHS AND WEAKNESSES

Assessment of the Self

Considerable research has shown that people seek accurate diagnostic information about their abilities (Trope, 1980, 1982). A recent experiment by Manion, Pacell, and Curtis (1990) demonstrates that people seek such information even when they believe it will be negative and when it is important to their self-views. This does not mean that people always prefer accurate information if it is expected to be negative rather than positive, however. Recently, the tendency for people in nonclinical sample to hold positive *illusions* of themselves has been well documented (Taylor & Brown, 1988; Taylor, 1989).

Only a few experiments have investigated whether people prefer accurate or positive information. Swann, Pelham, and Krull (1989), for example, found that participants preferred to interact with another participant who had offered an unfavorable but self-verifying evaluation, rather than a participant who had given them a favorable but non-self-verifying evaluation. Still, in another experiment, even participants with negative self-views rated the negative evaluator as less attractive and rated their affect as more unpleasant after a negative evaluation, although they rated the negative feedback as more self-descriptive and the negative evaluator as more competent (Swann, Griffin, Predmore, & Gaines, 1987). An attempt has been made to reconcile the motive to seek information that enhances self-esteem with the motive to verify already existing self-views when they are negative (Swann, 1990). Swann has suggested, for example, that people seek confirmation of their pre-existing self-views (as opposed to favorable feedback) to the extent that people hold negative self-views, to the extent that their self-views are salient, to the extent that they are certain of their self-views, to the extent that their self-views are not crucial to their goals and plans, and to the extent that they have plenty of time to make a decision.

Some recent research has also explored whether people assess themselves as distinct from others. McGuire and McGuire (1988) have found that children report distinct characteristics about themselves when asked the affirmational question, "Tell us about yourself," with minority children, for example, being more likely to report their race. Karniol (1990) has argued that ways in which the self is distinct affects judgments about others more than do self-schemas (Markus, 1977; Markus & Smith, 1981).

Knowledge of the Causes of One's Own Behavior

Research in social psychology has focused upon the ways in which people make causal attributions for behavior. According to Bem's (1967, 1972) theory of self-perception, of course, in the tradition of the British philosopher Ryle (1949), people learn about themselves the same way as they learn about others—through the observation of their own behavior. Although some differences in the attributions to self and others have been found (Jones & Nisbett, 1972), Nisbett and Wilson (1977) have reviewed many studies indicating that introspection leads to inaccurate reports of the causes of behavior. Nisbett and Wilson found that experimental participants were unaware of the situational variables that the data demonstrated to have influenced their behavior.

Clinical psychologists, of course, focus upon the variables affecting behaviors to which their clients are not attending (Curtis, 1991; Goldfried, 1991; Sullivan, 1953). Behaviorists focus upon reinforcing contingencies, analysts focus upon factors out of awareness, and experiential therapists focus upon affect. Both social and clinical psychologists agree that people are frequently unaware of the variables affecting their behavior. Both therapy and Eastern religious practices are designed to heighten awareness.

Knowledge of Others' Responses

Considerable research has now demonstrated that normal people overestimate the extent to which they are liked by others. In this regard, then, they are not accurate in their assessment of how they are coming across to others. Perhaps people are more accurate in perceiving the reactions of others when their own self-views are not involved.

Research regarding knowledge of the reactions of other people has come from the study of empathy. Infants show distress and cry in response to the sound of another infant's cry during the first week of life (Martin & Clark, 1982; Sagi & Hoffman, 1976; Simner, 1971). This reaction does not occur to a computer-simulated sound of equal intensity.

Although there appears to be little research regarding how accurate people are in perceiving the emotional reactions of others, there is considerable research demonstrating the effects of empathic reactions in both adults and children. In both groups, empathy leads to more altruistic behavior (Feshbach (1979, 1982; Iannotti, 1978; Leiman, 1978; Staub, 1971). Feshbach (1982, p. 320) concluded that empathy in children has many effects, including "greater emotions, competence, heightened compassion, caring, and religious behavior; regulation of aggression and other antisocial behaviors; increased self-awareness, enhanced communication skills, and greater cohesion between the cognitive, affective, and interpersonal aspects of the child's behavior." The capacity to react empathically appears to develop from a secure early attachment; parental affection; the availability of empathic models; parental encouragement of emotional perspective taking, of a perception of similarity to others, and of a positive self-concept; and discouragement of excessive competition (Barnett, 1987). Research shows that dispositional differences in empathy are related to the ability and readiness to take another's perspective, as well as to either general emotionality or a specific emotional reaction (Batson, Fultz, & Schoenrade, 1987).

The Role of Personality Characteristics

Although a very large quantity of research has been conducted demonstrating that depressed people and people with negative self-views spend more time looking at negative information about themselves and recall negative information better than do nondepressed people and people with positive self-views (see Kuiper, MacDonald, & Derry, 1983, for a review), there is little research examining the differences of persons with differing personality dispositions in the acquisition and avoidance of diagnostic information. Research regarding the positive illusions of nondepressed people shows that they may selectively remember positive information and suggests that they may seek out and attend to positive information. The only individual differences that have been found in the extent to which people seek accurate self-assessment are that people with high achievement motivation (Trope, 1980), people who tolerate and seek out high levels of uncertainty (Sorrentino & Hewitt, 1984), and people low in feelings of inadequacy (Manion & Curtis, 1989) have been found to seek out more diagnostic information about their abilities.

This body of research on the search for accurate diagnostic information leaves us with some interesting problems. How do we get people with negative self-views to attend to and recall positive information? And how do we get normal people to attend to and deal with negative information, such as the serious problems facing our globe, including global warming, deforestation, and the depletion of our ozone layer, largely from the use of air conditioning and the burning of fossil fuels (cf. Goleman, 1989)?

KNOWLEDGE OF ONE'S EMOTIONAL STATES

In this section, we first discuss social-psychological research regarding the self-inference of emotions, including research regarding the relative weight given to feelings, thoughts, and behaviors in the self-inference process. Then we discuss recent theory in clinical psychology on knowledge of one's emotions.

Social-Psychological Research on Self-Knowledge of Emotions and Inner States

According to Pennebaker (1980), emotions feelings, and illness are understood through an ongoing perceptual process of sensations. Individuals also are especially likely to attend to specific sensations when they have reason to believe that the sensations are characteristic of particular emotions, feelings, or illnesses. People select sensory input through the use of cognitive schemas or sets, which further help to define sensations. These schemas are confirmed or disconfirmed by the sensory input selected, or they are modified to interpret these sensations. Thus, the perceptual process is cyclical.

People may attempt to interpret what an emotion *is* in the sense of how they are *supposed* to feel physiologically when they have that emotion. That is, they may search their bodies for signs of a particular emotion (or illness). Most may attend to a specific internal sensations to verify emotions or illness. A given emotional label may be understood prior to a person's becoming aware of internal sensations, then temporarily seen from within a certain schema; this causes the person to attend to specific internal sensations to confirm or disconfirm the schema, set, or label. It is also the *way* in which one attends to particular sensations, rather than a generalized attention, that determines whether these sensations are interpreted as important or not.

If a situation is associated with a given emotional label, then, a person will interpret his or her internal sensations in regard to that label. The individual is searching for validating information in order to understand his or her emotions and inner states. Thus, people are more likely to "encode" label-relevant information than irrelevant or disconfirming information (Pennebaker, 1980).

Recently, Pennebaker (1989a) has conducted research of a quite different type regarding the perception of one's emotions. He has found consistently that disclosing traumatic events is associated with fewer illnesses and less subjective distress. For example, Pennebaker (1989a) has examined the self-reports of people who listened for several hours as Holocaust survivors recounted their experiences in concentration camps. He found that some listeners showed physiological changes at the same time as the Holocaust victims recounting their traumas experienced them. These listeners felt worse at the time of the interviews and immediately afterwards, but had fewer symptoms of physical distress, fewer visits to a physician, and fewer illnesses in the year that followed than listeners who did not exhibit the empathic physiological response during the interviews.

Schachter's (1964) attributional theory of emotion had led to an increasing interest in the study of expectations and "misattributions" of emotions. Ross and Olson (1981) recently proposed an expectancy–attribution model of the effects of placebos, which relates the causes for the misattribution of emotional symptoms to the wrong source. There are four preconditions on which they believe misattribution is contingent: (1) The reason for arousal is not apparent to the participants; (2) there is an obvious misattribution source; (3) the misattribution source is considered by the participants to be a possible cause for their arousal; and (4) participants believe that the impact of the misattribution source is stronger than that of the actual source. The most important point here is that an individual can attribute (or misattribute) emotions to a neutral source (placebo), simply because of a belief in the strength of that source to elicit arousal symptoms.

One very important addition to this theory is that the neutral source of arousal must occur at the same time and place as the arousal itself in order for it to be seen as a possible cause of that arousal. Support for the expectancy–attribution model was found in a number of studies (e.g., Nisbett & Schachter, 1966; Fries & Frey, 1980; Olson & Ross, 1988; Olson, 1988).

This model follows along the lines of Schachter's (1964) basic assumption that attributions about the causes of symptoms can influence emotions. Thus, self-inference processes, in the form of attributions, can have quite an effect on the experience of emotions. What a person infers as the cause of his or her own behavior may very well not be the true cause. Moreover, the person's cognitions and causal judgments about his or her own behavior may be the same ones used to understand the behavior of others.

Andersen and Ross (1984) observed that in hypothetical situations, participants experienced their own thoughts and feelings (over a 1-day period) as more informative and prototypical of the "true self" than their behaviors (observed over a long period). Participants were in an interview situation that stressed the importance of either cognitive–affective information (thoughts and feelings) or behavioral information. Hidden observers were told to rate the interview for its informativeness, as were the speakers. There was a main effect of interview conditions. The cognitive–affective interview was chosen by both speakers and observers as being significantly more informative. Thus, thoughts and feelings were seen to be more diagnostic of a speaker's self than were reported behaviors.

So Andersen and Ross might say that self-knowledge is defined more by thoughts and feelings than by overt behaviors. In addition, Andersen (1984) found that what appeared to be a correspondence between the accuracy of self-assessments and social assessments when speakers revealed thoughts and feelings: "Observers who heard speakers describe their thoughts and feelings, rather than their behavior, made inferences about speakers that were more accurate, or at least, more in accord with speakers' self-assessments and the assessments made by their friends" (p. 304). It was postulated that the inaccessibility of cognitive–affective information may have an affect on people's perceptions of its informativeness. Expectations of how a certain person should act may also affect the informativeness of behavioral information, because one person cannot form very reliable expectations about another's thoughts and feelings. Andersen (1984) conducted a subsequent experiment to eliminate the expectancy effects that may have resulted from the direct observation of a speaker in the study by Andersen and Ross (1984). Andersen attempted to reduce certain other factors as well that may have affected the results of previous studies. There is always a mixture of cognitive–affective and behavioral information in the interview situation, regardless of the fact that one kind is stressed above the other (at least they were in the two experimental conditions). Thoughts and feelings very often do not relate to overt behaviors, and vice versa. The language people use to relate behavioral information is decidedly different (when they are free experimental language constraints) from the language they use to relate thoughts and feelings.

Andersen, Lazowski, and Donisi (1986) created a situation in which participants were given a set of sentences about religiousness, written in such a way as to accommodate either behavioral *or* cognitive–affective information. The statements were not generated by the subjects themselves, but were given to them, thus making the manipulation of conditions much more salient. What was the impact of these statements on each participant's self-inferences? Cognitive–affective statements about religiousness were found to have a greater effect on each participant's future self-inferences than were simple behavioral statements. It was concluded that the specific content of thoughts and feelings that are salient for an individual at a particular time can change the precise direction of subsequent judgments about the attribute in question—in this case, religiousness—with regard to the inner self.

Andersen et al. (1986) attempted to explain this phenomenon—in light of the fact that differences in abstractness and overall content (for the statements used) were controlled for—by pointing out that thoughts and feelings differ in two distinct ways from behaviors. First, they differ in what Andersen et al. call "observability," or their potential visibility to others. That is, behaviors are much less private than thoughts and feelings, and theoretically *should* have more of an impact. Though the vividness of behaviors was more apparent in this study, subjects found thoughts and feelings to be of greater impact on self-knowledge. Second, thoughts and feelings have a much more individuating effect on a person because of their "inner" origin. This finding is supported by past studies (e.g., Andersen, 1984).

Clinical-Psychological Theory on Knowledge of One's Emotions

The clinical literature suggests that people avoid awareness of many negative emotions in order to avoid the experience of pain. According to psychoanalytic theory, people learn to avoid experiencing painful affect, especially when such affect would overwhelm the sense of identity and coherence of the young child and lead to the disintegration of a stable sense of self. People are able to experience painful affect to the extent that they have learned to regulate it through the internalization of a self-regulating other (Stern, 1985; cf. Stolorow, Chapter Two, this volume).

Thus, recent developments in psychoanalytic theory and infant research provide a different perspective on how people come to know what they are feeling. According to the theory advanced by Stolorow and his associates (Stolorow, Brandchaft, & Atwood, 1987), the caretaker either validates the affective experiences of the child by his or her own emotional attunement or fails to do so. Such validation is necessary in order for early affective experiences to be integrated into the self-state. Stern (1985) has described how such attunement is more than simple imitation, matching, or even "mirroring," which suggests temporal synchrony. It differs from empathy in that these attunements occur largely out of awareness. Affective attunement shares with empathy the initial process of emotional resonance (Hoffman, 1978). According to Stern, however, in attunement the caretaker takes the experience of emotional resonance and engages in a variation of the infant's own behavior, which the infant recognizes as corresponding to his or her own original feeling experience.

In research by Stern, Hofer, Haft, and Dore (1985), most attunements occurred across sensory modes; were matched in intensity with the infant's behavior; and were engaged in by the mother for reasons such as being with the infant or sharing in the experience, as opposed to reasons such as responding to the infant, quieting the infant, reinforcing the behavior, restructuring the interaction, or playing a game. The attunements of the caretaker do not result in changes in the infant's behavior. Rather, mis-attunements are what result in some alteration or interruption of ongoing behavior. Research regarding the "still-face" procedure (Tronick, Als, Adamson, Wise, & Brazelton, 1978), in which the caretaker is requested to remain impassive and expressionless, indicates that infants react with mild upset or withdrawal from a behavior in such situations. When the mother is asked to overshoot or undershoot the pitch, contouring, rate, and stress patterning of her standard response, the infant takes notice and looks, as if for further clarification.

When there is attunement, the affect is effectively regulated. Developmentally, this means that when there is an optimum level of arousal, as has been described, the affect is matched by the caretaker. When the arousal becomes too great and is aversive, the caretaker reduces the stimulation or attempts to provide circumstances that will reduce the stimulation. When the arousal is insufficient, the caretaker stimulates the infant or provides stimulating circumstances. The caretaker thus attends to the feeling of the infant and neither neglects the affect nor impinges (Winnicott, 1965) upon him or her. When the affect receives no validation from the external world—that is, it is ignored in the presence of another, or is impinged upon by the other and thus broken off prematurely—it is not assimilated into the experiential representational system.

Affective regulation is initially learned by an internalization of the regulatory processes of a "self-regulating other." As the rational conceptual system develops, however, another possibility for affective regulation develops. The infant may have cognitions that are soothing, such as "Mother always comes eventually," or "I'm starving but I won't starve to death."

SELF-KNOWLEDGE IN PSYCHOANALYTIC AND EXPERIENTIAL PSYCHOTHERAPIES, EXISTENTIAL PHILOSOPHY, AND ZEN BUDDHISM: THE DISINTEGRATION OF THE SELF

Self-knowledge has traditionally been one of the goals of psychoanalytic and experiential psychotherapies, of existential philosophy and of various forms of Eastern religions. In Freudian psychoanalysis, self-knowledge is gained by making the unconscious conscious and by the coming together of the unconscious wish with cognitive awareness of behavior or affect in the present moment. In self psychology, the person becomes aware of his or her true self in an empathic atmosphere; similarly, in experiential psychotherapy, self-knowledge is gained by feeling previously avoided feelings. In existentially oriented psychoanalysis, the patient gains self-knowledge after facing the inherent meaningless of existence, accepting his or her mortality, experiencing anxiety, confronting nothingness, and making choices and commitments to create meaning in life.

When confronted with the terror of the meaninglessness of existence, unlike existential philosophers who ended up in *angst* and trembling (Kierkegaard, 1849; Sartre, 1956), the Buddhist masters suggest a dissolution of the distinction between the self and the nonself. They do not rationally comprehend nothingness, but instead value "no-thing-ness"—that is, their experience of the nonmaterial world. So long as science investigates only the material universe, we shall have very little scientific self-knowledge of any import. And so long as we persist in our valuing of the experiences of "the self" over the experiences of the nonself, we shall have very little wisdom.

Although psychoanalysts have largely kept themselves apart from the academic and scientific mainstream, insisting that the psychotherapy session is the only appropriate data base for their therapy, this argument has made no sense for psychoanalytic theories of development and personality. Hypotheses generated from the psychoanalytic theory of development have long been investigated by researchers (Minturn & Lambert, 1964; Whiting, 1963; Whiting & Child, 1953), and hypotheses generated from object relations theory have been tested from the outset by analysts trained as psychologists (Mahler, Pine, & Bergman, 1975). Research related to hypotheses generated from psychoanalytic psychotherapy is slowly making its way into the scientific mainstream (Strupp & Binder, 1985; Weiss, 1990; Weiss, Sampson, & the Mount Zion Psychotherapy Research Group, 1986). Recently, social psychologists such as Hazan and Shaver (1990) have begun to investigate people's theories of relationships, based upon assumptions from Bowlby's theories and (1969, 1973, 1980) observations regarding attachment. Cognitive and social psychologists have again started to consider unconscious processes (Bowers & Meichenbaum, 1984; Kihlstrom, 1987; Sherman, 1987) and uncontrollable thoughts (Uleman & Bargh, 1989; Wegner, 1989). The time is now ripe to consider not only cognitive information about the self, but also experiential information. Epstein discusses these two types of knowledge in greater detail in Chapter Seven of this volume, but regardless of whether his ideas about two separate knowledge systems are accepted, certainly all of us should be able to accept the supposition that we have many different types of information about ourselves, including our thoughts, feelings, and our behaviors. And scientific psychology, having focused upon the study of behavior and then cognition, has now turned to the investigation of affect (Clark, 1982).

At the same time, the end of the pursuit of happiness largely through materialism and technology, and a recognition of the limits of the powers of reason to bring fulfillment, may be in sight. In the Orient, where the problem of self seems to have emerged long before it did in the West, a resolution also appears to have been apparent for many centuries. This resolution is discussed more fully shortly. For now, let it suffice to say that englightenment is believed to be a fusion of two types of knowledge: that of skillful action, associated more with men, and that of insight, associated more with women. Two recent films emphasize the finding of fulfillment through the triumph of what Epstein has called the "experiential conceptual system" over the rational conceptual system. In *The Hunt for Red October,* viewers are dazzled by the display of modern technology that guides American and Russian submarines beneath the surface of the oceans, through the narrow canyons of towering cliffs in the water's secret depths. Recent advances in technology have made it possible for the Russians' latest nuclear submarine, the *Red October,* to navigate undetected by electronic sonar systems within miles of the U.S. mainland, making likely a devastating Russian pre-emptive strike upon our country. The world is saved, however, by insight—the insight of the *Red October*'s captain into the absurdity of the situation, which the American, Dr. Ryan, has detected during a conversation at a diplomatic dinner. Dr. Ryan suddenly realizes that the Russian captain is planning to defect to the United States. And thus the exciting adventure begins. Throughout the film, human insight triumphs over the nightmare made possible by advances in technology.

In *Field of Dreams,* a baseball movie, one wonders whether the filmmaker has read Julian Jaynes (1976). A voice actually speaks to the main character (played by Kevin Costner) on several occasions, relaying obscure messages like those of the Greek gods. "Build it and he will come" is the first of these communications. The voice is so real that Costner's character actually inquires of the locals whether they have heard voices in the cornfield. He then sees a vision of a baseball diamond in his cornfield and proceeds to build it, driving his family close to bankruptcy. Throughout the film is the message that attunement to the experiential self, not to reason, is what brings happiness.

The wisdom of the ancient civilizations of the Orient has always emphasized the necessity of the attunement to such nonrational information. In one of the first stories of the Jataka (Davids, 1929), entitled "The Sandy Road Jataka," the Bodhisat (an incarnation of the Buddha) is a caravan leader with 500 carts. Traveling only at night, the caravan eventually becomes lost in the desert and runs out of water. The travelers are on the verge of giving up all hope when the Bodhisat spots a patch of dabba grass and begins to dig in the sand. When the workers hit a rock and give up, the Bodhisat tells them to keep digging. A boy attendant continues to dig, and underneath the rock is a stream that spurts forth water as high as a palm tree. The travelers are saved by nonrational "knowledge."

THE MAGICAL APPLES OF THE HUMAN PSYCHE

Many years ago, one of us (Curtis) had a dream about magic apples. In the dream, Curtis was in a foreign country waiting for a parade to pass. Having arrived early for the parade, she decided to walk up the hill she noticed behind her. She was delighted to discover on her right, as she ascended the hill, an archeological dig containing a Roman temple. Curtis had seen a photograph of the temple in her tourist guide, but did not know where it was and had missed it in her sightseeing. She was very happy to find this important monument on this accidental excursion. Then she noticed some apples on the ground and, being hungry, began to eat one. After she had eaten the skin off from all around (as is her habit sometimes), she noticed that embedded in the apple on all sides in bas-relief was an indentation of the scenery in the physical environment to which that surface of the apple had been exposed as it grew—a sort of Borgesian Aleph (Borges, 1949). On one side were houses; on the other was the archeological dig containing the Roman temple. Curtis threw down the partially eaten apple and descended the hill. There she inquired about the apple among three women waiting for the parade, whom she had met before ascending the hill. One of the women suggested calling her anthropology teacher. The teacher said there were reports of these apples in the past, but no one had seen any of them in recent years. At this point, Curtis realized that the apple was more important and valuable than she had thought before, and ascended the hill to see whether she could find it again.

An inquiry into self-knowledge cannot be meaningful if it is only an investigation of intellectual knowledge, for the tree of knowledge bears "magical apples," apples being a symbol of the totality of human experience (Circlot, 1962, p. 14). Tasting these apples leads to the knowledge of good and evil; this is not simply cognitive knowledge, but also the experience of pain when our actions lead to suffering in others. Because these apples do contain a physicial representation of all that they have experienced, we are beginning to observe and measure the types of experiential knowledge that were previously thought to exist only in the province of the mystical—that is, in a province neither apparent to the senses nor obvious to the intelligence. Thus, science is on the verge of displacing magic in one more area.

Although the realm of the spiritual—that is, the nonmaterial world—has always seemed mysterious and magical, beyond the domain of testable hypotheses and verifiable general laws, the progress of science has been such that more and more of what seemed beyond prediction and control has become the subject of scientific investigation. With studies of empathy, of brain waves and blood pressure (Alexander, Langer, Newman, Chandler, & Davies, 1989) during meditation, and of physiological responses to revelations of distress in others, we believe that the scientific inquiry into the human spirit has begun. According to the *Compact Edition of the Oxford English Dictionary* (1971), the spiritual deals with the "incorporeal . . . essence" and the "higher moral qualities" (Vol. 2, p. 2968). With this study, psychology finally reclaims its name and its origins in the myth of Psyche.

According to the legend, Psyche, a mortal, is taken away by Cupid, a supernatural being whom she has never seen before. Psyche is transferred by the West Wind to a faraway palace in a hidden valley; there she married Cupid, but she is forbidden to look at him. One night in disobedience, Psyche lights a lantern as Cupid sleeps, so as to see her mysterious husband, but a drop of oil falls on Cupid. He awakes and leaves her. The separated lovers are reunited as a result of Psyche's performing a series of apparently impossible tasks. When Psyche at last opens a supposed casket of beauty that contains instead a deathly sleep, she is overcome. Then Cupid intervenes in person, wins the consent of Jupiter to the marriage, revives Psyche, and unites her to him. And within the year, Psyche gives birth to a beautiful baby girl named Bliss.

So, we hope, the reunion of scientific psychology, the study of the rational and the observable, with the study of the meanings people make of their existence (as revealed in the records of consulting rooms, religious experiences, literature, legends, etc.) will lead to fruition in the eventual lessening of human misery. These meanings are often irrational and certainly hard, but not impossible, to observe and measure. This reunion should give birth to the scientific study of those issues most important to the human psyche. With consciousness of our own consciousness comes the potential of knowing good from evil. This knowledge cannot remain simply an intellectual knowledge unrelated to our behavior.

We have already seen, tasted, and analyzed many "apples" grown in the gardens of our laboratories. Let us now seek out, taste, and analyze the "magical apples" grown in the gardens of the human spirit—that is, in our feelings and in our dreams. In the impressions embedded in these "magical apples," we may find the secrets of more meaningful forms of self-knowledge that inform and guide our behaviors toward one another.

As people acquire self-knowledge, both rationally and experientially, they should have little difficulty differentiating their own needs and goals from those of others, but we believe that they will come to value the dissolution of the distinction between self and nonself as the master teachers of the Orient derived this value. Research shows that as empathy increases, so does altruism. To the extent that people acquire self-knowledge, both rationally and experientially, they shall come to care for others as much as for themselves. When this happens, let us hope that thoughts, affects, and behaviors will be in synchrony; the "self" will cease to be a major focus of attention; people's psyches will be aware of more information; and their problem-solving capabilities can be more effectively concentrated upon the challenges of the world beyond their "selves."

REFERENCES

Alexander, C. N., Langer, E. J., Newman, R. I., Chandler, H. M., & Davis, J. L. (1989). Transcendental meditation, mindfulness, and longevity: An experimental study with the elderly. *Journal of Personality and Social Psychology, 57,* 950–964.

Andersen, S. M. (1984). Self-knowledge and social inference: II. The diagnosticity of cognitive/affective and behavioral data. *Journal of Personality and Social Pscyhology, 46,* 294–307.

Andersen, S. M., Lazowski, L. E., & Donisi, M. (1986). Salience and self-inference: The role of biased recollections in self-inference processes. *Social Cognition, 4,* 45–95.

Andersen, S. M., & Ross, L. (1984). Self-knowledge and social inference: The impact of cognitive/affective and behavioral data. *Journal of Personality and Social Psychology, 46,* 280–293.

Barnett, M. A. (1987). Empathy and related responses in children. In J. Eisenberg & J. Strayer (Eds.), *Empathy and its development* (pp. 146–162). New York: Cambridge University Press.

Batson, C. D., Fultz, J. , & Schoenrade, P. A. (1987). Adults' emotional reactions to the distress of others. In N. Eisenberg & J. Strayer (Eds.), *Empathy and its development* (pp. 163–184). New York: Cambridge University Press.

Baumeister, R. (1986). *Identity: Cultural change and the struggle for self.* New York: Oxford niversity Press.

Bem, D. (1967). Self-perception. An alternative interpretation of cognitive dissonance phenomena. *Psychological Review, 74,* 183–200.

Bem, D. (1972). Self-perception theory. In L. Berkowitz (Ed.), *Advances in experimental social psychology* (Vol. 6, pp. 1–62). New York: Academic Press.

Borges, J. L. (1949). The Aleph. In *The Aleph and other stories, 1933–1969* (N. T. di Giovanni, Trans.). New York: Dutton, 1970.

Bowers, K. S., & Meichenbaum, D. (Eds.). (1984). *The unconscious reconsidered.* New York: Wiley.

Bowlby, J. (1969). *Attachment and loss: Vol. 1. Attachment.* New York: Basic Books.

Bowlby, J. (1973). *Attachment and loss: Vol. 2. Separation, anxiety and anger.* New York: Basic Books.

Bowlby, J. (1980). *Attachment and loss: Vol. 3. Loss.* New York: Basic Books.

Bucci, W. (1985). Serial coding: A cognitive model for psychoanalytic research. *Journal of the American Psychoanalytic Association, 33,* 571–608.

Bucci, W. (1989). A reconstruction of Freud's tally argument: A program for psychoanalytic research. *Psychoanalytic Inquiry, 9,* 249–281.

Cantor, N., Markus, H., Niedenthal, P., & Nurius, P. (1986). On motivation and the self-concept. In R. M. Sorrentino & E. T. Higgins (Eds.), *Handbook of motivation and cognition: Foundations of social behavior* (Vol. 1, pp. 96–127). New York: Guilford Press.

Circlot, J. E. (1962). *A dictionary of symbols* (J. Sage, Trans.). New York: Philosophical Library.

Clark, M. S. (1982). A role for arousal in the link between feeling states, judgments, and behavior. In M. S. Clark & S. J. Fiske (Eds.), *Affect and cognition: The seventeenth annual Carnegie Symposium on Cognition* (pp. 263–289). Hillsdale, NJ: Erlbaum.

Compact edition of the Oxford English dictionary (2 vols.). (1971). New York: Oxford University Press.

Curtis, R. (1991). Towards an integrative theory of psychological change in individuals and organizations: A cognitive–affective regulation model. In R. Curtis & G. Stricker (Eds.), *How people change: Inside and outside therapy* (pp. 191–210). New York: Plenum.

Davids, C. A. F. R. (Ed. & Trans.). (1929). The sandy road Jataka. *In Stories of the Buddha: Being selections from the Jataka* (pp. 1–4). New York: Dover, 1989.

Duval, S., & Wicklund, R. A. (1972). *A theory of objective self-awareness.* New York: Academic Press.

Federoff, N. A., & Harvey, J. H. (1976). Focus of attention, self-esteem, and the attribution of causality. *Journal of Research in Personality, 10*(3), 336–345.

Feshbach, N. D. (1979). Empathy training: A field study in affective education. In S. Feshbach & A. Fraczek (Eds.), *Aggression and behavior change: Biological and social processes* (pp. 234–249). New York: Praeger.

Feshbach, N. D. (1982). Sex differences in empathy and social behavior in children. In N. Eisenberg (Ed.), *The development of prosocial behavior* (pp. 315–338). New York: Academic Press.

Fishbein, H. D., Lewis, S., & Keiffer, K. (1972). Children's understanding of spatial relations: Coordination of perspectives. *Developmental Psychology, 7*(1), 21–33.

Fries, A., & Frey, D. (1980). Misattribution of arousal and the effects of self-threatening information. *Journal of Experimental Social Psychology, 16*(5), 405–416.

Gallup, G. G., Jr. (1979). Self-recognition in chimpanzees and man: A developmental and comparative perspective. In M. Lewis & L. Rosenblum (Eds.), *Genesis of behavior: Vol. 2. The child and its family* (pp. 107–126). New York: Plenum.

Gallup, G. G., Jr. (1982). Self awareness and the emergence of mind in primates. *American Journal of Primatology, 2*(3), 237–248.

Gallup, G. G., Jr. (1983). Toward a comparative psychology of mind. In R. L. Mellgren (Ed.), *Animal cognition and behavior* (pp. 473–510). New York: North-Holland.

Gallup, G. G., Jr., & Suarez, S. D. (1985). Alternatives to the use of animals in psychology research. *American Psychologist, 40,* 1104–1111.

Gallup, G. G., Jr., & Suarez, S. D. (in press). Toward a comparative psychology of self-awareness: Species imitations and cognitive consequences. In J. Strauss & G. Goethals (Eds.), *The self: An interdisciplinary approach.* New York: Springer-Verlag.

Goldfried, M. (1991). Transtheoretical ingredients in therapeutic change. In R. C. Curtis & G. Stricker (Eds.), *How people change: Inside and outside therapy* (pp. 29–37). New York: Plenum.

Goleman, D. (1989). What is negative about positive illusions? When benefits for the individual harm the collective. *Journal of Social and Clinical Psychology, 8,* 190–197.

Greenwald, A. G., & Pratkanis, H. K. (1984). The self. In R. S. Wyer & T. K. Srull (Eds.), *Handbook of social cognition* (Vol. 3, pp. 129–178). Hillsdale, NJ: Erlbaum.

Hamlyn, D. W. (1977). Self-knowledge. In T. Mischel (Ed.), *The self: Psychological and philosophical issues* (pp. 170–200). Totowa, NJ: Rowman & Littlefield.

Hazan, C., & Shaver, P. R. (1990). Love and work: An attachment-theoretical perspective. *Journal of Personality and Social Psychology, 59,* 270–280.

Hoffman, M. L. (1978). Psychological and biological perspectives on altruism. *International Journal of Behavioral Development, 1*(4), 323–339.

Hull, J. G., & Levy, A. S. (1979). The organizational functions of the self: An alternative to the Duval and Wicklund model of self-awareness. *Journal of Personality and Social Psychology, 37,* 756–768.

Iannotti, R. J. (1978). Effect of role-taking experience on role taking, empathy, altruism, and aggression. *Developmental Psychology, 14,* 119–124.

Jaynes, J. (1976). *The origin of consciousness in the breakdown of the bicameral mind.* Boston: Houghton-Mifflin.

Jones, E. E., & Nisbett, R. E. (1971). *The actor and the observer: Divergent perceptions of the causes of behavior.* Morristown, NJ: General Learning Press.

Karniol, R. (1990). Transformation rule model for prediction. In M. P. Zanna (Ed.), *Advances in experimental social psychology* (Vol. 23, pp. 211–247). San Diego: Academic Press.

Kierkegaard, S. (1849). *Fear and trembling and the sickness unto death* (W. Lourie, Trans.). Garden City, NY: Doubleday, 1955.

Kihlstrom, J. (1987). The cognitive unconscious. *Science, 237,* 1445–1452.

Kuiper, N. A., MacDonald, M. R., & Derry, P. A. (1983). Parameters of a depressive self-schema. In J. Suls & A. G. Greenwald (Eds.), *Psychological perspectives on the self* (Vol. 2, pp. 191–217). Hillsdale, NJ: Erlbaum.

Leiman, B. (1978, August). *Affective empathy and subsequent altruism in kindergartners and first graders.* Paper presented at the annual meeting of the American Psychological Association, Toronto.

Lewis, M., & Brooks-Gunn, J. (1979). *Social cognition and the acquisition of self.* New York: Plenum.

Mahler, M., Pine, F., & Bergman, A. 91975). *The psychological birth of the human infant: Symbiosis and individuation.* New York: Basic Books.

Manion, A. P., & Curtis, R. C. (1989, August). *Seeking on avoiding diagnostic information: The function of performance expectations.* Paper presented at the annual meeting of the American Psychological Association, New Orleans.

Manion, A. P., Pacell, D., & Curtis, R. C. (1990). *Self-enhancement vs. self-assessment in task selection when failure is expected.* Paper presented at the annual meeting of the Eastern Psychological Association, Philadelphia.

Markus, H. (1977). Self-schemata and processing information about the self. *Journal of Personality and Social Psychology, 35,* 63–78.

Markus, H., & Smith, J. (1981). The influence of self-schemata on the perception of others. In N. Cantor & J. Kihlstrom (Eds.), *Personality, cognition, and social interaction* (pp. 233–262). Hillsdale, NJ: Erlbaum.

Martin, G. B., & Clark, R. D. (1982). Distress crying in neonates: Species and peer specificity. *Developmental Psychology, 18,* 3–9.

Masangkay, Z., McCluskey, K. A., McIntyen, C. W., Sims-Knight, J., Vaughn, B. E., & Flavell, J. H. (1974). The early development of inferences about the visual percepts of others. *Child Development, 45*(2), 357–366.

McGuire, W. J., & McGuire, C. V. (1988). Content and process in the experience of self. In L. Berkowitz (Ed.), *Advances in experimental social psychology* (Vol. 21, pp. 97–144). San Diego: Academic Press.

Minturn, L., & Lambert, W. W. (1964). *Mothers of six cultures: Antecedents of child rearing.* New York: Wiley.

Nisbett, R. E., & Schachter, S. (1966). Cognitive manipulation of pain. *Journal of Experimental Social Psychology, 54,* 758–767.

Nisbett, R. E., & Wilson, T. D. (1977). The halo effect: Evidence for unconscious alteration of judgments. *Journal of Personality and Social Psychology, 35*(4), 250–256.

Olson, J. M. (1988). Misattribution, preparatory information, and speech anxiety. *Journal of Personality and Social Psychology, 54,* 758–767.

Olson, J. M., & Ross, M. (1988). False feedback about placebo effectiveness: Consequences for the misattribution of speech anxiety. *Journal of Experimental Social Psychology, 24,* 275–91.

Paivio, A. (1971). *Imagery and verbal processes.* New York: Holt, Rinehart & Winston.

Paivio, A. (1978). A dual coding approach to perception and cognition. In H. C. Pick & E. Saltzman (Eds.), *Modes of perceiving and processing information* (pp. 39–51). Hillsdale, NJ: Erlbaum.

Paivio, A. (1986). *Mental representations: A dual coding approach.* New York: Oxford University Press.

Pennebaker, J. W. (1980). Self-perception of emotion and internal sensation. In D. M. Wegner & R. R. Vallacher (Eds.), *The self in social psychology* (pp. 80–101). New York: Oxford University Press.

Pennebaker, J. W. (1989a). Confession, inhibition and disease. In L. Berkowitz (Ed.), *Advances in experimental social psychology* (Vol. 22, pp. 211–244). New York: Academic Press.

Pennebaker, J. W. (1989b, October). *Confronting vs. confronted by upsetting experience: Health risks of providing social support.* Paper presented at the meeting of the Society for Experiemental Social Psychology, Santa Monica, CA.

Ross, M., & Olson, J. M. (1981). An expectancy attribution model of the effects of placebos. *Psychological Review, 88,* 408–437.

Ryle, G. (1949). *The concept of mind.* London: Hutchinson.

Sagi, A., & Hoffman, M. L. (1976). Empathic distress in newborns. *Developmental Psychology, 12,* 175–176.

Sartre, J. P. (1956). *Being and nothingness* (H. E. Barnes, Trans.). New York: Philosophical Library.

Schachter, S. (1964). The interaction of cognitive and psychiological determinants of emotion state. In L. Berkowitz (Ed.), *Advances in experimental social psychology* (Vol. 1, pp. 48–81). New York: Academic Press.

Scheier, M. F. (1976). Self-awareness, self-consciousness, and angry aggression.

Journal of Personality, 44, 627–644.

Scheier, M. F., & Carver, C. S. (1977). Self-focused attention and the experience of emotion: Attracting, repulsion, elation, and depression. *Journal of Personality and Social Psychology, 35,* 624–636.

Sherman, S. J. (1987). Cognitive processes in the formation, change and expression of attitudes. In M. D. Zanna, J. M. Olson, & C. P. Herman (Eds.), *Social influence: The Ontario Symposium* (Vol. 5, pp. 75–106). Hillsdale, NJ: Erlbaum.

Simner, M. L. (1971). Newborn's response to the cry of another infant. *Developmental Psychology, 5,* 136–150.

Snyder, M. (1979). Self-monitoring processes. In L. Berkowitz (Ed.), *Advances in experimental social psychology* (Vol. 12, pp. 85–128). New York: Academic Press.

Snyder, M. (1987). *Public appearances, private realities: The psychology of self-monitoring.* San Francisco: W. H. Freeman.

Snyder, M., & Cantor, N. (1980). Thinking about ourselves and others: Self-monitoring and social knowledge. *Journal of Personality and Social Psychology, 39,* 222–234.

Snyder, M., & Kendzierski, D. (1982). Acting on one's attitudes: Procedures for linking attitudes and behavior. *Journal of Experimental Social Psychology, 18,* 165–183.

Sorrentino, R. M., & Hewitt, E. (1984). The uncertainty reduction properties of achievement tasks revisted. *Journal of Personality and Social Psychology, 47*(4), 884–899.

Staub, E. (1971). The use of role-playing and reduction in children's learning of helping and sharing behavior. *Child Development, 42,* 805–816.

Stern, D. N. 91985). *The interpersonal world of the infant.* New York: Basic Books.

Stern, D. N., Hofer, L., Haft, W., & Dore, J. (1985). Affect attunement: The sharing of feeling states between mother and infant by means of inter-model fluency. In T. Field & N. Fox (Eds.), *Social perception in infants* (pp. 249–268). Norwood, NJ: Ablex.

Stoetzel, J. (1963). *La psychologie sociale.* Paris: Flammarion.

Stolorow, R., Brandchaft, B., & Atwood, G. (1987). *Psychoanalytic treatment: An intersubjective approach.* Hillsdale, NJ: Erlbaum.

Strupp, H. H., & Binder, J. (1985). *Psychotherapy in a new key: A guide to time-limited dynamic psychotherapy.* New York: Basic Books.

Sullivan, H. S. (1953). *An interpersonal theory of psychiatry.* New York: Norton.

Swann, W. B., Jr. (1990). To be adored or to be known? The interplay of self-enhancement and self-verification. In R. M. Sorrentino & E. T. Higgins (Eds.), *Handbook of motivation and cognition: Foundations of social behavior* (Vol. 2, pp. 408–448). New York: Guilford Press.

Swann, W. B., Jr., Griffin, J. J., Predmore, S., & Gaines, B. (1987). The cognitive–affective crossfire: When self-consistency confronts self-enhancement. *Journal of Personality and Social Psychology, 52,* 881–889.

Swann, W. B., Jr., Pelham, B. W., & Krull, D. S. (1989). Agreeable fancy or disagreeable truth? Reconciling self-enhancement and self-verification. *Journal of Personality and Social Psychology, 57,* 782–791.

Taylor, S. E. (1989). *Positive illusions: Creative self-deception and the healthy mind.* New York: Basic Books.

Taylor, S. E., & Brown, J. (1988). Illusion and well-being: A social psychological perspective on mental health. *Psychological Bulletin, 103,* 193–210.

Tronick, E., Als, H., Adamson, L., Wise, S., & Brazelton, T. B. (1978). The infant's response to entrapment between contradictory messages in face-to-face interaction. *Journal of Child Psychiatry, 17,* 1–13.

Trope, Y. (1980). Self-assessment, self-enhancement and task preferences. *Journal of Experimental Social Psychology, 16,* 116–129.

Trope, Y. (1982). Self-assessment and task performance. *Journal of Experimental Social Psychology, 18*(2), 201–215.

Uleman, J. S., & Bargh, J. A. (Eds.). (1989). *Unintended thought.* New York: Guilford Press.

Wegner, D. (1989, October). *The suppression of exciting thoughts.* Paper presented at the meeting of the Society for Experimental Social Psychology, Santa Monica, CA.

Weinberger, J., & McClelland, D. (1990). Cognitive versus traditional motivational models: Irreconcilable or complementary? In E. T. Higgins & R. M. Sorrentino (Eds.), *Handbook of motivation and cognition: Foundations of social behavior* (Vol. 2, pp. 562–597). New York: Guilford Press.

Weiss, J. (1990). Unconscious mental functioning. *Scientific American, 261,* 103–109.

Weiss, J., Sampson, H., & the Mount Zion Psychotherapy Research Group. (1986). *The psychoanalytic process: Theory, clinical observations, and empirical research.* New York: Guilford Press.

Westen, D. (1985). *Self and society.* Cambridge, England: Cambridge University Press.

Whiting, B. (Ed.). (1963). *Six cultures—studies of child rearing.* New York: Wiley.

Whiting, J. W. M., & Child, K. L. (1953). *Child training and personality.* New Haven, CT: Yale University Press.

Wicklund, R. A. (1975). Discrepancy reduction or attempted destruction? A reply to Liebling, Seiber, and Shaver. *Journal of Experimental Social Psychology, 11*(1), 78–81.

Wicklund, R. A. (1978). Objective self-awareness: Three years later. In L. Berkowitz (Ed.), *Cognitive theories in social psychology* (pp. 509–521). New York: Academic Press.

Winnicott, D. W. (1965). *The maturational process and the facilitating environment.* New York: International Universities Press.

CHAPTER NINE

The Self in Cross-Civilizational Perspective: An Indian–Japanese–American Comparison

ALAN ROLAND

COMPARATIVE CONCEPTUALIZATIONS OF THE SELF

Once a psychoanalyst departs from Western shores to journey into the psyche of persons from other civilizations, such as India and Japan, a whole new comparative perspective arises that sheds quite different light on the nature and makeup of the self. Not only do the basic notions and assumptions regarding human nature and reality differ radically between civilizations—as do the flora and fauna of social patterns, symbolic codes and value systems, and child rearing—but the self also varies radically with the civilization. And this is true not only of indigenous cultural concepts of the self (Hallowell, 1955), which are often profoundly internalized into the psyche and influence behavior, but also of the observable manifestations of the self that emerge in the clinical psychoanalytic relationship.

From clinical psychoanalytic work in India and Japan, and with Indians and Japanese in New York City, I have formulated four different overarching conceptualizations of the self, all relevant to viewing the self from this comparative cross-civilizational perspective. I discuss these far more extensively in *In Search of Self in India and Japan: Toward a Cross-Cultural Psychology* (Roland, 1988), but need to give a sense of them here in abbreviated form. The first two emerge completely from a comparative perspective: the "familial self" of Indians, Japanese, and other Asians versus the "individualized self" of Westerners. I view the familial and individualized selves as supraordinate organizations of the self with a number of suborganizations. This theoretical perspective on the self relates to the work of Hartmann (1939), later developed in more sophisticated fashion by both Erikson (1963) and Lichtenstein (1977) in their work on identity, and elaborated still more in terms of suborganizations of the self by Klein (1976) and Gedo (Gedo & Goldberg, 1973; Gedo, 1979, 1981).

Still other psychoanalytic perspectives on the self have been extremely useful in formulating the familial and individualized selves, such as object relations theory and self psychology. In the former, social relationships and cultural symbols are filtered through and internalized into the psyche in affect-laden inner images of self and other(s) in complex interrelationships (Grinker, 1957; Jacobson, 1964; Kahn, 1974; Kernberg, 1975; Segal, 1964; Winnicott, 1965). The self is also related to issues of authenticity in terms of Winnicott's (1960) "true self" and "false self," and to related concepts of Kohut (1980), Loewald (1960), and Menaker and Menaker (1965).

In self psychology (Kohut, 1971, 1977), bipolar internalization processes involving empathic mirroring and idealization are intrinsically related to issues of self-regard and self-cohesiveness. Also relevant is Rank's notion of the self as encompassing individuation, will, and self-creation (Menaker, 1982). Naturally, the developmental models intrinsic to both object relations theory and self psychology also enter into my theorizing on the familial and individualized selves.

In this comparative civilizational perspective, the intrapsychic make-ups of the familial and individualized selves are profoundly interrelated with the emotional patterning of interpersonal relationships as they vary across civilizations. This calls for seeing the self in terms of social roles, presentations, and modes of communication (Goffman, 1959; LeVine, 1982; Parsons, 1964); taking into account those aspects of the self directly and consciously related to differing patterns of interpersonal relationships; and then seeing how this more socially related self enters into the configurations of the familial and individualized selves. I elaborate on the public and private selves of Indians and Japanese, both of which are deeply internalized into their familial selves. I particularly focus on how the familial selves of Indians and Japanese are rooted in the psychosocial dimensions of family and group hierarchical intimacy relationships, by contrast with the individualized self as it relates to social patterns based more on the egalitarian/contractual relationships of Western individualism.

I do, of course, duly note that the familial self of Asians varies significantly between different Asian societies such as India and Japan, while nevertheless maintaining a commonality when compared to the Western individualized self. Thus, I speak of the "familial–communal self" of Indians, which is primarily related to family and secondarily to community or caste (*jati*); and of the "familial–group self" of Japanese, which again is primarily related to family and secondarily to the varied groups run on familial principles of which Japanese tend to be long-term members. Similarly, the Western individualized self will vary from one Western culture to another—sometimes significantly, when one compares persons from Mediterranean cultures with those from northern European cultures—but the individualized self still maintains its commonality of structures across Western societies.

The third overarching conceptualization is that of the "spiritual self," a formulation that is completely denigrated in Freudian psychoanalysis, where it is relegated to regression to symbiotic modes of merger in early childhood or to psychopathology of one variety or another (Masson, 1976, 1980). However, the spiritual self is recognized to a somewhat greater extent by neo-Freudian psychoanalysts such as Karen Horney and Erich Fromm (Fromm & Suzuki, 1970); by Jung and many of his followers; and by English object relations theorists Wilfred Bion, Marjorie Brierley, and Marion Milner (Milner, 1973). Here I rely on a more Hindu conceptualization of the self—one that distinguishes between the finite self (*jiva*), which encompasses both the familial and individualized selves, and the infinite self (*Atman*)—with highly differing experiential components of consciousness and being in each (Bon Maharaj, 1963).

The cultural notion of the spiritual self is deeply ingrained in the preconscious of almost all Indians I have worked with, in a way that is simply not the case with most Americans today. Indian culture assumes a psychological process of self-transformation from grosser to more refined inner qualities. This does not mean that all Indians are involved in realizing the spiritual self, but they all assume that it can be tried. Spiritual disciplines and practices may vary considerably from one culture to another: In India there is an emphasis on different modes of yoga, whereas in Japan aesthetic disciplines tend to be more used (e.g., calligraphy, flower arranging, the tea ceremony, etc.).

The nature of the means of realizing the spiritual self will depend considerably on the makeup of the phenomenological self, whether familial or individualized; the person's own inner makeup; and the kinds of practices available in a particular culture. Thus, the spiritual self may be integrated in an entirely different way with a familial self than with an individualized one. As an instance, one popular spiritual discipline in India today is that of *bhakti*—devotional workship of Krishna, an incarnation of God, in which a man may sometimes take the role of Radha, a great female devotee of Krishna. *Bhakti* thus draws upon the much stronger maternal/feminine component in the makeup of an Indian man's self than is generally present in a Western man. Such a devotional approach would be unheard of in the West.

The fourth overarching conceptualization of the self is that of an "expanding self," to take into account how sociohistorical change profoundly affects the self, resulting in new integrations with not infrequent anxiety and inner conflict. Social change generating an expanding self can be affected from within a culture; an example of this would be the change resulting from the women's movement in the United States, where women have begun integrating traditional roles with new opportunities in careers and changing marital relationships over the last three decades. Or such sociohistorical change may be generated from contact with different civilizations, such as the British colonial occupation of India for two centuries and the American post-World War II Occupation of Japan. In these two instances, forces of Westernization/modernization were unleashed that have not only profoundly affected Indian and Japanese societies, but have also resulted in the new integrations of an expanding self, with painful conflict at times. In turn, as the result of a large influx of Eastern spiritual teachers into the United States over the last few decades—including Tibetan Buddhist lamas, Zen Buddhist masters, Sufi Pirs, Hindu gurus, and Burmese Buddhist monks—the individualized selves of some Americans have expanded to integrate a new psychological mode of functioning.

An expanding or bicultural self can be easily observed among Asians who have immigrated to the United States, or who have stayed here for prolonged periods. As they encounter a life style based on a value system, social patterns, and inner psychological makeup that is at times opposite to their own, considerable anguish and conflict frequently result. They gradually internalize the more individualized modes of functioning in American life while retaining basic facets of their own familial self, resulting in a new integration of a bicultural or expanding self.

What I would like to stress is that these four conceptualizations of the self resulting from a cross-civilizational perspective are not simply hypothetical, abstract constructs. Rather, they enter directly into psychoanalytic clinical work in terms of theory of personality and psychodynamics; in awareness of the influence of different developmental norms and modes; and in the nature of the psychoanalytic relationship, resistances, transferences, and countertransference. I have found that I can relevantly use all of the psychoanalytic categories of personality and of technique with Indians and Japanese, but I must first de-Westernize the content of each category as it is now elaborated in psychoanalytic theory, and recontextualize the content with the clinical data of Indians and Japanese. The same, of course, would be true of other Asians. As I elaborate different major dimensions of the Indian and Japanese familial, spiritual, and expanding selves, I cite clinical examples to illustrate them.

PSYCHOSOCIAL DIMENSIONS OF HIERARCHICAL RELATIONSHIPS

It is impossible to delve meaningfully into the various suborganizations of the familial self without first briefly describing the psychosocial dimensions of Indian and Japanese family and group hierarchical relationships in which the familial self is integrally related. Although these psychosocial dimensions vary across Asian cultures, they also assume a remarkable commonality (see Roland, 1988, for a fuller description).

There is first the "structural hierarchy" described at length by anthropologists, in which the formal social etiquette is observed by subordinate and superior (much more strictly in Japan than in India), and in which culturally spelled out reciprocal obligations and responsibilities of subordinate and superior toward each other are deeply internalized. Subordinates are to be loyal, deferent, and receptive to superiors, while the latter are to be nurturing and responsible to the former. In the second psychosocial dimension, "hierarchy by quality of the person," distinctions are quietly made between those who are in a formal superior position and those who are indeed superior persons, who may or may not be in a superior position. Thus, a husband is always a superior to a wife and must be deferred to, but she may at times be more respected as the superior person; this may be the case, too, between the oldest and younger brothers in a family. In hierarchy by quality, deference becomes transformed into respect and veneration. Aspects of structural hierarchy and hierarchy by quality of the person are central to understanding the mirroring and idealization processes of self psychology, as these are played out in Indian and Japanese social relationships in far more dominant modes than in the West.

The "qualitative mode of hierarchical relationships" highlights the intense intimacy relationships, the close emotional connectedness, and the stress on dependency and interdependence that have been elaborated in various ways by the anthropologist Frances F. L. K. Hsu (1971), and the psychoanalysts Takeo Doi (1973) and Sudhir Kakar (1978). This psychosocial dimension also emphasizes development of the capability for strong empathic resonance to others' feelings, moods, and wishes, and particularly to the nonverbal communication that is rife in Asian social interaction. A Chinese psychologist, for instance, confirmed that among the women of the extended family there are well over 100 different kinds of communicative silences. This was mentioned in response to an American writer, who observed in her husband's South Indian family that she could note down over 60 different kinds of silences that were operative.

It is the interaction of these three psychosocial dimensions of hierarchical relationships that results in the enormous subtlety of Asian relationships and communication. Thus, the formal social etiquette of the structural hierarchy is almost always observed, but gestures and actions may well communicate what the person is really feeling. Families and groups will always have superiors to be deferred to, but others may be looked up to as superior persons—sometimes a servant, younger brother, wife, or daughter-in-law. Or a relationship may change over the years from one based primarily on the structural hierarchy to being infused with the qualitative mode of intimacy, such as is common in mother-in-law–daughter-in-law relationships.

SUBORGANIZATIONS OF THE FAMILIAL SELF

Symbiosis–Reciprocity

The first suborganization of the familial self is what I have termed "symbiosis–reciprocity"—in contrast to separation–individuation—to deal with psychological realities that are simply not present to any significant degree in Western personality. This suborganization encompasses experiential and affective components of the self that are profoundly interrelated with the qualitative mode of hierarchical intimacy relationships.

First and foremost, self-experience is that of a we-self in contrast to the highly individualistic I-self of Westerners that forms a dualistic relationship between "I" and "you." The we-self always takes into account the other(s) in hierarchical relationships, and is profoundly identified with the family, community (*jati*), and work group. Moreover, the self is experienced not so much as an integrated identity that is relatively consistent with various others, as in the Western self, but is much more relational and varying according to the relationship. As an Indian woman artist put it, "Americans seem to have to be one thing. I and my Indian friends are able to be many different kinds of persons in different situations. I feel very comfortable slipping back and forth from being a professor to being a painter to being a mother and wife . . . I don't have to be one set self or have a single identity. In fact I avoid like the plague having a set identity." Thus, the Asian relational self is somewhat similar to the "relational morality" of Gilligan's (1982) and Bernstein's (1983) work on women, but is more accentuated for both men and women.

As another facet of symbiosis–reciprocity, ego boundaries are significantly differently constituted than in Western personality. Three ego boundaries must be taken into account to understand the familial self of Indians and Japanese, rather than the two described by Federn (1952). Outer ego boundaries between self and other(s) are far more permeable in Asians, with continuous affective exchanges and often warmly nurturing attitudes. Japanese generally seem to have vaguer outer boundaries than Indians, with more merger with others in the close family and group relationships. On the other hand, the innermost ego boundary between self and inner feelings, fantasies, and impulses differs considerably between Indians and Japanese. My impression is that Japanese are significantly less in touch with their inner world than Indians because of a much stricter conscience and observance of the formal social etiquette. Except in the area of anger and aggression, Indian patients seem more in touch with their inner world of feelings and fantasies than most of my American patients from a variety of ethnic backgrounds.

What distinguishes Asians from Westerners most strikingly in regard to ego boundaries is not only the more permeable outer boundary, but another inner boundary, which maintains a highly private self and inner psychological space that contains a variety of fantasies, thoughts, feelings, and such. This inner boundary is developed from early childhood to maintain a sense of inner privacy and individuality in an environment where there is little social privacy and the person is always closely emotionally enmeshed with others. An internationally noted Indian mathematician wrote two-thirds of his 120 published papers with children playing around him in the same room (A. K. Ramanujan, personal communication, 1980). In contemporary Western personality, where there is far more psychological space around oneself and one develops as a relatively autonomous monad with a variety of relationships and self-objects in the social world, there is far less need for such a well-developed private self.

In a "we-self" with more permeable outer ego boundaries, the inner representational world is also different from the individualized self of Westerners. There is far less separation of inner representations of self and other. Thus, self- and object-representations are in closer proximity in the familial self, and are more suffused with affect. Some Indian analysts I know were considering starting a journal called *The Feeling Mind,* a title that would be quite alien to Western analysts.

Dependence and interdependence are strongly fostered in all Asian societies. Children sleep next to their mothers until the next sibling is born, and then always sleep with another family member for a number of years; the youngest child may well sleep next to the mother until adolescence, as a couple of my Indian patients have done. There is a relative discouragement of separation: Indian and Japanese mothers tend to be more involved with their children when possible, giving a much greater degree of gratification and less frustration than would meet the current psychoanalytic norms of optimal frustration. Symbiotic modes of relating, dependence, and interdependence are present throughout life; this fact is the focus of Takeo Doi's (1973) *Anatomy of Dependence.* In Asian child rearing, individuation is fostered without the kinds of separation, autonomy, and limit setting that are the hallmarks and norms of current psychoanalytic developmental ego psychology.

It is within these highly interdependent hierarchical relationships that strong empathic capacities are fostered, including remarkable attunement to nonverbal communication. In fact, it is often considered crass or insulting to verbalize what one senses about another person, since the other senses that one knows. A Chinese psychologist reported that a teenage boy flew into a rage at her in a session because she verbalized what he sensed she knew; he considered her verbalizing it an insult and a denigration of him. In Japan there is a saying that nothing important should ever be communicated by words. Attitudes for receptiveness are cultivated much more than attitudes for assertiveness and mastery, which are cultivated in American children.

The last facet of symbiosis–reciprocity is a stronger wishing/wanting self—and, in the case of Indians, a libidinal/sensuous self—than is characteristic of most American patients I have had. This is manifested, however, in very different ways in Japanese and Indians. The former may only become aware of their strong needs and wants when a superior upon whom they are totally dependent and whom they count on to sense and fulfill their needs does not come through (Y. Idei, personal communication, 1982). Moreover, Japanese are highly restrained in their asking in relationships with outsiders, only confining it to intimate ones with insiders. By contrast, Indians are constantly asking and maneuvering in both insider and outsider relationships for what they want, being involved in a far greater degree of giving and asking than is characteristic of most Americans. Indians are constantly searching for a high level of exchange in intimacy relationships, and for a testing of intimacy in outsider relationships. Moreover, there is a strong cultivation of the sensual, which is contained in highly socially circumscribed behavior both within and outside the extended family.

Symbiosis–Reciprocity in Psychoanalytic Therapy

How do the various components of symbiosis–reciprocity manifest in the psychoanalytic relationship and in therapy? There are a variety of ways. First and foremost, Indians and Japanese (and, I would expect, other Asians as well) expect a far greater degree of emotional relatedness, involvement, and caretaking than is characteristic of most American patients I have seen. They expect a warmly nurturing relationship in which a "we-ness" is formed, where they can be fully dependent on the analyst to take care of them. In Japan, the expectation is for life. Japanese men relate to the analyst as a mentor or teacher in actuality, as a model superior from an extrafamilial group, above and beyond whatever other transferences there are (Taketomo, 1989). By contrast, Indians relate to the analyst as a kind of extended family elder to make up for what was missing in their families (Ramanujam, 1980). Both will tend to ask the analyst for all kinds of advice and guidance on everyday affairs, as they would a family elder or mentor. In turn, any anger or ambivalence toward the analyst is deeply inhibited, as it is toward other superiors in a direct relationship, so as not to interfere with the ambience of a warmly nurturing relationship and to risk abandonment. However, anger toward other superiors who have let them down in one way or another is usually vociferously expressed in session.

Naturally, the desire to be guided and given advice has to be handled tactfully, to enable the patients to begin delving into their minds and begin uncovering hidden patterns and motivations. I may convey that they have already been given reams of advice on their problems by concerned family members and others, but to no avail. Therefore, mutual exploration through the patients' saying what is on their minds will lead us in a better way to the sources of their problems and conflicts and to the resoltuion of these.

The private self plays a major role in psychoanalytic therapy, but in different ways with Indians and Japanese. I have found that once confidentiality is firmly established with Indian patients, and they sense the therapist is receptive and accepting of their problems, all kinds of feelings and fantasies will come pouring forth—more quickly than with most of my American patients. Indians tend to be very much in touch with their inner world. However, I have also seen Indian patients keep secrets for far longer periods of time than American patients. For example, Shakuntala, who was in therapy for over a year and a half with a psychoanalytic therapist in Bombay, kept the two most important inner struggles of her life from her therapist: (1) whether to continue a passionate love affair with a married man or to agree to an arranged marriage: and (2) whether to renounce all social life and go to her aunt's ashram to be groomed as a guru to succeed her aunt, as Shakuntala was deeply involved in meditation and spiritual experiences. She felt, and probably rightly so, that her first therapist would not be particularly receptive to either of these conflicts (see Roland, 1988, pp. 154–174). I have not seen any American patients who could keep their most central inner struggles completely out of an analysis for such a prolonged period of time.

A Japanese patient, on the other hand, expects an analyst to sense what is going on in his or her private self with a minimum of verbal and nonverbal communication, and to do this without actively inquiring or investigating. For the therapist to ask questions of the patient is considered to be intrusive at best and insulting at worst (M. Tatara, personal communication, 1981). The private self is simply not to be intruded upon in Japanese relationships, because it is an inner sanctum of individuality that often can only be minimally expressed in the rigorously observed social etiquette and obligations of hierarchical relationships. Traditional Japanese, in contrast to younger generations, tend to communicate what is in their private selves much more by innuendo; only at much later stages of the therapy do they become more open, as the analyst is only gradually transformed from an outsider to an insider on the basis of his or her sensitivity and concern. In turn, psychoanalytic therapy with more traditional Japanese patients takes place with a minimum of interpretation. The therapist similarly expects the patient to sense what is going on in the therapist's mind to an extent that is mind-boggling for Westeners.

In Hiroshima, I supervised a case of a woman who was seen in once-a-week psychoanalytic therapy for over a year and a half by Yoshiko Idei, an analyst trained at the William Alanson White Institute. It was patently clear to me from the process notes that enormous changes took place—changes that could easily be understood psychodynamically—but there were only a couple of interpretations during the entire period of therapy (see Roland, 1988, pp. 186–194). I subsequently learned that this is not unusual in Japanese psychoanalytic work with patients from more traditional backgrounds; in the homogeneity of Japanese society, each quickly senses what is on the other's mind. In the urban areas among the younger generations, there is a tendency to become much more verbally expressive—a result of the American Occupation and a gradual inculcation of Western norms and modes of functioning.

I have found in working with Japanese patients that it is important to empathize first with the pain, anxiety, or upset they are going through before making any connections or giving any interpretations. It is always important for them to experience the warmly nurturing relationship. Otherwise, the analyst is experienced as cold and critical.

We-Self Regard

Another major suborganization of the familial self involves "we-self regard." One cannot really speak of "self-regard" in Indians, Japanese, and other Asians because the experiential structure of the self-revolves around we-ness, and therefore issues of esteem are experienced in terms of a we-self. Self-regard is a more individualistic experience of Westerners.

We-self regard in Asians revolves a great deal around the reputation of the family, the community (caste) in India, and the work group in Japan. One is constantly sensitive as to how one's behavior reflects on the group, and in turn how other members also influence the family's and the group's reputation. We-self regard is also profoundly tied into hierarchical relationships, where both subordinate and superior reflect on each other.

One Indian patient, Ashis, kept his father's suicide secret from the most intimate of friends because of how it would reflect on himself; he quickly terminated therapy with me the first time I saw him, as soon as this secret surfaced through a dream (see Roland, 1988, pp. 25–47). Another Indian patient, Sunil, was in an unresolvable dilemma over issues of we-self regard and family reputation. He had come to the United States after doing only moderately well in college in India and not being able to get a job. He was sponsored by relatives who then thoroughly exploited him in their business, Sunil being unable to leave them because of his visa. To escape their exploitation, he married an American woman who was divorced and had a child. He was then free to open his own business, at which he did extremely well, sending considerable sums of money home. This not only raised his esteem in his family's eyes, but also reflected very well on them as having a son who had made good in America. On the other hand, marrying a divorced woman with a child was a serious blot on the family reputation. He was torn between staying with her as the one who had helped him make good and raise the esteem of his family, and separating from her as the divorced woman who was tarnishing his family's reputation—his own sense of esteem being profoundly identified with the family reputation.

The nature of self–selfobject relationships is of a significantly different order in both Indians and Japanese than in Westerners. Both mirroring and idealization processes are considerably more intense and pervasive than is characteristic of American life. Mirroring processes go on all the time in nonverbal gestures in structural hierarchical relationships, as superiors and subordinates in the family and group fulfill their reciprocal responsibilities and the complex social etiquette. This same nonverbal mirroring takes place in Asian child rearing to a considerable extent, and (as I have alluded to above) it is an integral part of the psychoanalytic relationship, especially with traditional Japanese.

The issue of maintaining high levels of we-self esteem is central to all Asians and is often spoken about in a more popular manner as "maintaining face." Cultural values and social patterns strongly support the bipolar internalization process of mirroring and idealizing self–selfobject relationships. Empathic attunement to others is universally emphasized in Asian societies, if not always observed; cultural attitudes constantly support idealization of elders and superiors throughout life, including mythic figures and the gods and goddesses.

Not only are levels of empathic resonance different in Asian societies from the West, but also what is empathized with differs. In Asian cultures, feelings of dependency, esteem, moods and feelings, wishes, and needs are empathically sensed—but not particularly any strivings to be more independent, assertive, or autonomous. These latter, on the other hand, are just what are most empathized with in American child rearing. Thus, Asians who immigrate to America often find the very values and modes of functioning to be vastly different and conflictual.

In Indian child rearing there are specific cultural injunctions against verbal praise. Praise of one's child is considered to be highly immodest, since the we-self includes the mother–child dyad. Furthermore, openly praising one's child can evoke the evil eye, or the envy of the other women of the extended family, which can then have untoward effects on the child. Moreover, culturally speaking, one does not want to have the child to have any inflated sense of oneself, since such egotism (*ahamkara*) distracts from knowing the true self or spirit (*Atman*). Nevertheless, through facial gestures of the adults, children well know when they are being warmly approved of.

If mirroring is the main self–selfobject relationship in structural hierarchical relationships, then idealizations taking the form of deep respect or veneration are central to hierarchy by quality of the person. Here, a subordinate who venerates superiors tries to get as close as possible to such superiors, to be like them or share in their respected qualities, and thus to become inwardly transformed into a more spiritual person with finer qualities—the ultimate psychological goal of Asian cultures. In India, just to share in the presence of a spiritual person, often silently, is called *darshan*.

In Japan, such idealizations, usually spoken of in terms of being with and becoming a mature, wise person, can be fraught with two difficulties. First, a culture where outer ego boundaries between self and other(s) can be rather vague, there is the threat of losing one's identity with the idealized person. Second, where hierarchical relationships (beginning with the mother–child dyad) involve very high levels of expectations for performance from the superior, being close to the idealized other may leave one feeling vulnerable to the other's expectations and evaluations.

In the psychoanalytic relationship, Japanese patients, especially men, tend to look to the analyst as a supportive teacher or mentor (Taketomo, 1989); as noted earlier, regardless of other transferences, this one will last throughout life. One analyst in Japan had a photograph of his own analyst enshrined in a sacred niche in his home. Americans, of course, may have a photograph or bust of Freud or an idealized founding father or mother of their institute, but not (so far to my knowledge) of their own analyst. In any case, both Indians and Japanese will expect the basic relationship with the analyst to last well beyond the analytic treatment.

The father–son relationship in both cultures, but more clearly evident in India, involves an extremely subtle reciprocal self–selfobject relationship. The father is the emotionally distant authoritative figure who gives structure and family leadership, in contrast to the mother's more symbiotic relationship with both boys and girls; however, he usually has an emotional tie that is much more covert with his sons and somewhat more open with his daughters. As a result, Indian sons, no matter what their age, strive to do well to gain their father's respect as well as to reflect well on their fathers, the father's esteem being very dependent on the sons. Older brothers are also deeply respected and deferred to by younger brothers. All elders are seen as being kinds of gods, or more accurately as partial manifestations of the gods and goddesses, since Indian metonymic thinking always allows for transcendent figures to have partial manifestations in the natural world. When fathers or older brothers are seriously deficient, the disillusionment can be very painful to sons and daughters, and to sisters and younger brothers. This was not only manifested in Ashis's response to his father's suicide (see above) but also in women patients who felt their older brothers had seriously let them down (Roland, 1988). In still another case, there was profound disillusionment with older brothers when the younger one began to see their problems and to realize that they were unable to guide him properly.

There is still another important, highly subtle issue in the intertwining of selfobject and dependency relationships in Indian and Japanese social interaction, and this too is frequently difficult for a Westerner to comprehend. In hierarchical relationships, a subordinate's asking and dependency actually constitute a form of giving to the superior. The superior is acknowledged as one who can give, and his or her esteem is further enhanced as he or she lives up to the ego-ideal of nurturing subordinates (M. Burg, personal communication, 1978; B. K. Ramanujam, personal communication, 1979). Americans often react negatively to the asking of Indians, experiencing it as an infringement on their autonomy rather than as a seeking of intimacy through exchanges of dependency and esteem.

This dynamic emerged in the case data of a Japanese man who was bitter at his stepfather for not sufficiently recognizing his contributions to the family business. He took out his anger at his stepfather by not requesting the kinds of expensive appliances that his brothers and sisters did. Thus, by refusing to be dependent on him, he hurt his stepfather's esteem by putting him in the position of one who was not able to give and nurture.

Ego-Ideal and Superego

Perhaps no other structure of the familial self is so different from the Western self and so difficult for Westerners to comprehend as the Asian conscience. The ego-ideal tends to be much stronger in Indians and Japanese than the superego (the opposite is true of Westerners), and it is different in both structure and content. It is highly contextual or situational rather than being based on relatively abstract, consistent principles; and it is governed by radar-like sensitivity to the norms of different groups and hierarchical relationships, rather than the gyroscopic consistency of the Western individualistic conscience.

Thus, Indians become acutely aware of the norms of whatever group or setting they are in, enabling them to adapt to highly foreign situations; furthermore, they can act and dress quite differently according to the situation, or can even say quite varying things on the same topic to different persons according to the relationship, while experiencing no inner conflict. As an example, an Indian psychoanalyst who was in two advanced psychoanalytic seminars in New York City espousing very different orientations felt absolutely no conflict about attending both. One seminar was highly academic and traditional in content, whereas the other innovatively emphasized the exploration of the therapist's countertransference from an object relations point of view. No other analyst I know would have considered being in these two groups simultaneously.

The Indian ego-ideal is consistent with culturally based principles, as in the laws of Manu and the concept of *dharma*, which contrast sharply with Western/Christian universalistic ethics based on the assumption of a universal human nature. In Manu, what is moral is to particularize, to see what is proper in a given situation, relationships, the differing natures of the persons involved, etc. Thus, each class of men or women has its own particularistic nature, and therefore its own particularistic ethics (Ramanunjan, 1990). *Dharma*, or proper moral behavior, is always contextual, and much more so than Gilligan's (1982) concept of women's morality.

The Japanese variation is a situational ego-ideal that is strongly perfectionistic in demanding very high levels of performance, both interpersonally and in tasks. This is originally inculcated by the mother's consistently high expectations and training. I have observed this ego-ideal in all of the Japanese patients I have worked with or supervised. As a result, Japanese patients are acutely sensitive to any criticism from others or indications of failure, which means that the analyst must be extremely tactful in pointing anything out. One patient, after a year and a half of four-times-a-week analysis, came 1 minute late to a session for the first time. He was very upset and afraid that I would be very critical of him. The fact that I was not infrequently late had nothing to do with his performance.

Both Indians and Japanese have a strong superego that arouses intense anxiety and inhibits any expression (sometimes even awareness) of anger at a hierarchical superior. It is well recognized by therapists in both countries that many of the frequent somatic and other symptoms are related to intense feelings of anger generated in family and group hierarchical relationships from which there is usually no exit—feelings that have to be inhibited or suppressed. I have found in longer-term intensive analyses with both Indians and Japanese that it is only after a considerable length of time, usually after at least a year and a half, that any direct manifestations of anger or criticism emerge toward me. In the beginning, these are very tentatively expressed. But even then, such expressions are inevitably followed by intense anxiety over whether I will retaliate by abandoning the patients—that is, by no longer being the concerned, nurturing superior. Not infrequently, when more intense anger emerges in the transference, it is acted out in one of the patient's close familial relationships and then has to be interpreted.

Sexuality, on the other hand, especially in Indians, is far less inhibited; instead, it is contained by strict social norms of behavior both in relationships outside of the family and in the complex kinship relationships within it. On the whole, the outside norms are stricter, so as not to sully the reputation of the family and thus affect the marriageability of the daughters. Within the family, however, more infatuations are permitted between first cousins (cousin-brothers and cousin-sisters), nieces and uncles, and such.

The Indian Oedipus is significantly different from the one predominating in the West. The son never loses his mother, and in effect looks to his father to offer a structuring identification from the more maternal symbiosis (Kakar, 1980). An Indian man's fear of impotence is not concerned nearly so much with castration anxiety as with engulfment by the woman. And, indeed, one of my Indian patients felt continuously vulnerable to being importuned by various women for sexual relationships and to becoming involved with them, regardless of how suitable he felt they were for him. The pull toward the maternal symbiosis became a major topic of the analysis.

THE SPIRITUAL SELF

As I have discussed at much greater length elsewhere (Roland, 1988, pp. 289–311), the spiritual self is totally different from what has been formulated in Freudian psychoanalysis. Rather than being a manifestation of a regressive pull to a maternal symbiosis, the spiritual self is in a highly paradoxical relationship to the familial self as both counterpoint and continuity. As counterpoint, it actually enables Indians and Japanese to individuate and emerge from more symbiotic emotional enmeshments with the inevitable frustrations generated by disappointed expectations or difficult superiors. R. K. Narayan (1967) poignantly portrays such counterpoint in the protagonist of his novel *Vendor of Sweets*. The effort made to realize the spiritual self is the most particularized and individualized part of Indian psychological functioning in a culture where there is careful, continuous observation of the social etiquette of hierarchical relationships. Such efforts depend a great deal on the particular psychological makeup, temperament, and inclinations of the person. For instance, different mantras are assigned, depending on the spiritual makeup of the person.

At the same time, there are modes of realizing the spiritual self that are continuous with the familial self and hierarchical relationships. The idealizations in hierarchy by quality of the person culminating with *darshan*, not only enhance inner esteem but are also oriented toward self-transformations. Exchanges and gifts in hierarchical relationships are also oriented toward self-transformation: The giving of subtle matter, such as education, is more transformative to finer qualities than the giving of grosser matter, such as food or clothing. Then, the devotional aspects of *bhakti* worship depend in part on a more maternal/feminine makeup in men, as alluded to above, and on the sensuous, symbiotic modes of relating of the familial self.

Still other orientations toward realizing the spiritual self include the magic–cosmic world of mythology, where the divine and the mundane are combined in mythic figures that guide persons (especially women) in their everyday relationship; of astrology, palmistry, numerology, and the like, which orient persons to their personal destiny in everyday decisions in the gradual development and unfolding of their spiritual nature; and of rituals that enhance the well-being of family members or others, or that modify destiny through self-transformations (Raheja, 1976).

In psychoanalytic practice, I have had three Indian patients where issues centered around the spiritual self played a major role in psychoanalytic therapy (Roland, 1988, pp. 25–47, 154–174), whereas with a number of other Indian patients it was present but much more in the background. One patient, a Moslem woman, simply stated that she knew that if she got up at 4 A.M. every morning and prayed and meditated, she would see God sooner or later. But she had three children, and she was just too tired to get up so early every day. In the three patients for whom this issue was dominant, a great deal of time in therapy was spent on conflicts and struggles related to the spiritual self. To have assumed that this was regressive or psychopathological would have made psychoanalytic work impossible with them—as had already occurred with Shakuntala in her sessions with her first therapist.

One woman patient, Veena, an artist, felt intensely cramped and inhibited by her husband in trying to realize her spiritual self, and was considering a separation. Through the analysis of her dreams, it emerged that Veena had unconsciously displaced similar inhibiting feelings onto her husband from her father's family, with whom she had gone to live during her adolescence; her earlier childhood had been under the influence of a maternal uncle, a revered holy man, who died when she was 12. Once she became aware of this displacement, she could continue living with her husband, only now more happily, while painting as her *sadhana* or spiritual discipline.

In all of my Indian patients, especially when they are Hindu, the magic–cosmic world of astrology and palmistry has played a major role in their lives. Ashis, for instance, consulted an internationally recognized scientist, who was also a noted local palmist, on any major decision he had to make. The scientist's advice coincided rather closely with psychoanalytic interpretations I made on a few occasions. Or Manoj, on considering marital choices, would always consult astrologers (both in the United States, where he lived, and in India), only giving them birth dates and times. Their readings of the women and the possible relationships between him and each of them seemed remarkably accurate on the basis of what I knew from sessions. However, the Indian astrologers in America commented more on the details of how Manoj and his prospective wife would get along, taking into account that Indian couples are much more on their own in America than in India. This whole magic–cosmic world is based on Indian metonymic thinking (Ramanujan, 1990), where there is continuity between everyday life events and the dual influences of the planets and of actions and experiences from past lives (*karma* and *samsara*).

THE EXPANDING SELF

In clinical psychoanalytic work with Indians and Japanese, it is often crucial to take into account the Westernizing/modernizing trends of social change, and the psychological processes involved that generate an expanding self as well as psychological conflict. This is equally true of working with Asians in America, because they encounter a radically different life style and psychology here that can also result in considerable inner conflict as well as a bicultural or expanding self. The very advent of psychoanalysis in India and Japan over the last half century or so is an integral past of these Westernizing/modernizing influences.

Three psychological processes related to social change are identifiable in India and Japan (for a fuller description, see Roland, 1988, pp. 17–54, 89–145). The first encompassses issues of identity, which are more pronounced in India than in Japan: India experienced two centuries of British colonial rule and denigration, compared to the relatively short period of the American Occupation in Japan, where radical changes were made in the society but essentially without denigration of the culture. In India, the effects of British colonialism were far more deleterious to the identity of Indian men than to that of women.

As alluded to above, the Indian father–son relationship is one in which the son does not rebel during adolescence, but rather tries to gain his father's respect and to reflect well on his father. When the father's values have changed to Western colonial ones that denigrate Hindu culture, sons identify with these attitudes in an upper layering of the self, but then devalue more deeply rooted layers of the self that are anchored in indigenous culture in the maternal matrix—which is so powerful in Indian men. This can result in intense inner conflict and psychological paralysis.

I have seen two Indian men in psychoanalysis who have had these psychodynamics. In both cases, the fathers were dominant figures in the family, were energetic and highly entreprenurial, and were closely identified with Western colonial attitudes that denigrated Indian culture and society. The first patient, Ashis, was an oldest son, completely within his father's sphere and closely identified with his father's values until the father committed suicide because of a scandal when Ashis was 19. Ashis then jettisoned his father's Westernized values, instead searching for new idealized selfobjects among some renowed relatives who were leaders of a major Hindu reform movement. Ashis came for therapy almost completely paralyzed in his functioning, feeling unresolvably caught between his father's Westernized sphere and his own turn to Hinduism until this psychodynamic was analyzed (see Roland, 1988, pp. 25–47).

The other man was a youngest son and was far more in his mother's emotional realm, though still greatly influenced by his father's Westernized attitudes and denigration of indigenous culture. This surfaced in conflicts in Bombay over what kind of woman to marry. Those from his mother's realm, whom he was much more attracted to and felt more comfortable with, were experienced as having little status and value; the women from the more elite, educated families were far more esteemed, but he could not get along with them very well. Like Ashis, this patient could only move forward as these two layers of the self were analyzed.

Japanese also have a double layering of the self as the result of social change. The upper layer is identified with Western values centering around independence, self-reflection, and rationality, whereas the deeper layers of the self are far more rooted in the empathic dependence/interdependence relationship with the mother (Nishizono, no date). These, too, have to be taken into account in analyzing Japanese patients. On the surface they may seem not unlike Americans, but actually they have far more intense dependency expectations.

The second psychological process involved in social change is the use of various aspects of the familial self in modernization, such as a more affiliative kind of achievement motivation, and contextualization of modern and traditional work and living settings. The third psychological process is greater individualization, especially in the urban areas. Individualization takes into account to a far greater extent an adolescent's wishes and inclinations, but does not go nearly as far as the individualism of Western societies, or the *Sturm und Drang* of American adolescent identity formation. Individualization in India and Japan is a key component in an expanding self, but can also be a source of considerable emotional distress when it conflicts with traditional hierarchical expectations.

In the United States, Indians and Japanese encounter a very different life style, dictated by a culture of individualism with egalitarian and contractual relationships. This can engender considerable conflict in several different areas that must be dealt with in psychoanalytic therapy. One area is hierarchical relationships: Both Indians and Japanese may feel deeply hurt when American superiors at work or in graduate school are not as nurturing as they expect them to be. Another problem area is the lack of intimate relationships of the kind that Indians and Japanese are used to. A third area is the degree of assertiveness and even confrontation that goes on in American work relationships, which may be completely foreign to Asians. Certainly, Japanese psychoanalysts have reported difficulty in being appropriately confrontative with American patients.

Yoshiko, a highly educated Japanese woman, was extremely upset when she was called upon to be highly assertive with her American company's clients. This went completely against the grain of her indigenous self, which called for politeness and communication by innuendo. Psychoanalytic therapy calls for an empathic response, acknowledging that one level of such a conflict is generated by the differences between the emotional responses of the indigenous cultural self and that of the American life style. This enables an Asian patient to choose and integrate which aspects of the indigenous self to keep and which aspects of American life to integrate into an expanding, bicultural self. It also enables the patient to delve deeper into problematic aspects of the indigenous self that are skewed by faulty familial relationships and development.

ACKNOWLEDGMENT

This chapter is substantially drawn from Chapters 1, 7, and 8 of *In Search of Self in India and Japan: Toward a Cross-Cultural Psychology* by A. Roland, 1988, Princeton, NJ: Princeton University Press. Copyright 1988 by Princeton University Press. Reprinted by permission.

REFERENCES

Bernstein, D. (1983). The female superego: A different perspective. *International Journal of Psycho-Analysis, 64,* 187–202.

Bon Maharaj, B. H. (1963). *Jiva atma or finite self.* Vrindavan, India: Institute of Oriental Philosophy.

Doi, T. (1973). *The anatomy of dependence.* Tokyo: Kodansha International.

Erikson, E. H. (1963). *Childhood and society* (2nd ed.). New York: Norton.

Federn, P. (1952). *Ego psychology and the psychoses*. New York: Basic Books.

Fromm, E., & Suzuki, D. T. (1970). *Zen Buddhism and psychoanalysis*. New York: Harper & Row.

Gedo, J. (1979). *Beyond interpretation*. New York: International Universities Press.

Gedo, J. (1981). *Advances in clinical psychoanalysis*. New York: International Universities Press.

Gedo, J., & Goldberg, A. (1973). *Models of the mind*. Chicago: University of Chicago Press.

Gilligan, C. (1982). *In a different voice*. Cambridge, MA: Harvard University Press.

Goffman, E. (1959). *The presentation of the self in everyday life*. Garden City, NY: Doubleday.

Grinker, R. (1957). On identification. *International Journal of Psycho-Analysis, 38*, 379–390.

Hallowell, I. A. (1955). *Culture and experience*. Philadelphia: University of Pennsylvania Press.

Hartmann, H. (1939). *Ego psychology and the problem of adaptation*. New York: International Universities Press, 1958.

Hsu, F. L. K. (1971). Psychological homeostasis and *jen*: Conceptual tools for advancing psychological anthropology. *American Anthropologist, 73*, 23–44.

Jacobson, E. (1964). *The self and object world*. New York: International Universities Press.

Kahn, M. (1974). *The privacy of the self*. New York: International Univesities Press.

Kakar, S. (1978). *The inner world: A psychoanalytic study of childhood and society in India*. Delhi: Oxford University Press.

Kakar, S. (1980). Observations on "the Oedipal alliance" in a patient with a narcissistic personality disortder. *Samiksa, 34*, 47–53.

Kernberg, O. (1975). *Borderline conditions and pathological narcissism*. New York: Jason Aronson.

Klein, G. (1976). *Psychoanalytic theory: An exploration of essentials*. New York: International Universities Press.

Kohut, H. (1971). *Analysis of the self*. New York: International Universities Press.

Kohut, H. (1977). *Restoration of the self*. New York: International Universities Press.

Kohut, H. (1980). Summarizing reflections. In A. Goldberg (Ed.), *Advances in self psychology* (pp. 473–552). New York: International Universities Press.

LeVine, R. (1982). *Culture, behavior, and personality: An introduction to the comparative study of psychosocial adaptation* (2nd ed.). Chicago: Aldine.

Lichtenstein, H. (1977). *The dilemma of human identity*. New York: Jason Aronson.

Loewald, H. (1960). On the therapeutic action of psychoanalysis. In H. Loewald, *Papers on psychoanalysis* (pp. 221–256). New Haven, CT: Yale University Press.

Masson, J. (1976). The psychology of the ascetic. *Journal of Asian Studies, 35*, 611–625.

Masson, J. (1980). *The oceanic feeling: The origins of religious sentiment in ancient India*. Dordrecht, The Netherlands: D. Reidel.

Menaker, E. (1982). *Otto Rank: A rediscovered legacy*. New York: Columbia University Press.

Menaker, E., & Menaker, W. (1965). *Ego in evolution*. New York: Grove Press.

Milner, M. (1973). Some notes on psychoanalytic ideas on mysticism. In D. Tuckett (Ed.), *The suppressed madness of sane men* (pp. 258–274). London: Tavistock, 1987.

Narayan, R. K. (1967). *Vendor of sweets*. New York: Viking Press.

Nishizono, M. (no date). *Problems imposed on psychotherapeutic intervention in traditional milieux: Acculturation in Japan and psychotherapy*. Unpublished manuscript.

Parsons, T. (1964). *Social structure and personality*. New York: Free Press.

Raheja, G. G. (1976, May). *Transformational processes in Hindu ritual: Concepts of "person" and "action" in the performance of a vrat*. Paper presented at the American Council of Learned Societies/Social Science Research Council Workshop on the Person and Interpersonal Relationships in South Asia: An Exploration of Indigenous Conceptual Systems, Chicago.

Ramanujam, B. K. (1980, October). *Technical factors in psychotherapy in India*. Paper presented at the annual meeting of the American Academy of Psychoanalysis, San Juan, Puerto Rico.

Ramanujan, A. K. (1990). Is there an Indian way of thinking? In M. Marriott (Ed.), *India through Hindu categories* (pp. 41–58). New Delhi: Sage Publications.

Roland, A. (1988). *In search of self in India and Japan: Toward a cross-cultural psychology*. Princeton, NJ: Princeton Universtiy Press.

Segal, H. (1964). *Introduction to the work of Melanie Klein*. New York: Basic Books.

Taketomo, Y. (1989). An American–Japanese transcultural psychoanalysis and the issue of teacher transference. *Journal of the American Academy of Psychoanalysis, 17*(3), 427–450.

Winnicott, D. W. (1960). Ego distortion in terms of true and false self. In D. W. Winnicott, *The maturational processes and the facilitating environment*. London: Hogarth Press and The Institute of Psychonalysis, 1965.

Winnicott, D. W. (1965). *The maturational processes and the facilitating environment*. London: Hogarth Press and The Institute of Psychoanalysis.

CHAPTER TEN

Cultural, Emotional, and Unconscious Aspects of Self

DREW WESTEN

In studying the Wintu Indians, anthropologist Dorothy Lee (1950) noted that the Wintu lack a concept of "self" similar to our own. Instead, the Wintu, like preliterate societies observed by many field workers, "conceive of the self not as strictly delimited or defined, but as a concentration, at most, which gradually fades and gives place to the other. Most of what is other for us, is for the Wintu completely or partially or upon occasion, identified with the self" (p. 134). One informant, asked to describe aspects of herself and her history, began with a story about her husband, and systematically described the lives of her kin. Whereas contemporary Westerners have little difficulty understanding the meaning of Polonius's advice to Hamlet, "To thine own self be true," this advice would have been undecipherable throughout much of human history to peoples such as the Wintu. To the extent that it carried any meaning for them, Polonius's advice would probably be interpreted as a cryptic way of saying, "Obey your duty to your family," "Do what nature decrees," or "Do not dishonor your kin," since kin and nature were inextricably bound up with selfhood.

The dichotomy between the views of "primitives" and "ourselves" is not, of course, so hard and fast. Where does the "self" to which Shakespeare refers come from? Is is entirely distinct from the "selves" of the significant others who reflected it to the young child? Are the aspirations and values embodied in it anything more or less than imperfect replicas of the standards of powerful parents the young child once admired and idealized? Some theorists of a Romantic bent of mind view the self, in Rousseauian fashion, as a pristine essence that, if untainted by a corrupting environment, will flourish. Rogers (1959), echoing Rousseau's lament that "man is born free and everywhere he is in chains," posits such a self destined for actualization if unfettered by externally imposed and then self-imposed "conditions of worth." Other theorists, following the symbolic interactionists, view this self as a product of social interaction and hence, like the Wintu self, not easily taken out of its social context.

Pathological failures in maintaining boundaries of self nevertheless can be seen in stark relief against the baseline of bounded selfhood characteristic of our culture. A recent research meeting grew hushed in sadness and discomfort as the participants read the transcript of a personality-disordered mother who described her sense of betrayal at her daughter's loss of virginity: The mother took this as an affront, deliberately perpetrated upon her (the mother) to make her suicidal. The daughter's sexuality belonged to the mother and was hers to dispose of when and if she saw fit. To this woman, who was profoundly embedded in her own perspective, there could be no explanation for the daughter's sexual behavior other than that she was trying to hurt her mother. The daughter, she explained in a later and equally disturbing vignette, was nothing but "my representative to the community."

What these examples suggest—a Wintu woman comfortably describing herself in her familial context, and a troubled mother struggling to define the limits of her own and her daughter's existence—is the importance of cultural and clinical factors in understanding the "self." This chapter argues that data from clinical observation point to important unconscious and affective aspects of self that need to be integrated with data from experimental investigations to provide a more comprehensive view of the "self." It concludes by noting as well the importance of anthropological data, and suggests that several processes related to technological development are producing a thoroughgoing revolution in the experience of self cross-culturally.

Before beginning it is important to note an issue of the philosophy of science that underlies this chapter. Philosophers sometimes distinguish between the context of scientific discovery, where new observations are made and theories are formed, and the context of justification, in which hypotheses are tested. Clinicians have argued for years that the clinical data base, while far less useful in the context of justification (hypothesis testing), is in many respects incomparable to the experimental data base in the context of discovery: The clinican observes many individuals in depth, over months or years, talking about real and affect-laden (rather than hypothetical and affectively neutral) life situations. Indeed, precisely what renders experiments useful in testing the validity of a hypothesis—the systematic control of variables and the constraining of subjects' response possibilities so that one can test the effect of independent on dependent variables—renders the experimental situation far less useful for discovery in psychology. The concept of "self" provides a good example of a construct that would never have been postulated or studied if researchers had not looked to their own experience or that of their patients for guidance on what to study and how to understand it.

Beyond the utility of clinical and other forms of nonexperimental data such as ethnographic observation in the context of discovery, there are two other ways in which such data are scientifically useful (see Westen, 1990a). First, as Kuhn (1970) and others have made clear, the hypotheses we test are always part of a broader theoretical perspective—implicit or explicit— that guides our thinking and our research agenda. In psychology this paradigmatic framework cannot and should not be based only on what has been observed to date in the laboratory (see Westen, 1988). In what one might call the *context of committed belief*, exclusive reliance on experimental data would provide a narrow and bizarre caricature of human beings— perhaps as creatures who in infancy hover over visual cliffs and suck on rubber nipples to make geometric designs appear, and as adults, that is, as 18-year-old middle-class caucasians, are motivated primarily by the desire to please experimenters, avoid cognitive dissonance, and fill out questionnaires.

Second, alongside the hypothetico-deductive context of justification described at length by philosophers of science such as Karl Popper is a second context of justification exclusive to the human sciences, which one might call an *interpretive context of justification*. Just as a good theory must lead to accurate predications, it must also lead to the ability to interpret the meanings of what people do and say in a way that competing theories and lay explanation cannot. If a theory of "self" cannot explain why television evangelists like Jimmy Swaggart and Jim Bakker preached against the evils of sex vehemently and with apparent conviction while simultaneously participating in illicit sex acts, it is not a good theory.

THE MULTIPLE MEANINGS OF "SELF": DISTINGUISHING CONSCIOUS AND UNCONSCIOUS ASPECTS OF SELF

One cannot read the literature on the self in psychology and psychoanalysis without being struck both by the richness of the phenomena being described and by the importance of clarifying precisely what we mean by different usages of "self" (see Offer, Ostrov, & Howard, 1981; Westen, 1985, 1990b; Horowitz, 1987). The most important distinction is between "self" and various hyphenated self-related terms, such as "self-concept," "self-system," "self-schema," and the like. If we were talking about a lamp in my bedroom, no one would claim that the lamp and my mental representation of it are the same thing, and hence no one would consider using the same word, "lamp," to describe them both. One is the actual lamp—knowable, imperfectly, through the senses (the Kantian "noumenal" reality)—and the other is my lamp representation, lamp schema, or specific instantiation of my lamp concept (Kantian "phenomenal" reality).

For some odd historical reason, this distinction has not been maintained in literature on the self, so that theorists of almost every theoretical persuasion have used the term "self" as a synonym for terms such as "self-concept," "self-representation," "ego," "self-schema," and the like. This has led to interminable theoretical confusions. The "self" can only mean the whole person as he or she really is, as when one says "herself" or "myself"; when one says, "She can take care of herself," one does not mean, "She can tend to her mental representation of her attributes." If "self" is simply used to denote the "real" person, then all derivative terms make logical sense. Thus, the self-concept is the person's concept of himself or herself; a "self-schema" is a schema about the person, about oneself. If, in contrast, one uses "self" and "self-schema" or "self-representation" interchangeably, as is commonplace in both psychoanalytic and social-cognitive literature—as if a lamp and its representation were the same thing—then one runs into an infinite regress: A self-schema is by definition a schema of the self, but if the "self" is defined as synonymous with "self-schema," the self-schema must be a schema of the self-schema (a psychologist's recursive nightmare!).

The self-concept is not a concept of a concept; it is a concept of a person, oneself. Thus, to ask a question such as "Do people have one self or many?" is largely an instance of muddled thinking brought about by linguistic confusion: There can only be one self, since each person only has one existence. The person may act differently in different situations or play multiple roles; the person may have many different representations of himself or herself; and the person may have difficulty seeing how the various sides of himself or herself fit together. Still, this individual is a single person—one self—whether he or she knows it or not. The lamp in my bedroom may be on or off, and I may represent it in my mind as sometimes on and sometimes off, but it is still one lamp.

One important complication is that representations of the self are, aside from being cognitions about the self, themselves part of the self. If the self includes everything about a person, body and soul, it includes the person's representations of himself or herself. Thus, a person's representations of self may include representations of these representations. Nevertheless, distinguishing between the self, the person's representations of self, and his or her representations of these representations can be critical clinically. One man, for example, agreed with me that he saw himself as evil and worthless, but he would have none of a treatment aimed at changing this self-perception: For him, the purpose of therapy was to change his actual evilness and worthlessness. Only then would he consider changing the way he saw himself.

Self as Subject and Self as Object

Several other distinctions regarding the self need to be made. James (1890) distinguished between self as subject (the experiencing subject or "I") and self as object (the mental representation of the self). The former is in many respects synonymous with the flux and flow of consciousness—the experience of thoughts, feelings, and intentions as they come into conscious focus. For Descartes, the experience of thinking—the exercise of subjectivity—demonstrated the reality of his existence. Similarly, the experiences of feeling and intending seem to establish the earliest sense of existential selfhood in infancy, even before the self is represented as an object located in time and space, with its own subjectivity in contrast to other subjectivities (Lewis & Brooks-Gunn, 1979; Stern, 1985).

The Jamesian "I" is best described as the "sense of self," although one could equally postulate an unconscious subjective self, since people act on the basis of feelings and intentions of which they are not consciously aware. A substantial body of literature documents the existence of unconscious emotional processes (Westen, 1985, Ch. 2; Westen, 1990a; Greenberg & Safran, 1987), which suggests that people feel things even without conscious awareness. For example, a study by Shedler, Mayman, and Manis (1990) isolated subjects with "illusory mental health," who were distinguished by a combination of self-reported psychological health and clinican-reported character pathology or severe defensive constriction. During a mildly stressful experimental procedure, these subjects demonstrated hyperreactivity relative to all other subjects on physiological indices related to stress and linked to cardiovascular disease, while simultaneously self-reporting significantly *less* distress than comparison subjects. Studies using different methods have yielded similar findings (see Weinberger, 1990). The affective response is obviously registering "somewhere" and influencing information processing. Although the person may have no conscious phenomenological experience of the feeling, it is nevertheless being subjectively experienced. Whether one wishes to call this "unconscious subjectivity" or "dissociated consciousness" is largely a matter of taste; the point is that the person may have subjective centers of experience that are not available to consciousness. When we resonate with the advice "To thine own self be true," we implicitly recognize precisely this distinction: Beneath a social facade and even a conscious sense of oneself while playing various roles, a person may or may not be true to his or her real desires, intentions, or values.

Unconscious Representations of Self

Most research related to the "self" focuses on the self as object—that is, on representations of the self. Several different forms of mental representations need to be distinguished. A "self-representation" (Sandler & Rosenblatt, 1962) or "self-schema" (Markus, 1977; Kihlstrom & Cantor, 1983) is a schema of the self—that is, an organized knowledge structure or enduring pattern of processing information about the self. Psychoanalytic theorists typically emphasize that self-representations include or integrate many representational modes other than semantic knowledge; they may, like all person schemas or object representations, include bodily/kinesthetic, emotional, and other sensory (such as visual and auditory) representations. The system of self-representations or self-schemas represented in memory and associatively connected with one another can be called the "self-system." Various schemas of the self may be organized hierarchically, with subschemas nested within superordinate categories (Taylor & Crocker, 1980).

A person's general concept of himself or herself—the view that comes to mind when the person reflects on the self in the abstract or is asked to describe the self by a psychologist—is the person's "self-concept." This may, like many concepts, be a prototype—that is, a general model abstracted from thousands of specific representations and not identical with any of them (Kihlstrom & Cantor, 1983). The self-concept is one of an infinite number of "working representations" of the self (specific representations that are active at a particular time). Working representations are constructed from current information as well as from enduring schemas. They are similar to the "internal working models" postulated by attachment theorists (Bowlby, 1969; Main, Kaplan, & Cassidy, 1985). The self-system is associatively linked with episodic memories, which include the self by definition (although people differ in the ways they represent the self in retrieving these memories—e.g., seeing vs. not seeing themselves in the mental "picture"). Also closely linked to the self-system are generalized event representations (Fast, 1985; Nelson, 1986), scripts involving the self (Abelson, 1981), and role relationship models of the self in interaction with others (Horowitz, 1987; Luborsky & Crits-Christoph, 1990).

All of these aspects of "self as object" have conscious as well as unconscious components. Like any cognitive structure or process, the self-system is only accessible to introspection to a limited degree, both because of cognitive limits to access to cognitive processes (Nisbett & Wilson, 1977) and because of defensive avoidance of painful self-knowledge. Because the distinction between conscious and unconscious mental representations of the self is so crucial clinically and so rarely noted in the experimental literature, I present two examples here to demonstrate its importance and to suggest ways in which an understanding of unconscious self-representations must have an impact on any sophisticated model of self structure (for a fuller elaboration applicable to social-cognitive theory more generally, see Westen, in press-a, in press-b).

The first example is the self-system in narcissistic personality disorders. People with narcissistic personality disorders are characterized by a sense of themselves as at the center of the universe: They experience their needs and desires as paramount; they respond with rage and shame when they are not admired and treated in accordance with their grandiose fantasies of themselves; and they manifest little empathy toward others (see Kohut, 1971; Kernberg, 1975). Narcissistic patients often make remarkable statements about themselves in therapy without pausing to reflect upon the way the therapist might react. One patient spoke of the "special dispensations" he received at his job because his work was "greater than great." Another, an artist, un-self-consciously stated that he was perfect but then corrected this: "No, not really perfect, but I could be." Narcissistic patients frequently either devalue the people around them to protect their own precarious self-esteem, or see all their friends and associates as remarkable because these people are in their orbit. Narcissistic patients or patients with prominent narcissistic dynamics often talk about falling in love with someone because "she's just like me"; Freud described this pattern in his classic essay, "On Narcissism: An Introduction" (1914).

Several aspects of the self-structure of narcissistic patients are worthy of note here. For example, these people tend to differentiate poorly between themselves and others and to form representations of other people that are highly egocentric, focused primarily on their relation to themselves and their needs. People often only seem to exist for narcissistic patients if they are in the patients' orbit as sycophants, admirers, potentially useful resources, or mirrors. Kohut (1971, 1977) observes that in psychoanalytic treatment a narcissistic patient often idealizes the therapist and identifies with the therapist's greatness; sees the therapist as a "twin" who has all the same thoughts and feelings as the patient (and who shares in the patient's magnificence); or treats the therapist as a "mirror" who is expected to reflect the patient's greatness. These forms of relatedness are mirrored in the patient's other relationships, and reflect both a problematic way of representing people mentally (they are incompletely differentiated from representations of the self; see Horowitz & Zilberg, 1983) and a pathological way of *investing* in people and relationships, in which others are only valued insofar as they are useful. The lack of differentiation of self and others in the narcissistic patient is illustrated in the remark of one such patient that "when you're involved with someone you just suck each other up"; the patient then gestured that a common boundary surrounded the two people like a coccoon. Similar phenomena have been documented empirically in patients with borderline personality disorders (Westen, Lohr, Silk, Gold, & Kerber, in press; Westen, Ludolph, Lerner, Ruffins, & Wiss, 1990). The fragility of the self-structure of the narcissistic patient and the need for mirroring are illustrated very concretely by the poignant story of one patient who frequently needed to slip into the bathroom in high school just to look at herself in the mirror and see her reflection.

Perhaps the most salient aspect of the self-system in narcissistic personality disorders is the presence of a defensively bloated self-concept and of working representations characterized by diametrically opposed conscious and unconscious components. Narcissistic people are at their most grandiose when their self-esteem is most threatened; that is, they are seemingly most inflated when they are unconsciously most deflated. The artist mentioned earlier flew into a frenzy of grandiose self-statements after losing a competition he had felt sure he would win. His conscious representation of self as extraordinary was a defensive transformation of the sense of self that was active unconsciously—namely, the self as totally worthless. If one were to speak, then, of his active or working self-schema or self-representation, one would have to say that he had a deflated representation active below consciousness that necessitated an inflated conscious representation. One need not have such malignant narcissistic pathology to make use of similar defenses, since relatively healthy people at times defend against perceived insults (typically with somewhat more basis in reality) or threats to self-esteem by defensively altering conscious representations.

Although researchers have pointed to numerous self-enhancing biases in social cognition (Greenwald & Pratkanis, 1984; Taylor & Brown, 1988), there have been no models proposed to account for the simultaneous presence of contradictory conscious and unconscious representations, where one is a defensive transformation of the other. Social-cognitive theorists have too often assumed that the *active* self-schema in "working memory" is simultaneously the conscious, accessible self-schema; the problem stems in part from inadequacies in cognitive models of "working memory," which have historically skirted the issue of consciousness. One might add that if a narcissistic patient were to complete the Rosenberg Self-Esteem Inventory, he or she would probably report tremendously high self-esteem—surely an inaccurate picture of someone whose self-esteem is polar, alternating between total inflation and total deflation.

A second example is the self-system of patients who have been treated with cognitive therapy for depression, whose self-structure should certainly be explicable by a social-cognitive account. Cognitive theorists of depression have assumed that "depressives" think in distorted ways and hence need to be taught to think normally (Beck, 1976; Ellis, 1962). Hollon and Garber (1988) have recently advanced the provocative thesis that depressed patients may exhibit cognitive distortions similar to those of normals (such as arbitrary inference, selective abstraction, false confirmation of schemas, etc.), but that the *contents* of their schemas are skewed negatively. The implication the authors suggest is that cognitive therapy may not teach such a patient to think like a normal person, but may instead teach the patient to utilize certain procedures, which are *not* used by nondepressed individuals, to counteract depressive ways of thinking. Along these lines, one might note that a study of remitted depressives (Hauri, 1976) found that depressive themes continued to be present in their dreams; this suggests that depressives' schemas (and presumably self-schemas) remain active despite remission of overt symptoms.

If Hollon and Garber's speculation were to be borne out, it would suggest that the therapeutic action of cognitive therapy stems not primarily from a patient's abandoning pathological cognitive processes or knowledge structures, but from the conscious activation of procedures used to circumvent or override schematic processes, including negative representations of the self. These procedures may then become automatized so that they, too, are carried out unconsciously. Thus, the patient may continue to have negative self-schemas, but these become less likely to be activated, are interfered with, or become less accessible to consciousness because the person has learned rules and procedures for blocking them and has come to associate them with aversive responses from the therapist (such as being told they are irrational).

In this view, then, a negative self-schema may be activated, but it has become associatively connected with a procedure that may itself come to be activated with or without conscious awareness, whose function is to block the schema from entering consciousness. Blocking the schema would presumably diminish conscious negative affective feedback that would normally exacerbate processes such as mood-congruent cognition, but it would not be likely to inhibit other concomitant depressive processes entirely, such as self-defeating behavior or the generation of depressive dreams.

With respect to models of self, the important point is that the person may come to have two active self-schemas, one negative and developed from years of experience, and the other positive (or antinegative) developed to counteract the more enduring one. How information is processed simultaneously through two different self-schemas—one activated for purposes of affect regulation because of the negative emotional impact of the other—is not clear, although such a possibility is certainly not incompatible with a parallel processing model of cognition.

Identity

One final self-relevant term is of note: "identity." When Erikson (1963, 1968) writes of "identity" and "identity crises," or when William James

(1890) writes of a "divided soul," something more is at stake than simply a prototypical self-concept. A sense of identity includes several components. It includes a sense of continuity of experience, of the Jamesian "I," as well as some stability to self-representation. It includes a self-concept with a hierarchical structure, which can integrate several important self-schemas. It also includes an affective weighting of various self-representations—that is, a stake in seeing oneself as a psychologist, a mother, an auto worker, a gang member, or a scapegoat. As these examples suggest, a person with a negative identity nonetheless has an affective investment in the identity he or she has chosen. Swann's (1987, and Chapter Eleven, this volume) work on identity negotation suggests that people actively attempt, behaviorally and cognitively, to maintain and get others to acknowledge important aspects of their identities, even negative aspects.

Part of the affective dimension of identity is a commitment to values and ideals, and hence to various ideal self-schemas. Clinically, a lack of a sense of coherent identity is almost always accompanied by a lack of meaning in life and sense of emptiness, related to an inability to invest in ideals (and in relationships) that make life worthwhile. Patients with severe character pathology, whom Kohut (1971) describes as suffering from a defective "self," may mask this lack of commitment with an intense pseudocommitment to particular ideals; they thus become nothing *but* their ideals, which they use to organize their experience in every situation. This defensive hyperinvestment in ideals is also seen in individuals in times of rapid social change, who adopt "totalistic" ideologies (Lifton, 1963) that define the world and the self in black-and-white terms, and hence circumvent painful ambiguity and ambivalence (see Westen, 1985, Chs. 12 and 13).

Identity thus includes a coherent self-concept, an investment in goals and standards that make life meaningful and worthwhile, a weighting of the importance of various aspects of self, and meaningful attempts to actualize one's ideal self-schemas. It also includes two other elements. The first is a commitment to a set of cognitive principles that orient one to the world; these may be largely unconscious but include ideological commitments typically related to values. In anthropological terms, this refers to a commitment to both an "ethos" and a "world view" (Geertz, 1973)—that is, to both a set of moral, esthetic, and evaluative principles that govern one's actions, and a "picture of the way things in sheer actuality are," including fundamental assumptions about the world, society, and the self. As Geertz notes, ethos and world view are typically intertwined:

> The ethos is made intellectually reasonable by being shown [by religion] to represent a way of life implied by the actual state of affairs which the world view describes, and the world view is made emotionally acceptable by being presented as an image of an actual state of affairs of which such a way of life is an authentic expression. (p. 127)

On a psychological level, Janoff-Bulman (1989) has similarly described the "assumptive worlds" that are disrupted with catastrophic events, and Epstein (1990, and Chapter Seven, this volume) has attempted to construct an inventory for assessing individual differences in broad-based assumptions about what one can expect from life and from other people.

As Erikson argues, identity also includes, finally, some recognition by the social and cultural milieu that one is indeed who one thinks one is. That is why social roles are often so important to a person's sense of identity, because they establish the identity of one's own and others' experience of self. The importance of this aspect of identity also accounts for the fact that the seeds of defective identity are often sown in the first years of life. During this time, appropriate attunement to the child's needs and feelings is necessary for the child to develop a consensually validated sense of self and attunement to his or her own experience. The "false self" described by theorists such as Rogers (1959), Winnicott (1971), and Laing (1959) refers to a developmental process in which the person is attuned primarily to the needs, feelings, and definitions of the self imposed by the needs and wishes of significant others (or, more accurately, the child's beliefs about those wishes). The result is that the person identifies with that version of self, attempts to actualize it, and is chronically left feeling (or leaves others feeling) as if he or she is a fraud—acting a part or donning a mask, rather than expressing any genuine feelings, desires, or identity. As noted above, the need to be recognized for who one believes one is has been studied empirically by Swann.

The Role of Others in the Self-System

Several theorists have recently suggested, as James did a century ago, that the self-system somehow includes representations of others (see Markus & Cross, 1990). As will be discussed below, this is particularly apparent in studying representations of self in nonindustrial societies, where a sense of distinct selfhood is neither valued nor typically emphasized as in our culture. It is also more apparent in studying women in our own society, whose self-concept has been described as more embedded in a relational context (Miller, 1986). This may have been particularly true and necessary for self-esteem maintenance in previous eras in which the only way a woman could attain any prominence was through the success of her husband or male children; her own self-esteem would thus be substantially influenced by the accomplishments not of herself but of her family members. (One could speculate, as well, on the evolutionary significance of the tendency of females to define themselves in more relational terms than males.) Tesser's work on self-esteem maintenance (Tesser & Campbell, 1983; Tesser, Pilkington, & McIntosh, 1989; and Chapter Thirteen, this volume) also focuses on the way self-esteem is enhanced by the accomplishments of significant others. This is, in fact, probably one of the major motivations for identification in childhood (Westen, 1985, Ch. 4; 1986).

The role of representations of others in the self-system is thus considerable, but it is important to specify precisely what that role is, so that the concept of "self" is not once again bloated to include all of social cognition (since anyone a person interacts with will be represented, at least momentarily, in relation to the self, and hence that representation could be taken as part of the self-system broadly construed). From a social-cognitive perspective, one source of confusion is a lack of theoretical clarity about the relationship between schemas and networks of association. My self-schema may be associatively linked to episodic memories of myself interacting with thousands of people; are these memories to be considered aspects of my self-schema? Even more problematic are the implications of hierarchical models of schemas or concepts: A person's self-schema may include a representation of self as intelligent, a subschema about one's intelligence in a particular domain, and several specific instantiations of situations in which one behaved intelligently. These instantiations include representations of others, of the setting in which the event took place, etc. Are all these details to be considered part of the self-schema? From a psychoanalytic perspective, a parallel source of confusion has been the failure of theorists to specify precisely what they mean by "boundary confusion" or poor differentiation of self and others. What, exactly, is happening to representations when a patient inappropriately attributes obvious aspects of the personality or subjective experience of the self to significant others?

The major way in which other people and social entities can meaningfully be said to be part of the self-system is that the person can define herself or himself in part on the basis of various social identity elements, reference groups, roles, or significant others, such as "a German," "a member of the First Baptist Church," "Mary and Jim's son," or "Bill's wife." Such representations may be activated momentarily or chronically, and they may be manipulated to enhance or protect self-esteem. For example, while watching my university's basketball team capture the NCAA championship last year, my most active representation was of "self as Wolverine," and I, like thousands of others, felt personally enhanced by the victory. When the same team was humiliated this year, they became "that damn team," and I had very little to do with them. In nonindustrial socieities, representations of self are largely socially dominated representations of this sort. The fact that so many aspects of identity are ascribed rather than achieved, and that ingroups are less voluntarily selected, probably renders manipulation of these identity elements somewhat more difficult.

The more a person invests emotionally in goals shared by significant others or groups, the more the person is likely to consider those others to be defining of the self, or to represent them as highly similar to the self, since the person will observe the self and these others to have similar goals and to have parallel emotional changes in the context of the same events. For example, a traditional housewife who derives much of her sense of efficacy from the accomplishments of her husband is likely to get emotionally invested in his "side" of battles at work and to be buoyed or depressed as he is at turns of events in his world—a world of which she may have little direct knowledge or contact. Through self-perception processes (Bem, 1972) she will come to believe and *feel* that his victories and defeats are hers, much as Tesser has pointed to the way people gain self-esteem through their identification with significant others.

Roles and scripts are not themselves aspects of the self-system. They contain elements that may be, but they may also have little or no relationship to self-definition. An example should make this clear. Therapists frequently find themselves involved in role-relationship enactments with patients, in which the patient casts the therapist in a role from the past, and the therapist unwittingly plays the part (see Wachtel, 1977). For example, in working with victims of sexual abuse, therapists can easily find themselves playing the role of a family member, denying the existence of the abuse and failing to help the patient bring it to consciousness and work through the experience. Conversely, the therapist may unwittingly take the role of the abuser, probing too deeply and too quickly or forcing meanings or insights onto the patient that feel untrue or unreal. In both cases the therapist is enacting a role, but "self as colluder" or "self as abuser" is surely not a role the therapist would consider self-definitional and may not even represent unconsciously. Role relationships probably always include some dimension of experiential selfhood—that is, what it feels like to be in that role—but it is precisely when that momentary sense of self becomes recognized and reconceptualized as part of a role-relationship model that the therapist may be able to use his or her "countertransference" reaction to benefit the patient—stepping out of the role, helping the patient become aware of the way this represents, in Freud's words, a new version of an old conflict, and collaborating with the patient to give the story a new, less painful and predictable ending.

Roles and scripts are thus things that *people* play out; they are not things that can be attributed to the self-system, although they may have *consequences* for self-representation and may be associatively linked to self-schemas. Scripts may be aspects of "procedural knowledge" that have no conscious or unconscious "declarative" analogues, and can be either enhanced or interfered with by their representation as aspects of self. (It would similarly make little sense to describe the neural systems involved in movement and in maintaining awareness of the body's position in motion as aspects of the self-system, since motoric "representations" of this sort, and the interactions among the parietal lobe, basal ganglia, cerebellum, and neural networks controlling movement in the frontal lobes, are as nonexperiential psychologically as the processes controlling regulation of heartbeat.)

Significant others may also play a part in identity through their associations with the person's sense of personal history. People who have lost spouses through death or divorce often report a sense that a piece of themselves and of their past has died or left with the departed spouse, since so many memories were shared only by the two of them. Spouses or intimate others also typically share rituals, private languages, and often private pet names, so that the end of the relationship spells the end of self-representations—including names—that were once important identity elements. Many patients with severe personality disorders report feeling as if their identities reside entirely in these shared experiences, so that their all too frequent experience of loss of relationships means to them a loss of identity and a sense of inner emptiness.

Other people may also be relevant to the self-system to the extent that the person activates self-representations and representations of others interchangeably or uses identical representational elements to represent them both. The kinds of "boundary confusions" described for years by clinicians reflect instances in which a person activates a self-representation in place of a representation of another person, or uses the same or highly similar representations to understand or describe two different people. The personality-disordered mother in the opening vignette of this chapter evidenced pathology not by representing herself as "mother of X" but by confusing her daughter's sexuality with her own and by confusing her own point of view (feeling tested by her daughter's experimentation with sexuality) with her daughter's intentions (attributing testing the mother's stability as a primary motive for the daughter's desire to have a sexual relationship). Similar pathology can be seen in the difficulty personality-disordered patients often demonstrate in momentarily differentiating representations of self from ideal and feared representations of self, as when a borderline patient believes that she actually *is* evil incarnate, as she fears, or when a narcissistic patient believes that he has met his ideal of being perfect.

These kinds of failures in differentiation are not, of course, always so pathological. Momentary failures in differentiation may occur in what Durkheim (1915) called "collective effervescence" in ritualized social events, in religious experiences (James, 1902), in sexually pleasurable experiences, in fantasy, in moments of feeling thoroughly understood, and in less pathological defensive processes. The attempt to alter the self-concept in accord with representations of a significant other is also an essential aspect of identification (Sandler, 1987; Westen, 1985).

Finally, representations of others can be important aspects of the self-system in relation to ideals and fears. For example, Higgins and his colleagues (Higgins, 1990) have documented empirically the way people's representations of what they think significant others want them to become (or fear they will become) are compared against their perceptions of the way those others actually see them (or the way they see themselves). This raises important questions about the role of the self-system in motivation.

AFFECT, DISCREPANCIES, AND SELF-SCHEMAS: THE MOTIVATIONAL PROPERTIES OF THE "SELF"

The "self" is typically implicated in motivation, but once again what this means depends on how carefully one defines one's terms. If "self" means the person, then of course all motivation stems from the "self." If one means self-schemas or self-representations, then the "self" has no motivational properties at all. My representation of my bedroom lamp does not motivate me to do anything, even if the room is dark. What motivates me is a wish to turn on the light or a fear of something in the dark. A representation of the light as off or on only becomes part of a motivational unit—a cognitive–affective schema that may itself come to be activated as a unit—in conjunction with an affective valuation of the light's being on. Thus, the structure of the *wish* regarding the light would include a representation of the current reality (namely, that the light is off) in relation to a representation of a desired state (the light is on) that has been invested with some kind of affect (e.g., I would feel less scared if it were on; I would be able to accomplish goals that would feel good or make me feel less anxious if the light were on; I have been conditioned to find darkness anxiety-provoking; etc.). My "lamp concept" or "lamp schema" thus becomes motivationally relevant to the extent that it is associated with affect. This affect may arise in a number of ways, such as through a discrepancy between wished-for and cognized reality (as in the example above) or through cognitively mediated conditioning and social learning processes (such as learning to associate a dark room with being left alone in one's room as a toddler).

The situation with self-representations is no different. If I see myself as a teacher, that has no motivational significance whatsover. It may take on motivational significance if I care what kind of teacher I am—good or bad. I could, however, represent myself as a poor teacher and still have no motivation to change the way I teach, if my affective investment in teaching well is zero. Since that is rarely the case, we are easily lulled into the view that the representation itself has motivational force. The representation, however, is only motivationally relevant when compared with a representation of a desired or feared state that is affectively significant.

In this regard, it is critical to distinguish between representations as models of reality as it is and representations as emotionally charged goal states or "set goals." The importance of the distinction can be most clearly seen in the case of self-defeating behavior. A delinquent boy with whom I worked denied any interest in schoolwork, and scoffed at the idea that it mattered to him one way or another whether he succeeded. He "put his money where his mouth was," since he failed all his classes one term. Most high school students in this situation would experience a discrepancy between a schema of "self doing poorly" and an emotionally invested ideal self-schema, set goal, or "possible self" (Markus & Nurius, 1986) of "self doing well"; because the set goal for most students is invested with considerable affect, this discrepancy would elicit an aversive emotion (guilt, lowered self-esteem, shame, anxiety, etc.), which would in turn motivate efforts to reduce the discrepancy. These efforts might include defensive distortions in cognition (e.g., "I'm only doing badly because my teachers are out to get me" or "I'm only doing badly because I'm not trying"), as well as behavioral efforts to reduce the discrepancy, such as doing more homework or listening more in class. (For a fuller elaboration of the model of affect and motivation behind this discussion, see Westen, 1985, Ch. 2; see also Higgins, 1990.)

For my budding sociopath, however, "self doing poorly" did not have any such motivational significance, as one would expect it would if representations can themselves be autonomously motivating. The reason was that this representation was compared with different set goals, and hence was part of very different cognitive–affective motivational units than would be the case with most students. For this boy, doing well in school was associated with two very different motivations. To do well would mean that other people would realize he could do so (as he would himself), and hence would come to expect more effort and greater success. Any failures, then, would become all the more painful because they would bring greater self-reproach and reproach from significant others. Thus, if the boy had minimal intrinsic interest in working hard at school, and if he had a representation of himself as not terribly competent, he would be motivated to avoid success because success would be associated with the likelihood of more intense negative affect in the future. I might add that none of these schemas, expectancies, or motivations was particularly accessible to this boy's consciousness.

My delinquent patient had another reason, however, not to strive for success despite failures at school that could have important negative consequences for him (such as failing to meet requirements of his probation). For this boy, succeeding at school meant accepting adult authority. The self-schema that was consequently activated by scholastic success was "self kissing ass"; when compared with his ideal self-schema of "self as his own boss," this elicited an intense feeling of shame that overrode any enjoyment at mastery or fulfillment of defensively denied wishes to feel competent and successful. The ultimate outcome of this combination of representations, wishes, and fears was that the costs of success far exceeded the benefits.

Experimental evidence corroborates the point. Cognitive-dissonance theory, like many discrepancy models and arguments about the role of self-schemas in motivation, tends to gloss over two kinds of discrepancies: those in which a person's understanding of a piece of information is discrepant from his or her enduring schemas, and those in which a person's understanding of a piece of information is discrepant from desires or emotionally invested goals. In one study (Westen, 1987), subjects were asked to describe situations in which they, significant others, and insignificant others violated an ideal of moral or appropriate behavior; to describe how they felt and how intensely they felt it; and to report how they responded and felt afterwards. Subjects were similarly asked to describe situations in which they and significant others did something unexpected and anomalous (i.e., cognitively discrepant but not "bad"), and to report how they felt and responded. As predicted, cognitive anomalies led to far less negative affect and a different set of responses than did cognitive–affective mismatches involving discrepancies between cognized reality and desired states. This occurred for both self and significant others: Violation of standards led to much more intense negative affect and more efforts to resolve the situation behaviorally or intrapsychically than did cognitive anomalies, whether it was the self or a significant other who violated an ideal self-schema or ideal other-schema.

What this analysis suggests is that the processes involved in self-discrepancies of various sorts (see, e.g., Rogers, 1959; Higgins, 1990; Tesser & Campbell, 1983; Tesser et al., 1989; Tesser, Chapter Thirteen, this volume) are general processes of motivation not limited to the domain of self. These occur whether the wish or discrepancy involves the self (such as violations of goals, morals, ideals, desires of significant others, comparisons with significant others, etc.), significant others (who can similarly violate standards), or the bedroom lamp (which can be off instead of on). Bowlby (1969) has pointed to similar processes involved in attachment, in which violation of set goals for proximity leads to negative affect and distress vocalizations; these are designed to bring the attachment figure back, and hence to minimize the discrepancy and shut off the aversive affective "feedback."

The considerations thus far suggest that although representations of the self are not themselves *motivating*, they can be *motivated*; in other words, a representation may reflect a compromise among competing psychological processes, including cognitive processes that normally lead to relatively veridical concept formation as well as wishes and fears that distort objectivity with respect to the self (see Brenner, 1982, on compromise formations). This is no different from cognitive and dynamic processes operative in the formation of all person schemas, particularly those of significant others, whom the person may be motivated to love, hate, idealize, or devalue.

The tendency of people to try to confirm, and to induce others to affirm, aspects of their identity, which Swann and his colleagues have documented in numerous studies (Swann, 1987), may be explicable in part by examining the particular set goals that may be violated if a salient aspect of the self-concept is threatened. Swann points out that stability to the self-concept, like stability to other important shemas (see Janoff-Bulman, 1989), provides some sense of existential security. The need to be affirmed and recognized is also itself a motive to which Kohut (1977), among others, has called attention. Swann also points to "pragmatic" considerations, such as the wish of a person who knows he or she lacks certain abilities to resist changes in self-representation that would lead him or her into various failure situations. As noted above, such beliefs about the self may at times be based less on rational acknowledgement of limitations than on neurotic beliefs established defensively or through identification in childhood, as one sees in many depressed patients. One patient who always felt criticized by his father as a child would never admit to himself any of his talents or abilities. To do so would have made him feel like a fraud, threatened his identification with his father, raised his hopes for success which he feared would not be realized, and activated frustrating wishes for his father's approval. In ways such as these, specific representations may become important emotionally to the person and thus defended, even if their affective consequences are objectively negative.

Distinguishing between various phenomena related to self as "schemas," "expectancies," or "set goals" would help eliminate confusion regarding various self-related constructs such as "self-efficacy" (Bandura, 1977, 1982). Gurin (1980) has proposed an important distinction between two components of self-efficacy: "competence" versus "system responsiveness" expectancies. Judgments of competence are assessments of one's ability to carry out an action. Assessments of system responsiveness are judgments of how much influence one's actions have on achieving outcomes. Gurin observed in her study of black youths (Gurin & Epps, 1975) that even if a person felt competent to perform certain actions, he or she could still lack a sense of personal control or self-efficacy because of an expectancy that the system would be unresponsive.

Bandura has often used the term "self-efficacy" as a synonym for "mastery" or "competence," even though, as Gurin (1980) suggests, that is only one component of self-efficacy judgments. Several other distinctions would render discourse in this area more coherent. When Bandura (1977) contrasts efficacy and outcome expectancies, he does not distinguish between outcome expectancies per se (judgments about whether things will work out as one desires—i.e., about whether a particular set goal will be met) and behavior–outcome expectancies (see Mischel, 1973—judgments about whether a particular behavior will achieve that set goal). These two kinds of expectancies are only similar in the kinds of experiments designed by researchers studying self-efficacy, which tend to have a heavy emphasis on achievement; in achievement situations, efficacy is the only way to achieve valued outcomes. The literature on self-efficacy also does not typically distinguish carefully between self-efficacy, competence, and outcome as *expectancies* and these same variables as *set goals* or desired states. Outcome set goals are the desired states that motivate action; outcome expectancies are beliefs about whether these set goals will be fulfilled. Similarly, a person may have wishes to be competent or efficacious, as well as beliefs about whether or not he or she is so.

These distinctions become particularly important in the myriad cases in human life in which outcome is to some degree independent of personal action, or in which competence or efficacy is desired (a set goal), even where it is not essential for a positive outcome with respect to some other variable (such as financial success). Many of our theories have been biased by the prevailing cultural view and ideal of our society as a meritocracy, in which what one gets is what one deserves; this view is, historically and cross-culturally speaking, a blip on the anthropological chart. As noted below, the importance of judgments of individual competence to our self-worth, and the belief that we control our own destiny, are ideas that have developed in large measure through the influence of industrialization and its various social concomitants and sequelae.

Without knowing about a person's specific outcome, competence, and efficacy set goals, one cannot predict the person's behavior or emotional state from a knowledge of the relevant expectancies. The delinquent boy described above was not particularly upset by his school failure because he did not invest in scholastic competence as a set goal. His major concern was with outcome—that is, with whether he kept his parole officer at bay. Whether he got passing grades through cheating, scaring his teachers, or luck made little difference to him; a positive outcome (passing grades) would have made him perfectly happy even if he felt he had learned nothing. In fact, positive outcome plus minimal competence might elicit the most positive affect, because he would have "ripped off the system." In contrast, students who are highly motivated to feel competent may be very upset if they do not understand the material, even if they receive good grades, because their competence set goal has been violated. Alternatively, another adolescent patient who was not sociopathic but was heavily invested in asserting his control and refusing to be controlled by authorities—that is, who had high (and highly invested) set goals for personal control—was very happy to sacrifice both competence and grade outcome by listening carefully in class but never doing homework. The result was a mediocre scholastic record and a feeling of uncertain competence about the material, but tremendous satisfaction at having exquisitely titrated the amount of his investment, interest, and effort in a way that allowed him to pass his classes but not to "give in" to his teachers by appearing interested in either the grades or what they had to offer.

Self-efficacy theory best applies to situations such as those involving achievement, in which efficacy judgments both influence action (because belief in one's ability to carry out an action influences one's willingness to attempt it) and affect (through comparison with competence or efficacy set goals). Self-efficacy theory becomes misleading, however, when applied to situations in which outcome is independent of efficacy. For example, Bandura (1984) asserts that "aerophobics" avoid airliners not because they are irrationally afraid of airplanes or of dying in an airplane, but because they lack a sense of efficacy (p. 236). The problem with this explanation is that *everyone* lacks efficacy in an airplane (except the pilot), and anyone who thinks he or she is efficacious in that circumstance is psychotic. The phobic's primary problem is the phobia; a secondary problem is the development of anticipatory fears of being afraid and unable to handle the situation (see Barlow, 1988). Only this latter problem is explicable (or optimally treatable) using a self-efficacy explanation, since the person has now developed expectancies about loss of control and needs help, as Bandura argues, in seeing that he or she has the ability to confront the fear.

The distinction between expectancies and set goals is also important in evaluating the claims of helplessness theories of depression, which have from the start confused expectancies of personal control, desires for personal control as a set goal, and desires for personal control as a way of achieving other desired outcomes. From the present perspective, the relationship between depression and personal control or efficacy expectancies can be reformulated as follows. Acute or chronic perceived nonfulfillment of highly valued set goals (such as proximity to a loved one, attainment of a long-standing fantasy or wish, or having friends)—including set goals for the ideal self (such as meeting internal standards for competence, beauty, intelligence, morality, and the like)—will produce negative affects including depression. Consequently, if outcome expectancies for these set goals are low, the person is likely to be vulnerable to depression. If the set goal does not involve competence or control and can be fulfilled without any action on the person's part, then negative competence or efficacy expectancies will have no impact on emotional state. A Republican who wants to see a Republican elected President but has no intrinsic interest in politics may be thrilled to take no part in an election and to find his candidate successful anyway. He may feel inefficacious and incompetent politically, but that makes no difference to him.

Recent reconceptualizations of helplessness theory are becoming more accurate in this regard, but in so doing they are diverging less and less from what most people (and certainly most clinicians) intuitively know about why many people become depressed. Abramson, Metalsky, and Alloy (1988), for example, have recently offered a "hopelessness" reinterpretation of helplessness theory, which states essentially that when bad things happen to people that they cannot control, they are likely to get depressed about them, particularly if they are characterologically susceptible to having negative thoughts about themselves and the world. Once again, however, one must separate the relative roles of control as a set goal and other outcome set goals. If something bad does not happen to a person (i.e., there is no major discrepancy between a highly invested set goal and cognized reality)—it does not make much difference what his or her expectancies of control are, unless, again, this person is one for whom control is terribly important in itself. Similarly, if a loved one dies, a person may be very upset that he or she cannot get the loved one back. However, the upsetting thing is not his or her inefficacy or helplessness per se (violation of an efficacy set goal)—but simply the loved one's absence (violation of an attachment set goal). Depression can be exacerbated if the person's history renders other negative events readily activated in this circumstance, makes other cognitive–evaluative mismatches salient (such as beliefs that the person somehow caused the loss or was not good enough to the loved one when alive), or activates depressive patterns of thought that emphasize discrepancies between wished-for and cognized states (such as negative beliefs about the self).

METHODOLOGICAL IMPLICATIONS

The arguments thus far have methodological implications for social-psychological research on the self. If representations of the self can be inaccessible to consciousness, and if the representations that reach consciousness can be defensively transformed negations of active unconscious self-schemas, then it follows that free-response and self-report methods are not useful for studying representations of the self that involve much evaluative content. Unfortunately, these comprise most representations of self. Reaction time measures of schematicity also become problematic if one acknowledges the existence of psychological conflict, since increased processing time can reflect either a relative lack of schematicity in some domain or emotional conflict regarding some highly schematized dimension of self.

Self-reports about the self are useful in three ways. First, they may provide some insight into the complexity of self-representations, since the complexity of a conscious free-response self-description is likely to bear some relation to the complexity of underlying unconscious schemas. My colleagues and I have obtained some empirical confirmation of this in research showing a significant correlation between complexity of free-response self-descriptions and complexity of representations of others, assessed from Thematic Appreception Test responses and from subjects' descriptions of interpersonal episodes (Leigh, Westen, Barends, & Mendel, 1989).

Second, free-response and questionnaire descriptions of self can be useful if one is interested in conscious self-representations as compromise formations, that is, as manifestations of the way the subject expresses conflicting needs, wishes, and fears in the context of trying to process information about the self in useful and adaptive ways. Self-reports can also be useful in the many instances in which people have relatively easy access to certain self-schemas, although researchers should never assume these to be the most important or motivationally most significant representations of self.

Third, self-reports about the self can be useful when people describe conscious representations that influence consciously guided behavior. McClelland, Weinberger, and colleagues (McClelland, Koestner, & Weinberger, 1989; Weinberger & McClelland, 1990) have marshaled considerable evidence supporting the distinction between two kinds of motives, which they call "self-attributed" (conscious motives, assessed by self-report) and "implicit" (unconscious motives, assessed projectively using instruments such as the Thematic Apperception Test). Each has different behavioral and developmental correlates. Essentially, where the person is exercising conscious control in taking action (or anticipating action, as in many studies of the predictive value of self-reported motives), self-attributed motives are better predictors of behavior. Where the person is not consciously choosing a goal-directed course of action, self-attributed motives contribute very little predictively, and implicit motives are much more predictive. Self-report methods are probably once again studying only a special case, in which conscious attention is directly focused on a consciously selected motive. We are likely in the years ahead to see the demise of serial-processing models of motivation, which assume that conscious decision makers are trying to obtain conscious aims one at a time (or bringing together two or three evaluative considerations simultaneously, as in expectancy–value theories). Conscious motives can be important in overriding, synthesizing, or clarifying unconscious ones, but as in models of parallel distributed processing in cognition, it is likely that at any point in time multiple motives are activated simultaneously and quasi-independently, and they may find compromised expression in the flow of thought and behavior.

The relative roles of self-attributed and implicit or unconscious motives should be obvious to many liberal academics involved in long-term relationships, who find that the male in the relationship does his share of the work and behaves more androgynously when he is deliberately focusing on his conscious ideology about gender roles, but reverts to gender-stereotyped behavior (as may his partner) when he is not thinking about it (or even when he is, as when he and his partner choose to have him continue to work full time after the birth of a baby while the woman adjusts her schedule). The positive and negative affects derived from fulfilling or failing to fulfill consciously held ideals may directly conflict with the fulfillment or lack of fulfillment of unconscious wishes or fears: The woman is such a relationship may feel satisfied and proud of her egalitarian relationship, but may unconsciously feel resentful toward her husband for not being "masculine" enough, or toward herself for not staying home with her child as her mother did. To what extent the processing of information through consciously accessed cognitive–affective schemas leads to changes in parallel processing through affectively imbued schemas developed in childhood is probably the most critical question at the interface of cognition and psychodynamics. It is also critical to understanding the therapeutic action of psychoanalytic and cognitive therapies, both of which attempt to alter or override previously active mental processes. One of the major goals of psychoanalytic forms of treatment is, of course, to help the person consciously schematize aspects of self that were previously only schematized, if at all, unconsciously; concurrently, the aim is to link these conscious representations to affective reactions and unconscious cognitive–affective motivational structures influencing behavior, so that the person can exercise more flexible conscious control over thoughts, feelings, and behavior.

CULTURE, SELF, AND THE ROLE OF TECHNOLOGICAL DEVELOPMENT

This chapter has focused on clinical observation as a window to unconscious and affective aspects of self that need to be integrated with experimental data to provide a more comprehensive view of self than either the consulting room or the laboratory can afford. Before I conclude, it is important to note the import of anthropological data for psychological theories of self as well.

The Wintu example with this chapter began is not atypical of reports from other preindustrial societies. All cultures have ways of representing the self, others, and personality more generally (see Mauss, 1938; Fortes, 1971), and different forms of social organization tend to have different forms of collective representations. From available evidence, it appears that before the rise of agriculture, and in the preagricultural societies that survived until the middle of this century, the self was not conceived as a separate category distinct from nature and society (see Shweder & Bourne, 1984; Westen, 1985).

Psychologists and anthropologists often contrast individualistic and collectivistic cultural orientations (Kluckhohn & Strodtbeck, 1961; Triandis, Bontempo, & Villareal, 1988), with concomitant views of self, and link this to differences between Eastern and Western cultures (for such cultural differences, see Marsella, DeVos, & Hsu, 1985; and Roland, Chapter Nine, this volume). Although there can be little doubt that cultural differences of this sort exist, cultural differences need to be carefully distinguished from the impact of more universal forces such as technological development. Western culture has not always been so individualistic, and rural and more traditional areas of Western countries such as Greece and Southern Italy have been shown by Triandis (Triandis et al., 1988) to resemble rural China in their collectivistic orientation. Baumeister (1987), relying on historical data and literature, has traced the evolution of the concept and experience of self in the West from a much less differentiated and individualistic form in the 11th century to its current shape that is typically contrasted with Eastern selfhood. Westen (1985) has marshaled historical, anthropological, and sociological evidence suggesting that selfhood has changed dramatically since the rise of agriculture and again since the Industrial Revolution in the West, and that this appears ultimately to occur everywhere similar social transformations occur. Indeed, available evidence suggests that technological development is associated with changes in self-structure and value orientations related to individualism in people maximally exposed to "modernizing" forces even in traditionally collectivistic cultures (Westen, 1985; see also evidence cited in Triandis et al., 1988; Triandis, 1989).

Distinguishing the impact of technological development, Westernization, and capitalism on self-structure is no easy task, since the three often occur together in developing countries. Nevertheless, technological development appears to have led to three major changes in self-structure. The first is a heightened differentiation of representations and emphasis on identity elements that are neither shared nor centered on social roles or reference groups, so that members of technologically developed societies or regions may see themselves first and foremost as individuals. The second is an increasing moral valuation of the pursuit of self-interest versus the needs of collectivities, where individual desire or self-definition may be seen as equal or superior goals to the needs of others or of social groups that were once paramount. The third, which is endemic to all periods of rapid social change, is that identity has become a problem that individuals may have to resolve, rather than something that is socially bestowed.

Several factors associated with technological development appear to be implicated in these changes in the experience and valuation of self. For example, geographical mobility no doubt influences all three, since the person may live far away from others whose interests and identities would once have been interlocked with his or her own. Literacy and the technological requisites of specialized learning also psychologically divorce knowledge from its previous social context, permitting and fostering the development of individual knowledge structures separate from traditional and less specialized knowledge. The fact that much of identity is achieved rather than ascribed, and that a man or woman may function occupationally in ways very different from his or her parents and extended family, probably has an impact on self-structure that cannot be overemphasized: When a man is a hunter or farmer like his father, for example, his representations of self and father will probably be highly similar, especially as he steps into the same social position in the same community as his father and grandfather did before him. Roles in such societies manifestly outlive their individual occupants.

Parental expectations of the likelihood that any given child will live may have ramifications for self-development, since parents of children in cultures with low infant mortality may have different attitudes toward the importance of a specific child or the way one invests in each child. Factors such as family size and whether children have their own rooms are likely of importance as well in fostering individualistic versus collectivistic conceptions of self. The presence of collective rituals, such as those emphasizing group solidarity and those that establish a socially bestowed identity in early adolescence, influence the nature of self-representations and identity. Further, as Triandis et al. (1988) observe, universalistic (e.g., monetary) rather than personalistic (e.g., service) exchange, and the presence of numerous ingroups from which to choose in more complex societies, may also foster a more individualistic orientation.

Particularly in periods of rapid change, as in the contemporary Third World, the demise of traditional values, world views, and ways of regulating relationships leads to tremendous difficulties for individuals attempting to form a coherent sense of identity. It may lead as well to defensively polarized representations of the self and of the social world, with people and institutions seen as either supporting or trying to destroy the way of life to which the person is committed. This is exacerbated by the apparent incompetence or seemingly atavistic beliefs and behaviors of parents and traditional leaders in the face of rapid social change. This makes childhood identifications that have been incorporated into all aspects of behavior and self-representation tenuous; these identifications may be intermittently embraced or defended against.

Given our unique historical circumstances, it is no wonder that many object relations theorists in psychoanalysis have come to see individuation as an endpoint of development, or that Kohut has placed the "self" at the center of psychological inquiry, arguing that all psychopathology is to some extent related to problems of narcissism and self-cohesion. It is similarly no wonder that Bandura has placed self-efficacy at center stage in his view of behavioral change, or that contemporary theories of depression stress maladaptive views of personal control and schemas about the self.

None of this is to suggest that these theories are all wrong or should be discarded. Although they are not always framed this way, they represent efforts to describe the nature of human beings at a particular historical epoch—and were developed by theorists who were influenced by the same confluence of socioeconomic, cultural, and historical factors as their subjects and patients. Our scientific theories are themselves individually and socially constructed compromise formations, reflecting a number of things other than the "noumenal" object they hope to describe. We are fundamentally constrained by cultural constructs that seem "natural," as well as by beliefs about ourselves, defenses against ideas that make us uncomfortable, biases imposed by our material interests, biases and limitations imposed by the nature of our information-processing system, and the source of data to which we are privy (clinical or experimental).

There is, unfortunately, no sanctuary to which one can escape for epistemological refuge. The best one can do is to recognize that self-knowledge starts at home: To understand the "self," we must understand ourselves.

REFERENCES

Abelson, R. P. (1981). Psychological status of the script concept. *American Psychologist, 36,* 715–729.

Abramson, L., Metalsky, G., & Alloy, L. (1988). The hopelessness theory of depression: Does the research test the theory? In L. Abramson (Ed.), *Social cognition and clinical psychology: A synthesis* (pp. 33–65). New York: Guilford.

Bandura, A. (1977). Self-efficacy: Toward a unifying theory of behavior change. *Psychological Review, 84,* 191–215.

Bandura, A. (1982). Self-efficacy mechanism in human agency. *American Psychologist, 37,* 122–147.

Bandura, A. (1984). Recycling misconceptions of perceived self-efficacy. *Cognitive Therapy and Research, 8,* 231–255.

Barlow, D. (1988). *Anxiety and its disorders.* New York: Guilford Press.

Baumeister, R. F. (1987). How the self became a problem: A psychological review of historical research. *Journal of Personality and Social Psychology, 52,* 163–176.

Beck, A. T. (1976). *Cognitive therapy and the emotional disorders.* New York: International Universities Press.

Bem, D. J. (1972). Self-perception theory. In L. Berkowitz (Ed.), *Advances in experimental social psychology* (Vol. 6, pp. 1–62). New York: Academic Press.

Bowlby, J. (1969). *Attachment and loss: Vol. 1. Attachment.* New York: Basic Books.

Brenner, C. (1982). *The mind in conflict.* New York: International Universities Press.

Damon, W., & Hart, W. (1988). *Self-understanding in childhood and adolescence.* New York: Cambridge University Press.

Durkheim, E. (1915). *The elementary forms of the religious life.* New York: Free Press.

Ellis, A. (1962). *Reason and emotion in psychotherapy.* New York: Lyle Stuart.

Epstein, S. (1990). Cognitive–experiential self-theory. In L. A. Pervin (Ed.), *Handbook of personality: Theory and research* (pp. 165–192). New York: Guilford Press.

Erikson, E. (1963). *Childhood and society* (2nd ed.). New York: Norton.

Erikson, E. (1968). *Identity: Youth and crisis.* New York: Norton.

Fast, I. (1985). *Event theory.* Hillsdale, Erlbaum.

Fortes, M. (1971). On the concept of the person among the Tallensi. In *La notion de personne en Afrique noire.* Paris: Colloques Internationales.

Freud, S. (1914). On narcissism: An introduction. *Standard Edition, 14,* 67–102. Hogarth.

Geertz, C. (1973). *The interpretation of cultures.* New York: Basic Books.

Greenberg, L. S., & Safran, J. D. (1987). *Emotion in psychotherapy.* New York: Guilford Press.

Greenwald, A. G., & Pratkanis, A. R. (1984). The self. In R. S. Wyer & T. K. Srull (Eds.), *Handbook of social cognition* (Vol. 3, pp. 129–178). Hillsdale, NJ: Erlbaum.

Gurin, P. (1980). *Sense of efficacy: Its dependence on judgments of the self and the world.* Unpublished manuscript, University of Michigan.

Gurin, P., & Epps, E. G. (1975). *Black consciousness, identity, and achievement: A study of students in historically black colleges.* New York: Wiley.

Hauri, P. (1976). Dreams in patients remitted from reactive depression. *Journal of Abnormal Psychology, 32,* 22–28.

Higgins, E. T. (1990). Personality, social psychology, and person–situation relations: Standards and knowledge activation as a common language. In L. A. Pervin (Ed.), *Handbook of personality: Theory and research* (pp. 301–338). New York: Guilford Press.

Hollon, S. D., & Garber, J. (1988). Cognitive therapy. In L. Abramson (Ed.), *Social cognition and clinical psychology: A synthesis* (pp. 204–253). New York: Guilford Press.

Horowitz, M. (1987). *States of mind: Configurational analysis of individual psychology* (2nd ed.). New York: Plenum.

Horowitz, M. J., & Zilberg, N. (1983). Regressive alterations of the self concept. *American Journal of Psychiatry, 140,* 284–289.

James, W. (1890). *The principles of psychology* (2 vols.). New York: Henry Holt.

James, W. (1902). *Varieties of religious experience.* New York: New American Library.

Janoff-Bulman, R. (1989). Assumptive worlds and the stress of traumatic events: Applications of the schema construct. *Social Cognition, 7,* 113–136.

Kernberg, O. (1975). *Borderline conditions and pathological narcissism.* New York: Jason Aronson.

Kihlstrom, J., & Cantor, N. (1983). Mental representations of the self. In L. Berkowitz (Ed.), *Advances in experimental social psychology* (Vol. 5). New York: Academic Press.

Kluckhohn, F., & Strodtbeck, F. (1961). *Variations in value orientations.* Evanston, IL: Row, Peterson.

Kohut, H. (1971). *The analysis of the self: A systematic approach to the treatment of narcissistic personality disorders.* New York: International Universities Press.

Kohut, H. (1977). *The restoration of the self.* New York: International Universities Press.

Kuhn, T. (1970). *The structure of scientific revolutions.* Chicago: University of Chicago Press.

Laing, R. D. (1959). *The divided self.* Harmondsworth, England: Penguin.

Lee, D. (1950). *Freedom and culture.* Englewood Cliffs, NJ: Prentice-Hall.

Leigh, J., Westen, D., Barends, A., & Mendel, M. (1989). *Assessing complexity of representations of people from TAT and interview data.* Unpublished manuscript. Department of Psychology, University of Michigan.

Lewis, M., & Brooks-Gunn, J. (1979). *Social condition and the acquisition of self.* New York: Plenum.

Lifton, R. J. (1963). *Thought reform and the psychology of totalism: A study of "brainwashing" in China.* New York: Norton.

Main, M., Kaplan, N., & Cassidy, J. (1985). Security in infancy, childhood, and adulthood: A move to the level of representation. In I. Bretherton & E. Waters (Eds.), *Growing points of attachment theory and research. Monographs of the Society for Research in Child Development, 50,* 1–2.

Markus, H. (1977). Self-schemata and processing information about the self. *Journal of Personality and Social Psychology, 35,* 63–78.

Markus, H., & Cross, S. (1990). The interpersonal self. In L. A. Pervin (Ed.), *Handbook of personality: Theory and research* (pp. 576–608). New York: Guilford Press.

Markus, M., & Nurius, P. (1986). Possible selves. *American Psychologist, 41,* 954–969.

Marsella, A. J., DeVos, G., & Hsu, F. (Eds.). (1985). *Culture and self: Asian and Western perspectives.* London: Tavistock.

Mauss, M. (1938). A category of the human mind. The notion of person, the notion of "self." In M. Mauss, *Sociology and psychology: Essays* (B. Brewster, Trans.). London: Routledge & Kegan Paul.

McClelland, D. C., Koestner, R., & Weinberger, J. (1989). How do self-attributed and implicit motives differ? *Psychological Review, 96,* 690–702.

Miller, J. B. (1986). What do we mean by relationships? *Work in Progress: Stone Center for Developmental Services and Studies, 22*, 1–23.

Mischel, W. (1973). Toward a cognitive social learning reconceptualization of personality. *Psychological Review, 80*, 252–283.

Nelson, K. (1986). *Event knowledge: Structure and function in development.* Hillsdale, NJ: Erlbaum.

Nisbett, R. E., & Wilson, T. D. (1977). Telling more than we can know: Verbal reports on mental processes. *Psychological Review, 84*, 231–259.

Offer, D., Ostrov, E., & Howard, K. I. (1981). *The adolescent: A psychological self-portrait.* New York: Harper & Row.

Rogers, C. (1959). A theory of therapy, personality, and interpersonal relationships, as developed in the client-centered framework. In S. Koch (Ed.), *Psychology: A study of a science* (Vol. 13). New York: McGraw-Hill.

Sandler, J. (1987). *From safety to superego: Selected papers of Joseph Sandler.* New York: Guilford Press.

Sandler, J., & Rosenblatt, B. (1962). The concept of the representational world. *Psychoanalytic Study of the Child, 17*, 128–145.

Shedler, J., Mayman, M., & Manis, M. (1990). *Illusory mental health.* Unpublished manuscript, University of California, Berkeley.

Shweder, R. A., & Bourne, E. J. (1984). Does the concept of the person vary cross-culturally? In R. A. Shweder & R. A. LeVine (Eds.), *Culture theory: Essays on mind, self, and emotion* (pp. 158–199). New York: Cambridge University.

Shweder, R. A., & LeVine, R. A. (Eds.). (1984). *Culture theory: Essays on mind, self, and emotion.* New York: Cambridge University Press.

Stern, D. N. (1985). *The interpersonal world of the infant: A view from psychoanalysis and developmental psychology.* New York: Basic Books.

Swann, W. B. (1987). Identity negotiation: Where two roads meet. *Journal of Personality and Social Psychology, 53*, 1038–1051.

Taylor, S. E., & Brown, J. D. (1988). Illusion and well-being: A social psychological perspective on mental health. *Psychological Bulletin, 103*, 193–210.

Taylor, S. E., & Crocker, J. (1980). Schematic bases of social information processing. In E. T. Higgins, P. M. Herman, & M. P. Zanna (Eds.), *Social cognition: The Ontario Symposium.* Hillsdale, NJ: Erlbaum.

Tesser, A., & Campbell, J. (1983). Self-definition and self-evaluation maintenance. In J. Suls & A. Greenwald (Eds.), *Psychological perspectives on the self* (Vol. 2, pp. 1–31). Hillsdale, NJ: Erlbaum.

Tesser, A., Pilkington, C. J., & McIntosh, W. D. (1989). Self-evaluation maintenance and the mediational role of emotion: The perception of strangers. *Journal of Personality and Social Psychology, 57*, 163–176.

Triandis, H. C. (1989). The self and social behavior in differing cultural contexts. *Psychological Bulletin, 96*, 506–520.

Triandis, H. C., Bontempo, R., & Villareal, M. J. (1988). Individualism and collectivism: Cross-cultural perspectives on self–ingroup relationships. *Journal of Personality and Social Psychology, 54*, 323–338.

Wachtel, P. (1977). *Psychoanalysis and behavior therapy.* New York: Basic Books.

Weinberger, D. (1990). The construct validity of the repressive coping style. In J.

Singer (Ed.), *Repression and dissociation*. Chicago: University of Chicago Press.

Weinberger, J., & McClelland, D. (1990). Cognitive versus traditional motivational models: Irreconcilable or complementary? In E. T. Higgins & R. M. Sorrentino (Eds.), *Handbook of motivation and cognition: Foundations of social behavior* (Vol. 2). New York: Guilford.

Westen, D. (1985). *Self and society: Narcissism, collectivism, and the development of morals*. New York: Cambridge University Press.

Westen, D. (1986). The superego: A revised developmental model. *Journal of the American Academy of Psychoanalysis, 14*, 181–202.

Westen D. (1987). *A psychodynamic–cognitive–behavioral approach to affect and affect regulation*. Unpublished manuscript, University of Michigan.

Westen, D. (1988). Official and unofficial data. *New Ideas in Psychology, 6*, 323–331.

Westen, D. (1990a). Psychoanalytic approaches to personality. In L. A. Pervin (Ed.), *Handbook of personality: Theory and research* (pp. 21–65). New York: Guilford Press.

Westen, D. (1990b). The relations among narcissism, egocentrism, self-concept, and self-esteem. *Psychoanalysis and Contemporary Thought, 13*, 185–241.

Westen, D. (in press-a). Social cognition and object relations. *Psychological Bulletin*.

Weston, D. (in press-b). The cognitive self and the psychoanalytic self: Can we put our selves together? *Psychological Inquiry*.

Westen, D., Lohr, N., Silk, K., Gold, L., & Kerber, K. (in press). Object relations and social cognition in borderlines, major depressives, and normals: A TAT analysis. *Psychological Assessment: A Journal of Consulting and Clinical Psychology*.

Westen, D., Ludolph, P., Lerner, H., Ruffins, S., & Wiss, C. (1990). Object relations in borderline adolescents. *Journal of the American Academy of Child and Adolescent Psychiatry, 29*, 338–348.

Winnicott, D. W. (1971). *Playing and reality*. New York: Basic Books.

PART FOUR

Integrative Approaches from Social and Personality Psychology

In the first chapter in this section, McNulty and Swann consider self-verification and self-concept changes. Given the tendency of people to choose friends and intimates who confirm their maladaptive self-views, these authors raise the question of how psychotherapy can hope to change behavior and self-conceptions without working with clients' social infrastructure. McNulty and Swann argue that therapists must address the interpersonal as well as intrapsychic antecedents of self-verifications, but suggest that therapists can focus clients' self-verification tendencies on strengths instead of weaknesses.

In Chapter Twelve, Baumeister provides an overview of people's attempts to escape self-awareness. He argues that people do so in order (1) to avoid the aversive emotions resulting from their faults or inadequacies; (2) to experience positive euphoric states such as love, mystical ecstasy, and flow; and (3) to avoid the stresses of modern life. He views masochism and suicide as means of escaping the self.

Tesser, in Chapter Thirteen, compares his model of self-esteem maintenance with Kohut's self psychology. Although the terms Tesser uses might suggest a different pairing of concepts, Tesser notes the similarities and differences between his "comparison" and Kohut's "mirroring" process, and between his "reflection" and Kohut's "idealization" process. According to Tesser's line of reasoning, poor self-evaluations do not necessarily come from a faulty self or faulty development, but may emanate from the environment or an individual's perception of the environment.

Ogilvie and Ashmore's research regarding "self-with-other" representations exemplifies the use of a self-report technique that can illuminate nonconscious hierarchical categories of the self-concept. Another advantage of their approach is that it elucidates changes and similarities in self-representations across relationships. Their research is an illustration of a promising type of inquiry resulting from consideration of both psychoanalytic concepts and situational variables over time.

CHAPTER ELEVEN

Psychotherapy, Self-Concept Change, and Self-Verification

SHAWN E. McNULTY
WILLIAM B. SWANN, JR.

When we undertake to cure a patient, to free him from the symptoms of his malady, he confronts us with a vigorous, tenacious resistance that lasts during the whole time of the treatment. This is so peculiar a fact that we cannot expect much credence for it. . . . Just consider, this patient suffers from his symptoms and causes those about him to suffer with him . . . and yet he struggles, in the very interests of his malady, against one who would help him. How improbable this assertion must sound!

—FREUD (1921, p. 248)

Improbable, perhaps, but the resistance phenomenon has daunted therapists since the time of Freud. Not surprisingly, then, many theorists and practitioners have struggled to lay bare the processes that underlie this phenomenon. The major purpose of this chapter is to present a novel perspective on resistance—one that grows out of recent research and theorizing on self-verification processes. Specifically, we suggest that out of a desire to make their worlds predictable and controllable, people strive to verify and sustain their self-views, even if those self-views are negative. We have devoted much of the chapter to a consideration of the implications of this assumption for the processes through which therapists strive to alter their clients' self-concepts.[1] Before addressing these issues, however, we place our arguments in context by contrasting them with two seemingly antithetical theoretical perspectives: the pleasure principle and self-enhancement theory.

THE PLEASURE PRINCIPLE AND
SELF-ENHANCEMENT PROCESSES

The notion that people work to maximize their outcomes is one of the few basic principles on which all behavioral scientists agree. Freud was among the first to endorse this position by proposing that the "pleasure principle" is the guiding force behind the id, the source of the basic motivations and energy (Freud, 1923). For Freud, the "pleasure" in the pleasure principle is derived from the reduction of unpleasant states of tension caused by basic physiological drives. In this tradition, neo-Freudians (e.g., Horney, 1958; Sullivan, 1953) and ego psychologists alike have accorded the desire to enhance or maximize perceptions of self-worth (i.e., self-enhancement) a central role in psychological functioning (Kohut, 1977; Patton, Connor, & Scott, 1982).

Social and personality psychologists have also clutched the self-enhancement assumption close to their hearts. That is, just as McDougall (1933) referred to self-enhancement as the "master motive," Allport (1955) gave "unabashed self-seeking" an influential role in his theory of personality. More recent, experimentally oriented social psychologists have treated the self-enhancement assumption as axiomatic (e.g., Jones, 1973; Schlenker, 1980). Jones and Pittman (1982), for example, have portrayed people as consummate self-presenters who work to maximize the appraisals of others. Similarly, Tesser and colleagues (Tesser, 1986, 1988; Tesser & Campbell, 1982; see also Chapter Thirteen, this volume) have offered a theoretical model and a wealth of evidence that illuminates some of the strategies through which people maintain positive self-evaluations. Finally, Taylor and Brown (1988) have claimed that self-serving biases and self-enhancing illusions not only are ubiquitous, but are actually conducive to mental health and proper functioning.

The intuitive appeal of the self-enhancement formulation cannot be denied; surely most people do indeed behave in ways that lead them to feel good about themselves and lead others to view them in a positive light. But this view of human nature cannot be complete, because it leaves unexplained one of the most vexing and, from a clinical perspective, important psychological phenomena: the persistence of negative views of the self and self-defeating interpersonal patterns. That is, a simple version of self-enhancement theory would predict that people's estimates of their own abilities and value as persons would continue to increase indefinitely. Yet the clinical literature is replete with case studies of clients with painfully and often unrealistically low estimates of their self-worth, who vigorously resist evidence that they are competent and likable. The pleasure principle and self-enhancement theory may characterize most people most of the time, but something more is needed to offer a complete picture of human motivation and behavior.

SELF-DEFEATING BEHAVIOR AND
SELF-CONSISTENCY STRIVINGS

Freud (1920), of course, came to recognize that the pleasure principle can not accommodate resistance and related phenomena:

> If we take into account observations such as these, based upon behavior in the transference and upon the life-histories of men and women, we shall find courage to assume that there really does exist in the mind a *compulsion to repeat* which overrides the pleasure principle. (p. 22, our italics)

Freud therefore proposed the repetition compulsion in an effort to reconcile evidence of resistance to therapeutic change with his belief that all human behavior is motivated and meaningful. He described the repetition compulsion as a primal striving to repeat old, familiar behavioral patterns that operates in conjunction with, and sometimes in conflict with, the pleasure principle. Unfortunately, Freud offered no explanation for the origins or function of the repetition compulsion; he simply presented it as an irreducible part of the psyche. This failure to articulate the mechanisms underlying the repetition compulsion relegated it to a relabeling of the basic phenomenon rather than an explanation for it. For this reason, the construct has come under fire from members of the psychoanalytic community (e.g., Wachtel & Wachtel, 1986).[2]

Many subsequent theorists have shared Freud's concern with explaining the tendency of people to resist improvements in their self-views and related self-defeating behaviors. Some have attempted to account for behaviors that tend to maintain negative self-views within an expanded version of self-enhancement theory. For example, several theorists have suggested that various self-defeating behavior patterns represent self-enhancement strivings gone awry (e.g., Horney, 1939; Strack & Coyne, 1983; Wachtel & Wachtel, 1986). This "ironic perspective" (Wachtel & Wachtel, 1986) suggests that people do not necessarily want to obtain social feedback that will confirm their negative self-views, but are caught in a vicious circle wherein their typical strategies for seeking positive feedback backfire. We have no doubt that some instances of self-defeating social behavior do indeed represent misguided efforts to elicit favorable reactions. Even so, empirical evidence that people with negative self-conceptions actually *seek* negative feedback (e.g., Swann, Hixon, Stein-Seroussi, & Gilbert, 1990; Swann, Pelham, & Krull, 1989; Swann & Read, 1981a, 1981b; Swann, Wenzlaff, Krull, & Pelham, in press) and flee from relationship partners who have overly favorable appraisals of them (Swann, Pelham, Hixon, & De La Ronde, 1990) indicates that there are some "self-defeating" behaviors that the ironic perspective simply cannot explain.

Other theorists have attempted to explain behaviors that tend to stabilize negative self-views by appealing to a motivational force that is quite independent of self-enhancement: self-consistency strivings. Erikson (1968), although not specifically dealing with resistance to therapeutic change or other self-defeating behaviors, emphasized the need to construct and maintain a self-identity that will insure a sense of continuity of experience over time and across situations. He explicitly granted the ego a crucial role in the maintenance of consistency in self-relevant knowledge structures: "[F]oremost among the complexities of human life is communication on the ego level, where each ego tests all the information received sensorily [sic] and sensually, linguistically and subliminally for the confirmation or negation of its identity" (p. 220). Erickson suggests that the ego's consistency-seeking activities are not limited to passive information processing, but extend to selecting relationship partners who will confirm the ego's identity. He contends, in fact, that the refusal to confirm a person's identity engenders hate and that the affirmation of one's identity is the foundation of love (p. 219).

Andrews (1977, 1989a, 1989b) has offered a more explicit and, in our view, richer account of how self-stability is maintained. His self-confirmation theory suggests that people's existing self-conceptions are integral aspects of a self-perpetuating negative feedback loop (e.g., Powers, 1973). According to Andrews, people's self-conceptions lead them to expect that they will be treated in a consistent fashion. These expectations guide their behavior, which in turn causes their partners to view and treat them in a manner consistent with their self-conceptions. In addition, people's perceptions of other people's behavior typically reinforce their self-conceptions by causing them to see the reactions of others as more compatible with their self-conceptions than is warranted by objective reality. Wachtel (1977) has provided a related account of the interpersonal processes by which people confirm their maladaptive self-conceptions.

We believe that both Erikson's self-identity theory and Andrews's self-confirmation theory offer more plausible accounts of resistance and related phenomena than Freud's repetition compulsion. Nevertheless, both stop short of answering a crucial question: *Why* is consistency and stability in the self so vitally important to human beings? Epstein's (1981, 1985, 1990; see also Chapter Seven, this volume) cognitive–experiential self-theory offers an intriguing response to this question.

Epstein argues that the most basic activity of the human mental system is the construction of theories about the self and the world (Epstein, 1973, 1981). In his cognitive–experiential self-theory, Epstein claims that people possess theories about themselves that are based on their conscious evaluation of their interactions with others, as well as theories that are based on emotionally significant events in their lives. He suggests that people form these self-theories to (1) aid them in finding ways to maximize pleasure and minimize pain; (2) translate the raw experiences of life into a coherent picture of the self; (3) maintain relatedness to others; and (4) enhance self-esteem (Epstein, 1990).

The first and last of these four functions for self-theories essentially define the self-enhancement motive mentioned earlier. The second function, interpreting the data of experience, provides the impetus for maintaining self-stability. That is, if a self-theory, or indeed any conceptual system, is going to fulfill its function of providing a coherent interpretation of reality, it must itself remain stable and consistent. Epstein argues that this need for self-theories to remain stable may in some cases mean perpetuating a negative view of the self, because people frequently prefer such a painful self-theory to the prospect of having no theory at all (Epstein, 1981). For Epstein, then, although stable negative self-views may be aversive at some level, they are preferred over confusion.

Cognitive consistency and balance theories (Aronson, 1968; Festinger, 1957; Heider, 1946, 1958; Lecky, 1945; McGuire, 1960; Secord & Backman, 1965) have also been used to explain self-defeating behavior. Most notably, cognitive dissonance theory (Festinger, 1957) asserted that cognitions that are logically inconsistent produce an aversive state of arousal in the person who holds them. Thus, people are motivated to reduce dissonance by altering or discarding one of the inconsistent cognitions or by constructing a superordinate "justifying" cognition that would subsume them both in a common framework.

Although dissonance theory dominated research in social psychology for many years, it suffers from two limitations as a theoretical explanation of self-destructive behavior. First, like many of the clinical theories reviewed above, cognitive dissonance theory failed to specify the functional significance of consistency. According to dissonance theorists, people sought consistency for its own sake. When researchers began conducting progressively more stringent tests of theory, however, it became apparent that a pristine desire for consistency could not of itself account for the full range of behavior that it was designed to illuminate. Something else, such as perceptions of choice, knowledge of consequences, or ego investment, was necessary to motivate participants to care about consistency (e.g., Abelson, 1983; Aronson, 1968; Cooper & Fazio, 1984; Greenwald & Ronnis, 1978; Jones, 1990).

The second problem with using dissonance theory to explain self-defeating behavior was that theorists and researchers steadfastly resisted taking people's enduring self-conceptions into account. Even when some researchers (Aronson, 1968; Aronson & Carlsmith, 1962) incorporated the self into their theoretical model, they decided to experimentally manipulate people's self-views, rather than examining the chronic self-views that participants brought with them into the laboratory. Aside from the inherent difficulty of attempting to manipulate a person's self-views in the laboratory, this approach made the dubious assumption that people would be highly invested in maintaining the consistency of a negative self-conception that they had just formed. We believe that this assumption was the major factor that led dissonance theorists to conduct demonstrations of self-defeating behavior (e.g., Aronson & Carlsmith, 1962) that proved exceedingly difficult to replicate (e.g., Dipoboye, 1977; Shrauger, 1975). In fact, recent research (Pelham, 1989) has shown that when people are uncertain of negative self-views (as they generally are when they have just formed such self-views), they work to *dis*confirm such views by seeking favorable feedback.

The tendency of dissonance theorists to ignore the chronic self-assessments of people provides a striking contrast to Lecky's (1945) early and extraordinarily inventive consistency theory. Lecky believed that the desire to confirm chronic self-views is *the* fundamental human motive, subsuming self-enhancement strivings and the pleasure principle. Contrary to dissonance researchers, however, Lecky proposed that people's idiosyncratic self-conceptions and life histories provided the raw materials that fueled their consistency strivings. In the latter respect, the theoretical model that is the focus of the remainder of this chapter—self-verification theory—can be viewed as an extension and refinement of Lecky's theory (see also Carson, 1969; Secord & Backman, 1965).

SELF-VERIFICATION THEORY

The self-verification formulation (Swann, 1983, 1987, 1990) assumes that people are motivated to verify their conceptions of self. Unlike many related theories, however, self-verification does not assume that consistency is valued for its own sake. Rather, people desire consistency and stability in their self-views because such stability furthers their goal of predicting and controlling their social environments (e.g., Heider, 1958; Kelly, 1955; Lecky, 1945; Rodin, 1986; Rotter, 1966).

More specifically, stable self-conceptions serve both "epistemic" (intrapsychic) and "pragmatic" (interpersonal) goals. Epistemically, a person's stable self-conceptions provide an anchor in worlds that sometimes change rapidly and unpredictably. The appeal of the familiar and safe is probably nowhere more evident that in the realm of the self. Thus, a man who has a well-defined image of himself as socially unskilled may take comfort in his well-articulated self-knowledge at the same time that it saddens him. Any evidence that he might be wrong in his estimate of his social competence is likely to be threatening to his belief in his ability to construct an accurate and useful picture of the social world. After all, if he does not know himself, what *does* he know?

These epistemic reasons for self-verification are complemented by pragmatic ones. Social interaction is to a large degree based on an implicit assumption that people will remain true to the identities they have "negotiated" with others (e.g., Goffman, 1959; Swann, 1987). As a result, people must make sure that the appraisals that others form of them are ones that they both want to and are able to live up to. Although a socially incompetent man may *want* to be the life of the party, he is apt to believe that he is *unable* to be witty and charming among strangers. Therefore, he should work to insure that his friends and associates recognize his social deficits, so he can rest assured that he will never be placed in an awkward and embarrassing position. He would follow this same logic, of course, even if his social ineptitude were merely self-perceived.

Self-verification theory holds that people use a variety of techniques to validate their self-views. One general approach is to create self-confirmatory opportunity structures (McCall & Simmons, 1966; Swann, 1987, 1990). This strategy is based on the assumptions that the social environments people inhabit are largely of their own making and that people work to construct environments that insure self-verifying feedback. First, people select interaction partners who are likely to confirm their self-conceptions (e.g., Swann, Stein-Seroussi, & Giesler, 1990; Swann, Pelham, et al., 1990; Swann et al., 1989; Swann et al., in press). Second, in any given setting, people display "identity cues" (e.g., the cars they drive, the clothes they wear, the titles they affix to their names) that tell others how they wish to be viewed (see also Goffman, 1959; Schlenker, 1980; Swann, 1983). Finally, once engaged in social interaction, people behave in ways that are designed to elicit self-confirming feedback from their partners (e.g., Curtis & Miller, 1986; Swann & Hill, 1982; Swann & Read, 1981b).

Even when people are not entirely successful in obtaining self-verifying feedback from their social world, they may still be able to verify their self-views. That is, there is considerable evidence that people process social feedback in ways that promote inflated estimates of the extent to which others see them as they see themselves. For example, people selectively attend to self-confirmatory feedback, selectively encode and retrieve it, and interpret it in ways that fit with their self-views (e.g., Shrauger & Lund, 1975; Swann & Read, 1981b; Swann, Griffin, Predmore, & Gaines, 1987).

In large measure, the epistemic and pragmatic consequences associated with failing to self-verify will determine the intensity of self-verification strivings. Thus, for example, people are more likely to verify self-conceptions of which they are relatively certain (e.g., Maracek & Mettee, 1972; Swann, Pelham, & Chidester, 1988; Swann & Ely, 1984; Swann, Pelham, et al., 1990), presumably because the more certain they are, the greater the epistemic and pragmatic threat associated with learning that they are mistaken. Similarly, being in a long-term marital relationship should make people more likely to verify their self-views than being in a dating relationship, because marriage partners tend to be especially credible and apt to discover a fraudulent identity. In support of this idea, Swann, Pelham, et al. (1990) found that married persons displayed more evidence of self-verification strivings than did persons who were dating.

Of greatest relevance here is evidence that people will seek feedback and information about the self that confirms their self-views even when those views are negative. In a series of experiments by Swann and Read (1981b), participants who were either high or low in social self-confidence were presented with two evaluations of their social skills (although participants were led to believe that the evaluations were from two psychology graduate students, in reality they were prepared in advance). One evaluation was relatively positive, and the other was relatively negative. Participants showed a clear preference for the feedback that they expected would confirm their self-conception. Most interestingly, participants with negative self-conceptions paid more attention to the negative feedback, spent more time examining it, and recalled it better than the positive feedback. Moreover, when given an opportunity to look at additional feedback from either a positive or a negative evaluator, participants with negative self-conceptions requested more feedback from an evaluator who harbored negative appraisals of them (Swann, Hixon, et al., 1990). Indeed, in one series of studies (Swann et al., in press), participants with negative self-views preferentially solicited unfavorable feedback even when they had reason to believe that it would make them depressed.[3]

Subsequent research extended these findings. Swann et al. (1989) found that negative self-conception participants preferred to interact with people who had evaluated them negatively. Similarly, Swann et al. (in press) found that highly depressed people (but not mildly dysphoric ones) preferred to interact with negative evaluators rather than positive ones. Depressed persons also behaved in a similar manner in the context of their ongoing relationships. For example, Swann et al. (in press) found that depressed persons were especially inclined to solicit negative feedback from their roommates. Moreover, the more negative feedback they sought, the more likely their partners were to reject them at the end of the semester!

Swann, Pelham, et al. (1990) showed that the tendency for people to prefer self-verifying social feedback influenced their choice of roommates and friends. For example, people with firmly held negative self-views preferred to remain in relationships with college roommates insofar as their appraisals were relatively unfavorable, and to drop roommates to the extent that their appraisals were favorable. Subsidiary analyses helped rule out several alternative explanations of this finding. For example, these effects were *not* due to a tendency for targets in congruent relationships to be more similar to each other or for targets with negative self-views to strive for self-improvement. Follow-up investigations of people involved in friendship relationships and of a group of married couples recruited at a local shopping mall provided further evidence that people with negative self-views tend to steer clear of partners who have favorable appraisals of them and to gravitate toward partners who have unfavorable appraisals of them. Once again, these results were not due to partner similarity or the hope of self-improvement. Nor were they driven by a desire on the part of negative-self-concept individuals to prove their partners' negative assessments wrong or to associate with partners who were seen as highly perceptive.

The implication of the foregoing studies is that people will attempt to surround themselves with friends and associates who view them as they view themselves, even when that means embracing unfavorable evaluators. This tendency is important because once a person with a low opinion of himself or herself has managed to find people to confirm this negative self-view, these people may provide active assistance in preserving his or her self-conceptions. Swann and Predmore (1985) found that participants who lacked social self-confidence and received a favorable evaluation on this dimension subsequently experienced an increase in self-confidence, but not if they had an opportunity to discuss the evaluation with an intimate (a dating partner) who viewed them congruently (i.e., consistently with their self-view). Hence, by entering into relationships with persons who share their negative appraisals of themselves, people enlist accomplices who assure them of a constant supply of self-verifying feedback (see also Wachtel, 1977).

The research reviewed thus far suggests that the desire for self-verification exerts a powerful channeling influence on a wide array of social behaviors. In particular, contrary to self-enhancement theory, people who view themselves negatively actively engage in interaction strategies and biased information processing that stabilize and thus sustain their negative self-conceptions and low self-esteem. Presumably, these same behaviors may account for some instances of resistance in therapy. We hasten to add, however, that this research has yielded two outcomes that support self-enhancement theory. First, although people with negative self-conceptions solicit negative feedback concerning those self-conceptions and view such feedback as more accurate than positive feedback, they are unhappy when they receive negative feedback (Swann et al., 1987; Swann et al., in press). In addition, when people with low self-esteem can solicit favorable feedback without violating their desire for self-verification (e.g., when feedback pertaining to a *strength* is available), they jump at the chance (Swann et al., 1989).

If people with negative self-views want favorable feedback at one level but self-verifying feedback at another, is it tenable to regard their self-verification activities as instances of self-defeating behavior? Consider that Curtis (1989) has defined "self-defeating behavior" as any action that leads to a lower reward–cost ratio than available alternatives. This definition suggests that self-verification strivings should be viewed as self-defeating *if* receiving negative feedback is more costly than receiving nonverifying feedback. Unfortunately, the information required to perform the relevant computation is seldom available. That is, just how costly is the unhappiness brought on by unfavorable feedback or the anxiety theoretically engendered by overly favorable feedback? Until we have answers to such questions, it will be difficult to determine whether it is appropriate to classify the verification of negative self-views as self-destructive.

Such definitional issues aside, the important point here is that people with negative self-conceptions are in an unenviable position. Torn between a desire to obtain favorable, self-enhancing feedback and a competing desire to obtain subjectively accurate, self-verifying feedback, they simply cannot have it both ways. This is why it is important for such persons to seek the help of therapists who will lead them out of the crossfire generated by their competing self-enhancement and self-verification motives.

THERAPY: ELUDING THE CROSSFIRE BETWEEN SELF-ENHANCEMENT AND SELF-VERIFICATION

To the extent that a client's negative feedback seeking is motivated by epistemic and pragmatic concerns, rather than by masochism or psychodynamic conflicts, self-verification theory has several specific implications for therapy. The most obvious way for people with negative self-conceptions to escape from the crossfire between self-enhancement and self-verification is for them to change their self-conceptions. For example, clients who believe erroneously that they are stupid or ugly or dislikable may be encouraged to revise such self-views so that they are able to satisfy their needs for positive and self-verifying feedback simultaneously. To clarify how such changes in self-evaluations might be produced, we present the hypothetical case of Todd K.

Todd seeks therapy because he is experiencing a general sense of failure and low self-esteem. In the initial interview, it becomes clear that Todd recognizes the fact that he is highly intelligent, but dismisses the importance of this trait. What concerns Todd the most is his (self-perceived) inability to make close friends or perform adequately in social interactions. Further complicating the picture is the fact that Todd's family and friends share both of these dysfunctional[4] (from Todd's perspective) attitudes. That is, not only do his primary interaction partners hold a low opinion of "eggheads," but they frequently provide Todd with feedback suggesting that he is not handling himself well socially. This latter feedback is not a deliberate attempt to hurt Todd; it is simply a response to his social behavior, which is characteristically awkward. Todd's social behavior is, in turn, a product of his relative lack of social skills (due to a history of avoiding situations where such skills could be practiced) and his occasional attempts at self-sabotage.

Changing Specific Self-Conceptions

Todd enters the therapeutic relationship with psychological baggage that includes not only his established beliefs about himself, but his established interaction patterns and techniques of self-verification as well. Thus Todd not only will deny assertions by the therapist that he is a socially competent person, but will also attempt to elicit confirmation of his negative belief about his social skills from the therapist. We suspect that this tendency for clients to employ with therapists the same self-verifying interaction strategies that they use outside the therapeutic relationship may partially underlie the phenomenon of transference (Freud, 1912, 1917, 1937; Gill, 1982; Westen, 1988). From the point of view of self-verification theory, it is of paramount importance that the therapist avoid "countertransference" (i.e., falling into the trap of reacting to the client's behavior in a way that provides confirmation of his negative self-conceptions). In fact, the most direct method of attacking a negative self-conception is for the therapist to assume the responsibility of providing positive, nonverifying feedback to the client. Thus, in the case of Todd K., the therapist may attempt to combat Todd's perceptions of social incompetence by giving him feedback on the positive aspects of his communication patterns and interpersonal style.

Of course, there is a problem with all of this, which is that Todd will only take such disconfirming feedback seriously if he views the therapist as a perceptive person. To avoid forfeiting his credibility in the interest of improving Todd's self-view, it may be wise for the therapist to provide some confirmation of Todd's (negative) view of his social skills, at least initially. This will both establish the therapist's competence and trustworthiness in Todd's eyes and diffuse some of the defensiveness that Todd may have adopted in anticipation of challenges to his self-views (Andrews, 1989a, 1989b). For similar reasons, it is important for the therapist to go about challenging the self-conception gently, starting with relatively innocuous questioning and gradually increasing the amount of disconfirming feedback. In fact, the earliest efforts should be aimed at reducing the certainty of Todd's negative self-view rather than directly challenging the self-view. Only after considerable doubt has been introduced should the therapist work to change the self-conception itself.

Throughout this process, the therapist must remain sensitive to the epistemic and pragmatic needs served by the negative self-conception. To minimize resistance, steps should be taken to insure that both sets of concerns are being dealt with within the framework of the newly evolving self-system. On the pragmatic side, the alteration of the client's self-evaluations should be accompanied by efforts to enable him to behave in accordance with his newly positive image. Often this may require the therapist to engage in explicit skills training and behavioral practice sessions (Wachtel, 1977). Attempts to alter the client's negative self-views without providing him with specific information about more effective behaviors may be especially counterproductive. This is because people who experience a pressure to behave differently without clear instructions concerning how to behave tend to fall back on their established behavioral patterns (e.g., Caspi, Bem, & Elder, 1989).

Dealing with the client's epistemic fears of being incapable of forming an accurate assessment of his own traits and abilities poses a stickier problem. There is no way of denying, after all, that Todd *is* being told that he is wrong about the self-conception in question. Perhaps the most useful strategy here would be to help Todd verify other self-conceptions while he is in the process of changing the target self-conception. To this end, the therapist can provide self-verifying feedback on the client's positive self-conceptions and, when necessary, even his other negative self-conceptions (these should be relatively unimportant ones, however). In addition, the therapist may also provide direct verbal assurances designed to bolster Todd's belief that he knows himself.

Another technique at the therapist's disposal is the use of leading questions. Implicit rules of conversation (Grice, 1975) lead people to answer leading questions in a manner that confirms their underlying premises, even when they do not agree with those premises (Snyder & Swann, 1978b; Swann, Giuliano, & Wegner, 1982). For example, a person who is asked, "What would you do to liven up a dull party?" is likely to provide an answer that subtly endorses the premise that he or she *would* do something to liven up a dull party. Most importantly, people not only follow the lead of leading questions; they also tend to modify their beliefs to bring them more into line with the answers they have given (Fazio, Effrein, & Falender, 1981; Bem, 1972). Thus, for instance, an introverted man who says he would start a conga line if he saw a party dying is likely to wind up seeing himself as a bit more extraverted than he did before.

The application of the leading questions technique to psychotherapy is fairly straightforward. In an attempt to alter Todd's negative opinion of his social skills, for example, the therapist may ask Todd some hypothetical questions based on the implicit assumption that he is a socially capable person. A bonus to this technique is that it is sufficiently subtle that respondents will be inclined to attribute their responses to their own personal characteristics, rather than to the questions that constrained their responses. This is important because people who perform behaviors that are incompatible with their existing beliefs or mood states are apt to experience change only insofar as they perceive such behaviors as self-initiated (e.g., Linder, Cooper, & Jones, 1967; Snyder & Swann, 1978a; Wenzlaff & LePage, 1990).

Unfortunately, a simple strategy based on leading questions or disconfirming feedback is unlikely to be effective in modifying the beliefs of clients who are extremely certain of their negative self-views. That is, high certainty has been shown to increase the degree to which people will work to verify a self-conception and resist self-discrepant feedback (Swann & Ely, 1984). Nevertheless, for clients who are highly certain of their self-views, a variation of the leading questions strategy may be effective. In particular, Swann et al. (1988) posed *superattitudinal* leading questions to participants. For example, they asked participants who had conservative sex-role beliefs questions such as "Why do you think men always make better bosses than women?" They found that participants who were highly certain of their beliefs strongly resisted the leading questions—even though the questions merely implied a somewhat more extreme version of their initial beliefs! Moreover, participants resisted these superattitudinal leading questions in the only way available: by providing answers indicating that they were really somewhat *moderate* in their beliefs. This, combined with a tendency for participants to infer their own beliefs from their behavior (e.g., Bem, 1972), caused participants to adopt more liberal beliefs.

One way of applying these findings to therapy with Todd would be for the therapist to ask questions and make comments implying an evaluation of Todd considerably more negative than his own. If Todd is very certain of his self-image, this should provoke a denial that may open the way for positive self-concept change. This technique of circumventing resistance by bringing self-verification motives into the service of change is clearly related to the paradoxical techniques championed by several earlier workers (e.g., Wachtel & Wachtel, 1986; Watzlawick, Weakland, & Fisch, 1974).

Maracek and Mettee (1972) have suggested an alternative strategy for changing highly certain self-conceptions. These researchers found that participants who were low in self-esteem and high in certainty resisted feedback that indicated that they were successfully performing a task, but not if they believed (incorrectly) that the task involved a large component of luck. In fact, participants who were certain of their self-views and who believed that they were lucky actually performed much better at the task when given a chance to engage in it again.[5] Apparently the noncontingent nature of the feedback diminished the extent to which it threatened their (negative) self-views, and they could accordingly benefit from the encouraging and energizing aspects of receiving such feedback.

How can these findings be applied to therapy? One possibility is that therapists could make positive feedback less threatening by convincing their clients that any given success should not be taken seriously and is irrelevant to their self-conceptions. Yet one might ask why a therapist would want to implement a technique that improves performance without altering the associated self-conception. The answer is that there are reasons to believe that positive feedback or success is likely to have a salutary impact on the self, even if it is initially disassociated from the relevant self-conception. First, and perhaps most importantly, noncontingent positive feedback may foster success by encouraging self-derogating persons to engage more frequently in activities that they might otherwise avoid. As such success experiences accumulate, it will become increasingly difficult for clients to maintain the position that they are incapable of performing well. By the time clients recognize the contingency between their actions and the successful outcomes, they are likely to have encountered too much success to dismiss or ignore it easily, and will be forced to modify their self-views accordingly.

Noncontingent successes will also be beneficial because they will encourage clients to engage in activities relevant to the negative self-conception and to benefit from the practice. A client such as Todd K., who has been avoiding interpersonal interactions for a long time, must become actively engaged in the social world to gain the experience and skills necessary to become more comfortable in social situations. Therefore, anything that could encourage Todd to get out and meet people may prove valuable, even if he attributes his success to good luck in the beginning.

As effective as the foregoing strategies may be, a therapeutic approach focused solely on the objective of altering people's specific self-views is inherently limited. For one thing, there are some negative self-views that therapists should *not* alter. For example, convincing dull-witted people that they are contenders for a Nobel prize or uncoordinated people that they should consider trying out for the Olympics will not help them and may be highly disadvantageous. In addition, when people with low global self-esteem encounter favorable feedback pertaining to a particular negative self-conception, they may attempt to compensate by seeking evidence to support other negative self-views (that were *not* targeted by the feedback; Swann & Tafarodi, 1990). These data suggest that attempting to improve self-esteem by altering any given self-view will be fruitless if recipients of favorable feedback are bent on maintaining low self-esteem. Finally, changing people's negative self-conceptions without increasing their self-esteem may result in clients who are better able to function in certain specific areas but who continue to experience considerable distress. For these and related reasons, therapists may sometimes need to implement techniques that will help raise their clients' global self-esteem.

Raising Global Self-Esteem

Before suggesting how therapists may bolster self-esteem, we should briefly explain what we mean by "self-esteem" and how specific self-views are related to global self-esteem. William James (1890) was the first psychologist to point out that a single person has a myriad of "selves" or identities. A woman, for example, may think of herself in terms of the roles she occupies (e.g., real estate agent, wife), the groups to which she belongs (e.g., professional organizations, political party), the personality traits that she displays (e.g., extraversion, dominance), the abilities that she possesses (e.g., intelligence, musical talent), on so on. The beliefs that such a woman holds about herself will have a variety of implications, both for her actions in the belief-relevant domains and for her overall sense of self-worth. In the spirit of James, we refer to such cognitive, propositional representations of abilities, traits, and identities as "self-conceptions." Examples of self-conceptions are "I am intelligent," "I am an extravert," and "I am a Republican." Although the theory of self-concept change discussed above could in principle be applied to any type of self-relevant belief, some self-conceptions clearly have more potential significance from a clinical perspective than others. For example, self-conceptions that have evaluative implications for the person characteristically become central concerns in therapy.

The notion of evaluative significance provides the link between specific self-conceptions and self-esteem. "Self-esteem" refers to one's global feelings of self-worth or worthlessness. In one sense, self-esteem can be viewed as a highly abstract, higher-order self-conception (i.e., a person's belief about himself or herself *qua* person). But self-esteem differs from more specific self-conceptions in three important ways. First, self-esteem is more affectively charged than any other self-conception. This is easily seen in our emotional reactions to praise or criticism. Being complimented by a friend on one's wit or skill on the tennis court does not produce nearly the joy that comes from being told that one is an outstanding human being. Likewise, being told that one is not terribly attractive does not have the same crushing impact as learning that one is viewed as having no redeeming value.[6]

Second, both the epistemic and pragmatic stakes are particularly high when it comes to self-esteem. Because people's global self-evaluations subsume their specific views, a change in self-esteem would have the broadest possible implications for the self-system. And global evaluations have far greater pragmatic implications than any piece of specific feedback. The opinion that a woman's friends hold of her athletic prowess, for example, may have consequences for her participation on a softball team, but the opinions they hold of her as a person have consequences for their acceptance or rejection of her across most situations.

Finally, because of its abstract nature, self-esteem poses unique difficulties for a change agent such as a therapist. Whereas a specific negative self-conception might be profitably attacked by giving the client inconsistent feedback and contradictory evidence (e.g., "You seem to be conducting yourself quite competently in this interaction. Perhaps you are not as socially unskilled as you think"), assurances of one's worth as a person are more readily dismissed because global self-views are multiply and complexly determined. Some of the principal determinants of global self-esteem were illuminated by Pelham and Swann (1989).

Pelham and Swann (1989) had a large sample of college students complete Rosenberg's (1965) measure of global self-esteem, some measures of specific self-conceptions, and a measure of the tendency to experience positive and negative affective states (Watson, Clark, & Tellegen, 1988). The self-conception measure asked the respondents to rate themselves relative to other college students on 10 specific attributes. In addition, respondents also indicated how certain they were of their self-conceptions and how important each attribute was to them. A regression analysis revealed that each of these variables made an independent contribution to the respondents' self-esteem. Positive affectivity was associated with high self-esteem, and negative affectivity was associated with low self-esteem. Furthermore, an abundance of positive self-conceptions was associated with high self-esteem. This relationship was qualified, however, by the certainty and importance of the specific self-conceptions, in that specific self-conceptions were more likely to influence self-esteem when they were high in both certainty and importance. That is, beliefs about the self that were held with a great deal of hesitation or doubt were unlikely to be intimately linked with a person's self-system. Likewise, abilities or deficits that seemed trivial or unimportant to the person possessing them were not seen as having many implications for self-worth.

An intriguing finding from this same investigation concerned those participants who possessed a large number of negative self-conceptions. For these people, the self-perceived importance of their most positive attribute was highly correlated (.61) with self-esteem, provided that they were relatively certain of the positive attribute. Thus, having even one positive attribute may enable a person to maintain a somewhat positive self-view, as long as the person is able to convince himself or herself of the value of the attribute.

What implications does this research have for therapeutic efforts to improve self-esteem? More specifically, how might Todd K.'s therapist go about altering his general sense of failure and worthlessness? Given the relationship between self-conceptions and self-worth, a useful approach in many cases would be to raise self-esteem by changing as many of Todd's negative self-conceptions as possible, using the techniques suggested in the preceding section of this chapter.

Another approach would involve altering the *evaluative significance* of Todd's self-conceptions. Insofar as people's self-esteem is related to both the certainty with which self-conceptions are held and the importance that is accorded to them (Pelham & Swann, 1989), it should be possible to increase self-esteem by maximizing the certainty and importance of the client's positive self-conceptions and minimizing the certainty and importance of his negative self-conceptions. Thus, for example, increasing the certainty of Todd's positive self-conceptions would involve affirming his abilities and positive traits (e.g., intelligence). The therapist could also point to evidence supporting these self-views that Todd may have given little weight to or overlooked. In similar fashion, the therapist could introduce uncertainty into Todd's negative self-conceptions (e.g., social incompetence) by providing him with disconforming feedback and drawing attention to contradictory evidence from his life.

Increasing the perceived importance of Todd's positive self-conceptions could be accomplished in several different ways. First, the therapist could point out the practical significance of his positive attributes and elaborate on what they enable him to do. Second, he could emphasize Todd's uniqueness by pointing out that not everyone possesses Todd's gifts. Finally, the therapist might recommend that Todd become involved with certain groups or activities where his positive attributes would be more valued. Although completely changing one's social environment is rarely an option, exposure to other reference groups can be invaluable in reinterpreting one's strengths and weaknesses. It is probable, for example, that Todd would experience a substantial gain in self-esteem if he were to enter a social environment where his intelligence was seen as a valuable commodity. Naturally, the techniques for lowering the perceived importance of negative self-evaluations are the inverse of those used for elevating importance.

These two general strategies—changing negative self-conceptions and changing the way self-conceptions are framed—are clearly complementary. Indeed, the processes of changing the self-conception or lowering its certainty, although conceptually distinct, are difficult to discriminate in practice. A more unified account of these processes would include a phase wherein the certainty of a negative self-conception is progressively lowered until the self-conception actually becomes positive, followed by a phase in which the client's confidence in this newly positive self-conception is gradually bolstered. In principle, the therapist can increase the perceived importance of positive self-conceptions at any point in the sequence. Nevertheless, it may be advisable to refrain from stressing the importance of a particular domain until after a positive self-conception has been firmly established, since clients will be more inclined to resist changes to important self-conceptions.

Making Intrapsychic Changes Stick: The Role of the Social Environment

A client's interpersonal environment can pose considerable difficulties for the therapist. In the case of Todd K., for example, his family and friends share his view that the one thing he is good at (intellectual matters) is not terribly important. Moreover, they have provided him with signals (based both on his actual behavior and on their expectations of him) that he is deficient in the highly valued arena of social skills. In this case, any effort to convince Todd that his one saving grace is indeed a laudable characteristic is certain to meet with resistance from the important people in his life. Likewise, unsophisticated efforts to improve Todd's negative self-view in areas in which there are obvious deficiencies will fail because of the negative expectations of others.

Such considerations illustrate that people with negative self-views are not just suffering from an intrapsychic conflict. Rather, their maladaptive self-conceptions have become externalized into the worlds in which they live—worlds that now validate and sustain their negative self-views (Andrews, 1989a, 1989b; Swann & Predmore, 1985; Wachtel, 1977). Any attempt to alter such self-conceptions must recognize that resistance to change is likely to come not only from the client, but from the client's friends and intimates as well (e.g., Wachtel & Wachtel, 1986). For this reason, any attempt to produce lasting change must enlist the help of the client's primary interaction partners in validating and sustaining the new self-conceptions.

In many respects, the dilemma faced by therapists is similar to that faced by religious groups who seek to change the beliefs of potential converts (Swann, 1983). Studies of such groups have shown that belief change tends to be permanent only insofar as the initial change attempt is supported by a religious community that sustains the converts' newly formed belief system (e.g., Berger & Luckman, 1966). The creation of such a social infrastructure is emphasized by some religious groups to the point of actually removing new converts from their usual environment and seeing to it that they only come into contact with believers during the "indoctrination" period.

In light of the powerful social forces that may undermine desired changes in self-conceptions, it is tempting to conclude that all therapy should be family therapy. Although a family systems approach is necessary in some cases, there are a variety of ways to integrate systemic or interpersonal techniques into an individual therapy session (Wachtel & Wachtel, 1986). At a minimum, the therapist should attempt to gain some insight into *how* clients' interaction partners support their self-conceptions. Bringing clients to recognize these interpersonal mechanisms may enable them to find ways of circumventing, altering, or nullifying these mechanisms; at the very least, heightened awareness may give them new ways of categorizing and discounting negative feedback. For example, once he understands the specific aspects of his behavior that tend to elicit negative social evaluations, Todd will be better equipped to break the self-verification cycle playing itself out in his social world. Even if Todd were able to completely eliminate his socially awkward behaviors through skills training and practice, however, he would probably continue to receive negative feedback for some time, because of the distorting properties of others' expectations of him. Knowing this will help Todd to discount such "residual" negative feedback when he receives it.

In some cases, it may be helpful for the therapist to meet the significant people in a client's life (Wachtel & Wachtel, 1986). Such meetings may not only help the therapist understand the self-verifying patterns at work in the client's social milieu; they may also be opportunities to modify the social environment by involving family and friends in the therapeutic process. The overall goal of such modifications is to prepare these people to alter their behavior patterns "in sync" with changes in the client's interpersonal behavior and self-conceptions.

Specific goals would include discussing with family members the nature and extent of the changes the therapist hopes to effect in the client's self-views; the specific behavioral changes they might expect to see as a result of improvements in these self-conceptions; and the necessity of making changes in their expectations of, and behavior toward, the client. For the family and friends of Todd K., an important goal would be to convince them that they have played an unwitting but influential role in maintaining Todd's negative views of himself and that they can play an equally influential role in improving his emotional health. Another goal may be to impress upon them the importance of viewing Todd in terms of his strengths rather than his weaknesses. Finally, the therapist may want to warn Todd's loved ones that Todd's transformation into a socially adept person will not be instantaneous and that his first efforts at acting out his new self-view are likely to be halting and clumsy. Such a warning may prevent Todd's early attempts at verifying his positive self-conception from initiating a feedback loop that would trap him once again in the self-verifying cycle that he is seeking to escape.

SUMMARY AND CONCLUSIONS

The question of why people stubbornly cling to negative views of themselves that cause them obvious pain is a vital one for theorists and psychotherapists alike. In this chapter, we have suggested that people cling to their negative self-conceptions for the same reason they cling to their positive self-conceptions: because having stable and reliable self-knowledge affords a sense of epistemic security, as well as the practical benefits associated with living in a predictable social world. But for people with negative self-evaluations, predictability and control may be purchased at the price of low self-esteem and emotional distress.

In the broad view, the goal of psychotherapy with such clients is not to convince them to eschew the pursuit of self-verification, but rather to change the manner in which their self-verification strivings gain expression. This may mean changing specific self-conceptions or altering the focus of self-verification strategies from weaknesses to strengths. In either case, any permanent solution to the clients' difficulties must also address the interpersonal as well as intrapsychic antecedents of self-verification by helping to introduce change in the clients' social behavior and environment. Clearly, the efficacy of such efforts will hinge on a recognition that the tendency of people with negative self-views to resist self-concept change is the product of a characteristically adaptive propensity for self-verification. The ability of therapists to help such clients balance their self-verification strivings with their self-enhancement strivings may well be a key to the success of therapy.

NOTES

1. We claim only that our framework offers *one* window on resistance phenomena—a window that lends insight into the cognitive origins of resistance. We view approaches that emphasize the affective antecedents of resistance as complementary to our own.

2. Ultimately, Freud himself realized the inadequacy of the repetition compulsion as an explanatory construct. The solution he proposed was to attribute the repetition of maladaptive behaviors to a death instinct. Perhaps because of the rather

intuitive assumption that all instincts must have adaptive value, the concept of the death instinct has never been very influential in psychoanalytic thought.

3. In our discussion of these and similar experiments, results are reported in terms of what participants with low self-esteem or negative self-conceptions did. Unless otherwise indicated, the results for positive self-conception participants may be assumed to be symmetrical (i.e., where negative self-conception participants solicited *negative* feedback, positive self-conception subjects solicited *positive* feedback). The behavior of people with positive self-conceptions has fewer implications for clinical populations and is of less theoretical interest, since both self-enhancement and self-verification models would predict that they should seek positive feedback.

4. "Dysfunctional" here refers to a self-conception or belief that results in low self-esteem or causes the client distress. Thus Todd's discounting of his intelligence may be considered dysfunctional, whether or not it interferes with his daily life.

5. Participants who were uncertain of their low self-esteem responded better to positive feedback if they believed that it reflected skill.

6. This is true only if the feedback on global and specific self-views is matched for credibility. Feedback concerning one's overall worth as a person is typically relatively vague and subjective, and thus easier to dismiss than feedback about specific traits or abilities.

REFERENCES

Abelson, R. P. (1983). Whatever became of consistency theory? *Personality and Social Psychology Bulletin, 9,* 37–54.

Allport, G. W. (1955). *Becoming.* New Haven, CT: Yale University Press.

Andrews, J. D. W. (1977). Personal change and intervention style. *Journal of Humanistic Psychology, 17,* 41–63.

Andrews, J. D. W. (1989a). Psychotherapy of depression: A self-confirmation model. *Psychological Review, 96,* 576–607.

Andrews, J. D. W. (1989b). *Interpersonal self-confirmation and challenge psychotherapy.* Unpublished manuscript, University of California at San Diego.

Aronson, E. (1968). A theory of cognitive dissonance: A current perspective. In L. Berkowitz (Ed.), *Advances in experimental social psychology* (Vol. 4, pp. 1–34). New York: Academic Press.

Aronson, E., & Carlsmith, J. M. (1962). Performance expectancy as a determinant of actual performance. *Journal of Abnormal and Social Psychology, 65,* 178–182.

Bem, D. J. (1972). Self-perception theory. In L. Berkowitz (Ed.), *Advances in experimental social psychology* (Vol. 6, pp. 1–62). New York: Academic Press.

Berger, P. L., & Luckman, T. (1966). *The social construction of reality.* Garden City, NY: Doubleday/Anchor.

Carson, R. C. (1969). *Interaction concepts of personality.* Chicago: Aldine.

Caspi, A., Bem, D. J., & Elder, G. H., Jr. (1989). Continuities and consequences of interactional styles across the life course. *Journal of Personality and Social Psychology, 57,* 375–406.

Cooper, J., & Fazio, R. H. (1984). A new look at dissonance theory. In L. Berkowitz (Ed.), *Advances in experimental social psychology* (Vol. 17, pp. 229–266). New York: Academic Press.

Curtis, R. C. (1989). Choosing to suffer or to . . . ? Empirical studies and clinical theories of masochism. In R. C. Curtis (Ed.), *Self-defeating behavior: Experimental research, clinical impressions and practical implications* (pp. 189–210). New York: Plenum Press.

Curtis, R. C., & Miller, K. (1986). Believing another likes or dislikes you: Behavior making the beliefs come true. *Journal of Personality and Social Psychology, 51,* 284–290.

Dipoboye, R. L. (1977). A critical review of Korman's self-consistency theory of work motivation and occupational choice. *Organizational Behavior and Human Performance, 18,* 108–126.

Epstein, S. (1973). The self-concept revisited: Or a theory of a theory. *American Psychologist, 28,* 404–416.

Epstein, S. (1981). The unity principle versus the reality and pleasure principles, or the tale of the scorpion and the frog. In M. D. Lynch, A. A. Norme-Hebeisen, & K. J. Gergen (Eds.), *Self-concept: Advances in theory and research* (pp. 27–37). Cambridge, MA: Ballinger.

Epstein, S. (1985). The implications of cognitive–experiential self-theory for research in social psychology and personality. *Journal for the Theory of Social Behavior, 15,* 282–309.

Epstein, S. (1990). Cognitive–experiential self-theory. In L. A. Pervin (Ed.), *Handbook of personality: Theory and research* (pp. 165–192). New York: Guilford Press.

Erikson, E. (1968). *Identity: Youth and crisis.* New York: Norton.

Fazio, R. H., Effrein, E. A., & Falender, V. J. (1981). Self-perceptions following social interaction. *Journal of Personality and Social Psychology, 41,* 232–242.

Festinger, L. (1957). *A theory of cognitive dissonance.* Evanston, IL: Row, Peterson.

Freud, S. (1912). The dynamics of transference. *Standard Edition, 12,* 97–108.

Freud, S. (1917). *Introductory lectures on psychoanalysis.* New York: Norton, 1977.

Freud, S. (1920). Beyond the pleasure principle. *Standard Edition, 18,* 3–64.

Freud, S. (1921). *A general introduction to psychoanalysis.* New York: Boni & Liveright.

Freud, S. (1923). The ego and the id. *Standard Edition, 19,* 3–66.

Freud, S. (1937). Analysis terminable and interminable. *Standard Edition, 23,* 209–253.

Gill, M. (1982). *The analysis of transference: Vol. 1. Theory and technique.* New York: International Universities Press.

Goffman, E. (1959). *The presentation of self in everyday life.* Garden City, NY: Doubleday/Anchor.

Greenwald, A. G., & Ronnis, D. L. (1978). Twenty years of cognitive dissonance: Case study of the evolution of a theory. *Psychological Review, 85,* 53–57.

Grice, H. P. (1975). Logic in conversation. In P. Cole & J. L. Morgan (Eds.), *Syntax and semantics* (Vol. 3, pp. 41–58). New York: Academic Press.

Heider, F. (1946). Attitudes and cognitive organization. *Journal of Psychology, 21,* 107–112.

Heider, F. (1958). *The psychology of interpersonal relations*. New York: Wiley.

Horney, K. (1939). *New ways in psychoanalysis*. New York: Norton.

Horney, K. (1958). *Neurosis and human growth*. New York: Norton.

James, W. (1890). *The principles of psychology* (2 vols.). New York: Henry Holt.

Jones, E. E. (1990). *Interpersonal perception*. San Francisco: W. H. Freeman.

Jones, E. E., & Pittman, T. S. (1982). Toward a general theory of strategic self-presentation. In J. Suls (Ed.), *Psychological perspectives on the self* (Vol. 1, pp. 231–262). Hillsdale, NJ: Erlbaum.

Jones, S. C. (1973). Self and interpersonal evaluations: Esteem theories versus consistency theories. *Psychological Bulletin, 79,* 185–199.

Kelly, G. A. (1955). *The psychology of personal constructs*. New York: Norton.

Kohut, H. (1977). *The restoration of the self*. New York: International Universities Press.

Lecky, P. (1945). *Self-consistency: A theory of personality*. New York: Island Press.

Linder, D. E., Cooper, J., & Jones, E. E. (1967). Decision freedom as a determinant of the role of incentive magnitude in attitude change. *Journal of Personality and Social Psychology, 6,* 245–254.

Maracek, J., & Mettee, D. R. (1972). Avoidance of continued success as a function of self-esteem, level of esteem certainty, and responsibility for success. *Journal of Personality and Social Psychology, 22,* 90–107.

McCall, G. J., & Simmons, J. L. (1966). *Identities and interactions: An examination of human associations in everyday life*. New York: Free Press.

McDougall, W. (1933). *The energies of men: A study of the fundamentals of dynamic psychology*. New York: Scribner.

McGuire, W. J. (1960). Cognitive consistency and attitude change. *Journal of Abnormal and Social Psychology, 60,* 345–353.

Patton, M. J., Connor, G. E., & Scott, K. J. (1982). Kohut's psychology of the self: Theory and measures of counseling outcome. *Journal of Counseling Psychology, 24,* 268–282.

Pelham, B. W. (1989). *On confidence and consequence: The certainty and importance of self-knowledge*. Unpublished doctoral dissertation, University of Texas at Austin.

Pelham, B. W., & Swann, W. B., Jr. (1989). From self-conceptions to self-worth: On the sources and structure of global self-esteem. *Journal of Personality and Social Psychology, 57,* 672–680.

Powers, W. T. (1973). *Behavior: The control of perception*. Chicago: Aldine.

Rodin, J. (1986). Aging and health: Effects of the sense of control. *Science, 233,* 1271–1276.

Rosenberg, M. (1965). *Society and the adolescent self-image*. Princeton, NJ: Princeton University Press.

Rotter, J. B. (1966). Generalized expectancies for internal versus external control of reinforcement. *Psychological Monographs, 80* (1, Whole No. 609).

Schlenker, B. R. (1980). *Impression management*. Belmont, CA: Wadsworth.

Secord, P. F., & Backman, C. W. (1965). An interpersonal approach to personality. In B. Maher (Ed.), *Progress in experimental personality research* (Vol. 2, pp. 91–125). New York: Academic Press.

Shrauger, J. S. (1975). Responses to evaluation as a function of initial self-perceptions. *Psychological Bulletin, 82*, 581–596.

Shrauger, J. S., & Lund, A. (1975). Self-evaluation and reactions to evaluations from others. *Journal of Personality, 43*, 94–108.

Snyder, M., & Swann, W. B., Jr. (1978a). Behavioral confirmation in social interaction: From social perception to social reality. *Journal of Experimental Social Psychology, 14*, 148–162.

Snyder, M., & Swann, W. B., Jr. (1978b). Hypothesis testing processes in social interaction. *Journal of Personality and Social Psychology, 36*, 1202–1212.

Strack, S., & Coyne, J. C. (1983). Social confirmation of dysphoria: Shared and private reactions. *Journal of Personality and Social Psychology, 44*, 798–806.

Sullivan, H. S. (1953). *The interpersonal theory of psychiatry*. New York: Norton.

Swann, W. B., Jr. (1983). Self-verification: Bringing social reality into harmony with the self. In J. Suls & A. G. Greenwald (Eds.), *Psychological perspectives on the self* (Vol. 2, pp. 33–66). Hillsdale, NJ: Erlbaum.

Swann, W. B., Jr. (1987). Identity negotiation: Where two roads meet. *Journal of Personality and Social Psychology, 53*, 1038–1051.

Swann, W. B., Jr. (1990). To be adored or to be known? The interplay of self-enhancement and self-verification. In R. M. Sorrentino & E. T. Higgins (Eds.), *Handbook of motivation and cognition: Foundations of social behavior* (Vol. 2, pp. 408–448). New York: Guilford Press.

Swann, W. B., Jr., & Ely, R. J. (1984). A battle of wills: Self-verification versus behavioral confirmation. *Journal of Personality and Social Psychology, 46*, 1287–1302.

Swann, W. B., Jr., Giuliano, T., & Wegner, D. M. (1982). Where leading questions can lead: The power of conjecture in social interaction. *Journal of Personality and Social Psychology, 42*, 1025–1035.

Swann, W. B., Jr., Griffin, J. J., Predmore, S., & Gaines, B. (1987). The cognitive–affective crossfire: When self-consistency confronts self-enhancement. *Journal of Personality and Social Psychology, 52*, 881–889.

Swann, W. B., Jr., & Hill, C. A. (1982). When our identities are mistaken: Reaffirming self-conceptions through social interaction. *Journal of Personality and Social Psychology, 43*, 59–66.

Swann, W. B., Jr., Hixon, J. G., Stein-Seroussi, A., & Gilbert, D. T. (1990). The fleeting gleam of praise: Behavioral reactions to self-relevant feedback. *Journal of Personality and Social Psychology, 59*, 17–26.

Swann, W. B., Jr., Pelham, B. W., & Chidester, T. (1988). Change through paradox: Using self-verification to alter beliefs. *Journal of Personality and Social Psychology, 54*, 268–273.

Swann, W. B., Jr., Pelham, B. W., Hixon, J. G., & De La Ronde, C. (1990). *The self-concept and preference for relationship partners*. Manuscript submitted for publication.

Swann, W. B., Jr., Pelham, B. W., & Krull, D. S. (1989). Agreeable fancy or disagreeable truth? Reconciling self-enhancement and self-verification. *Journal of Personality and Social Psychology, 57*, 782–791.

Swann, W. B., Jr., & Predmore, S. C. (1985). Intimates as agents of social support: Sources of consolation or despair? *Journal of Personality and Social Psychology, 49*, 1609–1617.

Swann, W. B., Jr., & Read, S. J. (1981a). Acquiring self-knowledge: The search for feedback that fits. *Journal of Personality and Social Psychology, 41,* 1119–1128.

Swann, W. B., Jr., & Read, S. J. (1981b). Self-verification processes: How we sustain our self-conceptions. *Journal of Experimental Social Psychology, 17,* 351–372.

Swann, W. B., Jr., Stein-Seroussi, & Giesler, B. (1990). *Why people self-verify.* Manuscript submitted for publication.

Swann, W. B., Jr., & Tafarodi, R. W. (1990). *Embracing criticism in the wake of praise: Compensatory self-verification among people with negative self-views.* Manuscript in preparation.

Swann, W. B., Jr., Wenzlaff, R. M., Krull, D. S., & Pelham, B. W. (in press). Seeking truth, reaping despair: Depression, self-verification, and selection of relationship partners. *Journal of Abnormal Psychology.*

Taylor, S. E., & Brown, J. D. (1988). Illusion and well being: Some social psychological contributions to a theory of mental health. *Psychological Bulletin, 103,* 193–210.

Tesser, A. (1986). Some effects of self-evaluation maintenance on cognition and action. In R. M. Sorrentino & E. T. Higgins (Eds.), *Handbook of motivation and cognition: Foundations of social behavior* (Vol. 1, pp. 435–464). New York: Guilford Press.

Tesser, A. (1988). Toward a self-evaluation maintenance model of social behavior. In L. Berkowitz (Ed.), *Advances in experimental social psychology* (Vol. 21, pp. 181–227.) New York: Academic Press.

Tesser, A., & Campbell, J. (1982). Self-evaluation maintenance and the perception of friends and strangers. *Journal of Personality, 50,* 261–279.

Wachtel, P. L. (1977). *Psychoanalysis and behavior therapy.* New York: Basic Books.

Wachtel, E. F., & Wachtel, P. L. (1986). *Family dynamics in individual psychotherapy: A guide to clinical strategies.* New York: Guilford Press.

Watson, D., Clark, L. A., & Tellegen, A. (1988). Negative affectivity: The disposition to experience aversive emotional states. *Journal of Personality and Social Psychology, 54,* 1063–1070.

Watzlawick, P., Weakland, J. H., & Fisch, R. (1974). *Change: Principles of problem formation and problem resolution.* New York: Norton.

Wenzlaff, R. M., & LePage, J. P. (1990). *The role of affective–cognitive dissonance in depression and mood change.* Paper presented at the Second Annual Convention of the American Psychological Society, Dallas, TX.

Westen, D. (1988). Transference and information processing. *Clinical Psychology Review, 8,* 161–179.

CHAPTER TWELVE

The Self against Itself:
Escape or Defeat?

ROY F. BAUMEISTER

The purpose of this chapter is to provide an overview of my work on self-defeating behavior and escaping from self. It is centrally concerned with the paradox of self-destructive behavior. People engage in a variety of behaviors that seem inimical to the self, including suicide, masochism, and religious participation (especially meditation aimed at ego dissolution). It seems ironic to find such patterns in a culture that has placed great positive emphasis on the self. Western culture has created and defined the individual self to be regarded as unique, special, entitled to enjoyment of various rights and privileges, and endlessly fascinating. Indeed the self has to some extent replaced divine figures as a source of ultimate moral justifications. Given this emphasis on and fascination with self, why would people engage in self-destructive behavior?

The answer is somewhat complex. First, this chapter covers what is known about self-defeating behaviors among nonclinical groups, based mainly on laboratory work. These studies indicate that people are rarely if ever motivated by a desire to harm or thwart the self; rather, people are often engaged in the pursuit of various benefits, and the risk or harm to self is accepted as a by-product of these benefits, as in a tradeoff. One major class of benefits behind these behavior patterns is escape from self-awareness.

Next, this chapter considers why people would want to escape from self-awareness. Three groups of reasons can be cited: the aversive emotion that results from awareness of the self's faults or inadequacies; the positive euphoric states that sometimes accompany a loss of self-awareness (love, mystical ecstasy, flow); and the stressful nature of modern selfhood per se. Lastly, this chapter takes a direct look at some of the major patterns of escape from self, including suicide and masochism.

ROOTS OF SELF-DEFEATING BEHAVIOR

Why do people engage in self-defeating behaviors? Do they, in fact, engage in them? Clinicians have long observed such patterns in their patients and have hypothesized a variety of causes, including a death instinct, internalized hostility, and a desire to suffer punishment to relieve guilt feelings.

Many of these hypotheses would seemingly apply to people in general (i.e., not just therapy patients or mentally ill individuals). This raises the question of whether normal people do show general patterns of self-defeating behavior. If so, one would expect these to have been studied in experimental social psychology, for social psychologists have long been eager to examine the paradoxical aspects of human behavior.

Steve Scher and I set out to survey the social psychology research literature to find out what is known about self-defeating behavior patterns among normal individuals. We did indeed find quite a few studies showing patterns of this sort. Our review can be briefly summarized as follows (for more details, see Baumeister & Scher, 1988).

Self-defeating behaviors can be sorted into three broad types that differ in the level of intentionality. Obviously, intentional self-destruction is the most paradoxical form, for it requires the person to want to bring harm, failure, or frustration to himself or herself. Thus, the first category may be called "deliberate self-destruction," for it involves cases in which harm to self is the person's primary goal. If the individual's actions are based on foreseeing and desiring harm to self, it seems appropriate to speak of deliberate self-destruction.

At the opposite extreme, people may engage in self-defeating behaviors in which the harm to self is neither desired nor foreseen. In these cases, people do not want to defeat themselves, but their actions lead systematically to that outcome contrary to their goals. This category can be labeled "counterproductive strategies," for it denotes achieving harm to self without any intention of doing so. In a sense, the harm to self is accidental, although for these to be general patterns (capable of being shown in a laboratory study), they must be systematic, regularly occurring accidents.

The third category lies in between the other two. It refers to harm to self that is foreseen but not desired. In such cases, the person can tell (or at least should presumably be able to tell) that a certain course of action could lead to some harm to self, but the person undertakes it anyway. Presumably the reason is that the course of action offers benefits that the person wants very much. The risk of harm to self is thus accepted as the cost that accompanies the benefits. This category can be labeled as "trade-offs," for harm to self is brought about in the course of pursuing various positive consequences.

What, then, did the research literature tell us in that framework? We found ample evidence of many self-defeating behavior patterns, but none of them really fell into the first category (i.e., deliberate self-destruction). There were a few studies suggesting that sometimes people will deliberately choose to suffer, especially studies in which people will volunteer to eat a worm or receive electric shocks (e.g., Comer & Laird, 1975); however, choosing to suffer in these contexts often appears to have certain hidden benefits (such as a belief that it will reduce future suffering; Curtis, Rietdorf, & Ronell, 1980), and so it deserves to be classified as a tradeoff rather than as deliberate self-destruction. There are a few cases in which people will apparently try to fail, or at least not try very hard to succeed, but these appear also to have hidden benefits, such as avoiding the burden of expectations for future performance (Baumgardner & Brownlee, 1987). In short, people to not seem to be substantially motivated to harm themselves, at least not under any conditions that can be reproduced in the laboratory.

One additional comment about deliberate self-destruction deserves mention. Guilt has often been suggested as a motivating factor in self-destructive behavior. It is possible that laboratory studies are generally ineffective at inducing guilt, but at present there is precious little evidence to support the view that guilt motivates people to want to suffer. The hypothesis that guilt motivates self-defeating behavior, such as a wish to suffer punishment, must be regarded as very doubtful at present, based on the lack of laboratory research support for it. Of course, we are not confined to the laboratory here. A look at the criminal justice system provides ample insight into how people act when they are indeed genuinely guilty. The behavior of guilty criminals provides very little support for the view that they desire punishment. In fact, usually they seem to do everything they can to avoid punishment, even if they acknowledge their guilt. They hire lawyers, make plea bargains, appeal sentences, seek probation or parole, and so forth. Arlene Stillwell and I have recently conducted several studies on interpersonal transgressions, including ones that people feel very guilty about, and we have found little evidence of any desire to suffer (e.g., Baumeister, Stillwell, & Wotman, 1990).

I have referred to the middle category of self-defeating behavior as "tradeoffs." Here, people are seeking benefits, and they accept certain costs or risks that accompany these benefits. Many varieties of self-defeating tradeoffs have been demonstrated. Getting drunk may be a paradigmatic example. Alcohol abuse is clearly self-destructive, for it involves damage to the brain and central nervous system; harm to the liver; stress on the digestive system, kidneys, and other bodily parts; and the risk of social embarrassment and even addiction. People clearly engage in alcohol abuse despite these risks. Yet it is apparent that the appeal of alcohol lies not in the harm to self, but rather in the benefits, such as feelings of well-being, reduction in various unpleasant feelings, and willingness to enjoy oneself in an uninhibited fashion. The same could be said of drugs, about which our society is currently so concerned. They do carry significant risks, but people accept these risks because the drugs make them feel good.

There are other tradeoffs. Self-handicapping is an important one. Berglas and Jones (1978) showed that people place obstacles to their own performance in order to achieve attributional benefits: Failure is blamed on the obstacle, and success confers added credit. They suggested alcohol use and underachievement as self-handicapping strategies (Jones & Berglas, 1978). Tice (in press) has recently shown that people with low self-esteem engage in self-handicapping to protect themselves from failure, whereas people with high self-esteem engage in self-handicapping to enhance their credit for success.

Shyness represents a familiar pattern of self-defeating behavior. In the cycle of shyness, the individual fails to approach others or to form relationships because of a fear of rejection, and so the person ends up lonely and unhappy. This cycle represents a tradeoff in which long-term loneliness is suffered in return for immediate freedom from the intense anxiety associated with approaching others. The willingness to sacrifice long-term gains for the sake of short-term safety from painful affective experiences is also apparent with embarrassment: Several studies have shown that people will literally trade off tangible benefits such as money in order to avoid losing face or to repair damage to their public images (Brown, 1968; Brown & Garland, 1971).

Research on health psychology provides one last tradeoff. It is apparent that many people fail to take medicines, keep medical appointments, or otherwise comply with a prescribed regimen of health care (e.g., Sackett & Snow, 1979). Such negligence often contains substantial risks to health, and in some cases failure to comply with medical procedures can lead to death. Research has increasingly shown that the reasons for these low rates of compliance involve short-term benefits, especially freedom from immediate discomfort or pain.

Thus, a variety of patterns of self-defeating behavior fit into the "tradeoff" category. In such patterns, people do sabotage their projects or bring harm to themselves, but that is not their goal. Rather, the harms or risks are accepted as costs of attaining various benefits, such as feeling good and avoiding pain, discomfort, or negative feelings about the self.

The final category of self-defeating behavior is that of counterproductive strategies. People seek a positive goal or outcome, but because of errors in judgment or other miscalculations, they adopt strategies that backfire. Thus, people persist in losing causes or endeavors, with the result that they end up losing all the more. On important performances, they monitor themselves closely, which impairs skilled performance and causes "choking" under pressure (Baumeister, 1984). They adopt bargaining strategies that lead to deadlocks or to nonoptimal outcomes (e.g., Bazerman, 1986), and they adopt ingratiation strategies that backfire (Jones & Wortman, 1973). In short, people are vulnerable to various judgment errors that lead them into maladaptive approaches to their goals.

What, then, can be concluded from this survey of self-destructive patterns? People do engage in a large variety of self-defeating behaviors, but harm to self rarely seems to be the goal. Rather, harm to self is an unforeseen and unwanted outcome of counterproductive strategies, or it is a by-product of the pursuit of appealing, desirable goals.

Many of these goals appear to involve escaping from unpleasant awareness of self—that is, from awareness of the self's shortcomings or inadequacies. Alcohol reduces self-awareness (Hull, 1981), and people consume it in response to failure, in order to help them avoid reflecting on how the failure reflects on self (Hull & Young, 1983; Hull, Young, & Jouriles, 1986). Self-handicapping protects a person from failure's implication that the self is incompetent or inadequate. The shy person's avoidance of others prevents the acutely painful self-awareness associated with interpersonal rejection. Costly revenge-seeking behaviors help one recover from a loss of face (Brown, 1968).

Thus, it appears that many *apparently* self-destructive behaviors are actually motivated by a desire to escape from awareness of the self. People want to forget the self, not to harm it. Understanding why people want to escape from self may provide an important key to understanding many self-defeating patterns.

THE BURDEN OF SELF

Why would people want to forget themselves? Probably there is more than one reason. Three broad classes of reasons can be suggested.

Self as Bad

The first motivation to escape from self has to do with unpleasant awareness of the self's deficiencies and the negative affect that may accompany them. Self-awareness involves comparing oneself against standards (Duval & Wicklund, 1972; Carver & Scheier, 1981), and inevitably people will sometimes fall short of their goals and ambitions. These shortfalls produce unpleasant emotional reactions (Higgins, 1987). People are motivated to avoid or escape from unpleasant emotions, so when events cast the self in a bad light they may become motivated to avoid self-awareness in order to stop the painful emotions (Baumeister, 1990a, 1990b).

Thus, people may escape from self in order to bring an end to an unpleasant state. Experiments have confirmed that people avoid self-focusing cues in response to aversive self-awareness. Situations that motivate people to escape from self-awareness include receiving a bad evaluation (Duval & Wicklund, 1972), receiving an interpersonal rejection or put-down (Gibbons & Wicklund, 1976), having a failure experience (Dixon & Baumeister, in press), learning that one's flaws cannot be ameliorated (Steenbarger & Aderman, 1979), and performing in a counterattitudinal fashion (Greenberg & Musham, 1981).

Ecstasy

The second reason holds that the absence of self-awareness is often a positive, pleasant, desirable state. Indeed, the word "ecstasy" is derived from roots meaning "to stand outside oneself," implying a loss of self-awareness. And, indeed, the removal of the ordinary sense of self is often described as accompanying some of the most powerfully pleasant states people experience, including mystical ecstasy or the bliss of religious experience (as in merging with God); merging with another human being in passionate love; immersion in some activity ("flow"—see Csikszentmihalyi, 1982); and so forth. Evidence also shows that awareness of self can prevent people from enjoying certain experiences. Sex therapists, for example, have long found that people who maintain self-awareness during sexual intercourse have greater difficulty enjoying sex and reaching orgasm (Masters & Johnson, 1970). And the use of alcohol for celebrations is probably attributable in part to its capacity to enable people to forget themselves, which leads them to shed inhibitions and enjoy the events.

Self as Stressor

These first two reasons for escaping from self are fairly specific. Escape from awareness of the self's deficiencies may be limited to circumstances in which events have just cast the self in an unflattering light. Desire to experience an ecstatic loss of self-awareness may be limited to certain individuals or to certain occasions. In contrast, the third motivation may be much more pervasive and common. The third reason holds that the self, especially the complex modern self, is a source of stress, and that escape from self is periodically desirable as a relief from that stress.

To explain how the self is a stressor, let me return to the point that unpleasant emotional states are caused when the self falls short of standards. Higgins (1987) has explicated several different kinds of negative affect that can arise from different types of failures to surpass standards: guilt, anxiety, disappointment, dejection, sadness, depression, and so forth. To have a self with high standards is to be constantly vulnerable to a variety of unpleasant emotional experiences.

True, these shortfalls may only arise on occasion, and even when people fail to reach goals they are apparently adept at avoiding the implications. The unpleasant emotional states may therefore only occur occasionally. But stress research has shown over and over that people can be under great stress even if nothing bad ever happens. Stress resides in the threat of negative outcomes, not their actual occurrence. Stress involves living with the possibility that something bad might happen: It is the anticipation, not the occurrence, of aversive events that creates stress. Indeed, one study of physiological responses to stress found that responses were nearly identical, regardless of whether the likelihood of electric shock was presented as 5%, 50%, or 100% (Monat, Averill, & Lazarus, 1972). People can experience considerable stress just worrying about what might go wrong, even if nothing ever does go wrong.

To have a self, then, is to be constantly vulnerable to negative outcomes and thus to unpleasant emotional states. Selves cause stress to the extent that they are defined in connection with demanding standards and expectations. An important corollary concerns which selves will be most stressful, and hence from which a person is most likely to need escape. That is, the higher the standards associated with the self, the greater the vulnerability to falling short, and hence the greater the stress.

Of course, there are many sorts of standards, but two very major sources must be mentioned. One is the expectations of others. The self exists very substantially in the minds of others (Baumeister, 1982), and people are very concerned with maintaining a favorable image in others' minds. The more these others expect, the greater the danger of falling short. The other source of standards involves the status quo. As adaptation-level theory has taught us, the present is always a basis for comparison for future states and changes. With the self, too, the status quo is always an important baseline. As long as people are improving, they are likely to feel good about themselves even if their absolute level of performance is not especially good, because they are surpassing an important standard—namely, how well they have done in the past. By the same token, if people are doing worse than they have done in the past, they are likely to become upset even if their absolute level of performance is good. In short, selves may cause stress, especially selves that are associated with high standards or some other heavy burden of expectations.

One other finding from stress research is relevant here, and that concerns the time distribution of stress. It is apparent that the subjective effects of stressful circumstances are greatly reduced if there are periods of respite—that is, of freedom from vulnerability. This has been called the "safety signal" hypothesis. Brady's (1958) "executive monkey" experiment attracted considerable attention by proving that it was possible to kill a monkey by making it press a button to avoid electric shock, even though hardly any shocks were actually received by the monkey. Weiss (1971a, 1971b) showed, however, that one extremely stressful feature of the executive monkey's situation was the absence of any feedback except shock. No news was the best news that the executive monkey could receive, and apparently this was a very stressful situation. When Weiss provided his subjects with a tone to indicate successful avoidance, the rate of ulcers declined sharply. The reason was presumably that a subject could relax until the next tone. Similar effects have been found with human beings. Predictable events, even very unpleasant ones, produce much lower levels of stressful and harmful effects than unpredictable events, presumably because a person is able to relax during the safe intervals (e.g., Glass, Singer, & Friedman, 1969).

These findings indicate that what is often most stressful about stressful events is the sense of constant vulnerability, of never being able to relax and feel safe. This can be applied to the self. If one feels constantly vulnerable to falling short of many standards, then one is likely to feel a high degree of stress. This is the burden of self at its worst: constant pressure to live up to high expectations and maintain a highly favorable image of self in the face of unending threats.

But if the person is able to escape from the burden of self, even just briefly and occasionally, the stressful aspects of self are likely to be greatly reduced. Accordingly, brief periods of escape from self-awareness may function like the safety signal in stress research. For a brief time, the person does not have to be striving to sustain an inflated image or to live up to high expectations.

These three motivations for escaping from the self make somewhat different predictions about patterns of escape. The first, involving escape from acute negative feelings about the self, may be most likely to occur after major personal setbacks or failures. The second, involving the pursuit of ecstatic states, may not necessarily be associated with personal crises, but rather may occur in comfortable circumstances among people who have the leisure and motivation to cultivate intense personal satisfactions. The third, involving relief from stress, is likely to show up as chronic or recurring patterns among people whose ordinary lives contain recurrent or constant demands for maintaining a favorable image of self, or contain various and frequent threats to personal esteem.

Cultural and social changes may affect these three reasons differently. For example, the recent shift in Western cultures toward increasing emphasis on selfhood and individuality may have increased the third reason by making the maintenance of a self that much more demanding and stressful. This may be reflected in an increase in masochistic sexuality (see Baumeister, 1988a, 1989) and possibly in an expansion of binge eating (Heatherton & Baumeister, in press).

These three causes are not necessarily rival hypotheses, for they may all operate. If they do indeed all lead to escapist tendencies, then probably people will use a large assortment of behaviors to escape from self-awareness.

VARIETIES OF ESCAPE

Having described the motivations to escape, I now turn to a direct examination of several of the methods people use to escape from self. I begin with two that other theories have often construed in terms of self-defeating motivations—namely, masochism and suicide.

One general theme needs to be explained. It is not easy to turn off self-awareness. Obviously, one cannot monitor one's efforts *not* to attend to oneself, for that would be a paradoxical exercise. Instead of direct suppression (cf. Wegner, Schneider, Carter, & White, 1987), many escapes seem to rely on a strategy of cognitive narrowing—that is, of refusing meaningful thought. The individual focuses narrowly on the here and now, and so broader implications are avoided.

Identity is a set of definitions that tie the person to past and future events, across time and space. If attention is restricted to the immediate present, identity is deconstructed, and the self is reduced to a mere physical body. This is sufficient for most escapes. It is the meaningful aspects of self that are to be escaped, especially the comparison of inferred attributes with important standards—which is obviously a very meaningful calculation. A person who stops comparing stops noticing that he or she falls short. Deconstruction of this sort replaces meaningful action with mere bodily movement (cf. Vallacher & Wegner, 1985, 1987), and it replaces meaningful experience with mere sensation. In the process, emotion is prevented.

Masochism

The term "masochism" was coined by Krafft-Ebing (1922) to refer to a pattern of sexual behavior involving submission to another's will and typically containing acceptance of pain and humiliation. Later theorists used sexual submission as a metaphor and extended the usage of the term to nonsexual patterns of behavior, although these usages have frequently provoked controversy (Franklin, 1987; Caplan, 1984).

Masochism is a highly paradoxical behavior pattern, for it denotes the pursuit of pain, humiliation, and loss of control, all of which seem to contradict psychology's accumulated knowledge about human behavior and the self. To unravel this puzzle, I felt it necessary to return to a close examination of the core phenomena and original form of masochism— namely, sexual masochism. I might add that while doing the research I gradually became persuaded that usages of the term to refer to nonsexual behavior patterns have created more confusion than clarity, as well as offending and possibly stigmatizing individuals; therefore, my recommendation is that the usage of the term "masochism" be restricted to sexual masochism.

The essence of masochism appears to be an escape from self (see Baumeister, 1988a, 1989). Masochism is not self-destructive; in fact, most masochists apparently are extremely careful to avoid any harm or injury, and they seem able to live quite normal and well-adjusted lives. They seek escape, not harm. To understand how masochism provides escape, it is necessary to consider the three main features of masochism: submission or bondage, humiliation, and pain.

Submission, or loss of control, is a common feature of masochism. It often takes the form of being tied up or blindfolded. Masochists also submit to rules, commands, and other infringements on their freedom of action. It becomes impossible for the self to exercise one of its functions—namely, decision, initiative, control. The individual is forced to become passive, and thus the scope of the self is diminished.

Humiliating or embarrassing experiences are common in masochism. They take a wide variety of forms, ranging from insults to symbolic degradations (such as being put on a leash or commanded to kiss someone's feet) to being displayed nude in the presence of fully dressed others. (This is an area in which there are important sex differences; see Baumeister, 1988b, 1989.) This contradicts the esteem-maintaining function of the self, which is one of its most pervasive functions. Identity requires a certain amount of dignity, and masochistic humiliations seem explicitly designed to be incompatible with that. For example, our image of a male U.S. senator is not compatible with his dressing up in women's lingerie and licking a prostitute's feet while she calls him insulting names. These actions simply make that identity radically impossible, so they provide an effective escape from that identity. And, indeed, researchers have found an unusually high frequency of masochistic activity among politicians and other power figures in our nation's capital (see Janus, Bess, & Saltus, 1977). At the time this was surprising, although nowadays it has become very difficult to surprise people about anything regarding the sexual antics of our politicians!

Lastly, masochism involves pain. Masochists use pain in a peculiar way: They strip it of its natural function, which is to warn of injury, and indeed they seem very concerned to receive pain without injury. Limited, safe doses of pain are used as a kind of narcotic. Pain has a powerful capacity to focus the mind on immediate sensations and to prevent abstract thought; pain effectively *deconstructs* the world (see Scarry, 1985). It is thus an important tool in focusing the mind on the here and now. Indeed, masochists often rely on merely the threat of pain, rather than the actual sensation, to accomplish this manipulation of attention. As one woman, who has experienced both dominant and submissive sexuality, describes it, "A whip is a great way to get someone to be here now. They can't look away from it, and they can't think about anything else!" (Califia, 1983, p. 134).

In short, masochism is a set of techniques for escaping from awareness of one's ordinary identity. Most masochists apparently use these experiences as respites from their ordinary, everyday selves, which often seem to be of the more stressful sort. Thus, masochism appears to be more common among the upper classes and among more successful and powerful people than among the downtrodden. (Indeed, being humiliated or subjected to another's will might not be much of an escape for society's real victims.) Janus et al. (1977) pointed out, for example, that politicians' lives are dominated by the constant need to maintain a highly favorable image of self, especially in the public's eyes, despite constant threats from the media or from political opponents who may desire to reduce their esteem. This professionally mandated egotism can become highly stressful, and so the escape of sexual submission may be quite appealing.

Although entering a life of full-time sexual slavery is a common and popular fantasy among masochists, it is very rarely attempted in reality. Masochism remains a temporary respite from identity.

Suicide

Suicide is in many ways the ultimate in self-destructive behaviors, for it does often succeed in destroying the self. Yet research on suicide indicates that escape often seems to be the main goal. The harm to self is often merely a means to achieving escape. Indeed, people often seem to achieve the escape without harming the self, such as in failed suicide attempts.

My research on masochism was hampered by a lack of available data, but suicide more than made up for this; there are literally thousands of publications dealing with suicide. Here I can provide just a cursory overview (for more details, see Baumeister, 1990b).

Suicide is associated with high standards and favorable expectations, and this link accounts for a number of the seeming paradoxes in the suicide literature—particularly evidence that favorable circumstances often produce higher suicide rates than unfavorable circumstances. For example, suicide rates are higher in developed and industrialized countries than in poorer countries; higher in places with better weather; higher in U.S. states with higher standards of living; higher among college students than among people of the same age who are not in college; and so forth. Of course, many unfavorable circumstances are also associated with high suicide rates, such as divorce, job loss, financial catastrophe, and so forth. In general, suicide appears to be most common when customary expectations and standards are high, but recent events fall short of them.

The causal chain leading from these recent disappointments to suicide has multiple steps, as one would expect in view of the fact that most people who experience setbacks and failures do not attempt suicide. The presuicidal process involves attributing the setbacks or failures to oneself, so that the self is seen as guilty or deficient. The person is thus aware of himself or herself in a very painful or aversive fashion (and, indeed, evidence suggests that levels of self-awareness are unusually high among suicidal individuals); this creates various unpleasant emotional states.

To escape from the aversive self-awareness and the associated negative affect, the individual resorts to cognitive narrowing (Baumeister, 1990b; see also Henken, 1976). Action and experience are deconstructed, meaningful thought is avoided, a passive attitude is taken toward all meaningful actions or decisions, and so forth. This deconstructive response also removes inhibitions, for inhibitions are based on meaningful evaluation of potential actions in light of various norms and standards. (The reduction of inhibitions is also apparent in masochism; see Baumeister, 1989.) The person's normal internal restraints against taking extreme actions, including killing himself or herself, are thus disengaged.

Normally, a major setback or trauma is followed by this cognitive narrowing, but then the person finds new sources of meaning to replace them, and life can be resumed. In other words, the normal structure of coping involves deconstruction followed by the construction of new meanings. Suicide attempts occur when the second, constructive phase fails to take place. The deconstruction is accomplished, but the person is unable to replace what has been lost, unable to evolve new definitions of self and world. The individual remains stuck in the narrow, deconstructed state, alternating between a boring and empty awareness of the immediate present, and an acutely painful awareness of the recent failure and its catastrophic implications.

The suicide attempt thus can be seen as an escalation of the person's efforts to escape from the definition of self that has evolved from the recent problems or setbacks. The old self is no longer tenable, and no new definition of self has emerged to replace it. The person can neither let go of the past meanings nor accept them. In such circumstances, the appeal of suicide is mainly oblivion. It is not an aggressive catharsis, or whatever, but rather simply an ultimately effective form of escape. It makes the world stop.

It is worth noting that unsuccessful suicide attempts may often be successful escapes (Baumeister, 1990b). A person who tries to kill himself or herself is typically removed from the life context and setting that caused the problems. The person may be taken to a hospital or other institution; the problems are kept away; family or acquaintances may pay extra attention to the individual and shield the individual from the painful, disturbing circumstances; and so forth. All of this does not really solve any of the problems, but it does temporarily make them go away. And in the cognitively narrow mental state typical of the presuicidal individual, time is restricted to the immediate present, so temporary solutions are sufficient. To the suicidal individual, the short run is all that matters.

Alcohol Use

Alcohol use is an important form of escape. I have already covered it to some extent in the section on self-defeating behaviors. Although alcohol use is literally self-destructive in that it brings harm and risk to the user, it is not ordinarily sought for this self-harmful outcome. Rather, it appears to be sought mainly for its capacity to enable the individual to escape from self-awareness (Hull, 1981).

Alcohol use appears to fit all three of the hypothesized motivations for wanting to escape from self-awareness. Experiences of failure increase people's desire to escape from self-awareness, presumably in order to avoid the unpleasant awareness of the failure's implications about the self. Thus, sometimes alcohol is used to get away from unpleasant self-awareness. At other times, people seem to be positively attracted to the intoxicated state and desire to experience it for its pleasant aspects. Lastly, and perhaps most commonly, many people seem to like to have a drink or two as a means of providing relief from the stress of daily life. In this connection, it is noteworthy that not all forms of stress contribute to alcohol consumption, but only self-related stress (see Hull, 1981; Hershenson, 1965).

Alcohol appears to facilitate cognitive narrowing, or "alcoholic myopia," as Steele and Josephs (1988) have termed it. Abstract and complex thought becomes increasingly difficult as one consumes alcohol, and so attention is refocused on immediate sensations (including the pleasant sensations of drunkenness) and movement. Thus, once again, the complex and meaningful aspects of identity are removed.

Binge Eating

Binge eating is a pattern of behavior that has attracted increasing attention in recent years. Binge eating can be literally self-destructive, in that it carries various medical risks. But it is more specifically self-defeating in the context of the individual's efforts to lose weight. Most binge eaters are dieters concerned with becoming slimmer, and episodes of binge eating make it much harder to achieve that goal.

Still, a sizable amount of evidence fits the view that binge eating, too, is often a form of escape from self (see Heatherton & Baumeister, in press, for a review). Binge eaters suffer from high standards and expectations; in particular, they are acutely sensitive to what they perceive as the very high expectations of others. These include expectations for thinness, as well as expectations for superior performance in work and school. Indeed, evidence indicates that bulimia occurs most frequently among high-achieving women (Barnett, 1986), and bulimics are unusually likely to have unrealistic expectations for performance and achievement (Butterfield & Leclair, 1988). Inevitably, they sometimes fall short of these standards, and the result is a sharply painful awareness of self as deficient. Bulimics, obese individuals, and dieters are well known for having low self-esteem and unfavorable body images (see Heatherton & Baumeister, in press, for a review), and there is even evidence that dieters with low self-esteem are more likely to engage in binge eating than are dieters with high self-esteem (Polivy, Heatherton, & Herman, 1988). Dieting has been shown to correlate with high self-awareness, especially public self-awareness (Blanchard & Frost, 1983).

These painful recognitions of the self's shortcomings are often accompanied by emotional distress, including depression and anxiety. To escape from these unpleasant states, binge eaters apparently resort to cognitive narrowing, which in turn disengages some of their inhibitions—including the ones against eating. Evidence for the cognitive narrowness in binge eaters is scattered but consistent; for example, bulimics score unusually low on scales that measure meaningful, existential thinking (Keck & Fiebert, 1986).

One area of uncertainty in the literature on binge eating is whether the heavy eating is a result or a means of escaping from self. For example, evidence suggests that during a binge, dieters have ceased to monitor their food intake (Polivy, 1976); this indicates successful escape from self-awareness, but it also explains why they may end up eating so much. However, it is also plausible that focusing attention on the simple, immediate, bodily processes of biting, chewing, tasting, and swallowing food may be a powerful technique for cognitive narrowing. Such a focus restricts awareness to the simplest sensations and bodily movements, away from broadly meaningful issues and concerns. Still, it seems quite clear that escape from high levels of aversive self-awareness is centrally involved in binge eating.

Meditation

Thus far, I have emphasized escapes that have some undesirable connotation or danger associated with them. Suicide is extremely maladaptive; binge eating and alcohol abuse involve the risks of disapproval and personal danger; and sexual masochism is stigmatized. Not all escapes have negative aspects, however. Indeed, meditation is often regarded as a constructive and beneficial activity.

Escape from self is a central aspect of meditation. Religions that emphasize meditative practice generally speak of the need to break free of the self. Often they phrase this in terms of dissolving the ego or overcoming the barriers of selfhood. The ecstasy associated with peak religious experiences may well be a direct result of this overcoming of selfhood. Perhaps more importantly, spiritual disciplines from all over the world tend to regard the self as an impediment to spiritual progress.

Meditative techniques use cognitive narrowing in order to deconstruct the self. The beginner's exercise in Zen is an excellent illustration for this. Beginners are instructed to focus their attention on their breathing. They count their breaths up to 10 and then start over. Breathing is of course one of the most basic and minimal bodily functions, so focusing attention on it is a clear example of reducing self from a complex identity to a mere body. Restricting the count to 10 breaths narrows one's temporal focus by removing anything farther away than the current minute. The goal of rejecting meaningful thought is epitomized in the attempt to reduce one's mental process to counting to 10 over and over. Other thoughts spring up in one's mind, but the novice is instructed to abandon them gently and return to his or her breathing.

CONCLUSION

Modern Western society has placed great emphasis on the self, and indeed the cultivation and aggrandizement of self are central to many of the goals and purposes that shape the activity of the modern citizen. Still, not everything is consistent with the aggrandizement of self. There is a substantial subset of activities that seem designed to undermine, thwart, or remove the self.

There is no basis at present for concluding that normal human beings are motivated by a desire to bring harm, failure, or misfortune to themselves. People do self-destructive things, but these harmful results appear either to result from mistakes in judgment or to be by-products of the pursuit of desirable goals.

There is, however, substantial reason to believe that normal people are sometimes motivated by a desire to escape from themselves. These escapes take the form of reductions in self-awareness, especially awareness of the full, complex, symbolic, temporally extended identity. Escape often takes the form of narrowing attention to the immediate present and reducing awareness of self from identity to body. Attention is restricted to immediate movement and sensation. This relieves the burden of selfhood and allows people to experience the benefits that accompany a suspension of self-awareness.

In most cases, the desire to escape from self appears to be temporary. People may imagine it as permanent, such as in masochistic fantasies of identity change, but in practice they pursue it only as an occasional relief from the burdens of identity. The main exception to this temporariness is suicide, which if successful is of course permanent. But there is some reason to think that the suicidal mental process is often so restricted in time that the person is not really thinking about the distant future. Instead, the person is focused on the immediate present and the pressing desire for relief (through oblivion) from immediate suffering. Moreover, if the person survives the suicide attempt, the escape generally turns out to be temporary, for very few people show chronic patterns of suicidal behavior. Suicidal behavior is rare or at most intermittent, consistent with the hypothesis that people mainly desire occasional escapes from self.

The hypothesis of escape from self is thus capable of shedding light on some of the most enigmatic and paradoxical behavior patterns seen among normal individuals, including suicidal activity, sexual masochism, and binge eating. Recent increases in such behaviors may well reflect cultural shifts in the construction of selfhood. As our culture places increased demands on the self, the need to escape from self may also be increasing.

REFERENCES

Barnett, L. R. (1986). Bulimarexia as symptom of sex-role strain in professional women. *Psychotherapy, 23*, 311–315.

Baumeister, R. F. (1982). A self-presentational view of social phenomena. *Psychological Bulletin, 91*, 3–26.

Baumeister, R. F. (1984). Choking under pressure: Self-consciousness and paradoxical effects of incentives on skillful performance. *Journal of Personality and Social Psychology, 46,* 610–620.

Baumeister, R. F. (1988a). Masochism as escape from self. *Journal of Sex Research, 25,* 28–59.

Baumeister, R. F. (1988b). Gender differences in masochistic scripts. *Journal of Sex Research, 25,* 478–499.

Baumeister, R. F. (1989). *Masochism and the self.* Hillsdale, NJ: Erlbaum.

Baumeister, R. F. (1990a). Anxiety and deconstruction: On escaping the self. In J. M. Olson & M. P. Zanna (Eds.), *Self-inference processes: The Ontario Symposium* (Vol. 6, pp. 259–291). Hillsdale, NJ: Erlbaum.

Baumeister, R. F. (1990b). Suicide as escape from self. *Psychological Review, 97,* 90–113.

Baumeister, R. F., & Scher, S. J. (1988). Self-defeating behavior patterns among normal individuals: Review and analysis of common self-destructive tendencies. *Psychological Bulletin, 104,* 3–22.

Baumeister, R. F., Stillwell, A., & Wotman, S. R. (1990). Victim and perpetrator accounts of interpersonal conflict: Autobiographical narratives about anger. *Journal of Personality and Social Psychology, 59,* 994–1005.

Baumgardner, A. H., & Brownlee, E. A. (1987). Strategic failure in social interaction: Evidence for expectancy disconfirmation processes. *Journal of Personality and Social Psychology, 52,* 525–535.

Bazerman, M. H. (1986, June). Why negotiations go wrong. *Psychology Today,* pp. 54–58.

Berglas, S. C., & Jones, E. E. (1978). Drug choice as a self-handicapping strategy in response to non-contingent success. *Journal of Personality and Social Psychology, 36,* 405–417.

Blanchard, F. A., & Frost, R. O. (1983). Two factors of restraint: Concern for dieting and weight fluctuations. *Behaviour Research and Therapy, 21,* 259–267.

Brady, J. V. (1958). Ulcers in "executive" monkeys. *Scientific American, 199*(4), 95–100.

Brown, B. R. (1968). The effects of need to maintain face on interpersonal bargaining. *Journal of Experimental Social Psychology, 4,* 107–122.

Brown, B. R., & Garland, H. (1971). The effects of incompetency, audience acquaintanceship, and anticipated evaluative feedback on face-saving behavior. *Journal of Experimental Social Psychology, 7,* 490–502.

Butterfield, P. S., & Leclair, S. (1988). Cognitive characteristics of bulimic and drug-abusing women. *Addictive Behaviors, 13,* 131–138.

Califia, P. (1983). A secret side of lesbian sexuality. In T. Weinberg & G. Kamel (Eds.), *S and M: Studies in sadomasochism* (pp. 129–136). Buffalo, NY: Prometheus.

Caplan, P. (1984). The myth of women's masochism. *American Psychologist, 39,* 130–139.

Carver, C. S., & Scheier, M. F. (1981). *Attention and self-regulation: A control-theory approach to human behavior.* New York: Springer-Verlag.

Comer, R., & Laird, J. D. (1975). Choosing to suffer as a consequence of expecting to suffer: Why do people do it? *Journal of Personality and Social Psychology,*

32,92–101.

Csikszentmihalyi, M. (1982). Toward a psychology of optimal experience. In L. Wheeler (Ed.), *Review of personality and social psychology* (Vol. 2, pp. 13–36). Beverly Hills, CA: Sage.

Curtis, R., Rietdorf, P., & Ronell, D. (1980). "Appeasing the gods?" Suffering to reduce probable future suffering. *Personality and Social Psychology Bulletin, 6,* 234–241.

Dixon, T., & Baumeister, R. F. (in press). Escaping the self: The moderating effect of self-complexity. *Personality and Social Psychology Bulletin.*

Duval, S., & Wicklund, R. A. (1972). *A theory of objective self-awareness.* New York: Academic Press.

Franklin D. (1987, January). The politics of masochism. *Psychology Today,* pp. 52–57.

Gibbons, F. X., & Wicklund, R. A. (1976). Selective exposure to self. *Journal of Research in Personality, 10,* 98–106.

Glass, D., Singer, J., & Friedman, L. (1969). Psychic cost of adaptation to an environmental stressor. *Journal of Personality and Social Psychology, 12,* 200–210.

Greenberg, J., & Musham, C. (1981). Avoiding and seeking self-focused attention. *Journal of Research in Personality, 15,* 191–200.

Heatherton, T. F., & Baumeister, R. F. (in press). Binge eating as escape from self-awareness. *Psychological Bulletin..*

Henken, V. J. (1976). Banality reinvestigated: A computer-based content analysis of suicidal and forced-death documents. *Suicide and Life-Threatening Behavior, 6,* 36–43.

Hershenson, D. B. (1965). Stress-induced use of alcohol by problem drinkers as a function of their sense of identity. *Quarterly Journal of Studies on Alcohol, 26,* 213–222.

Higgins, E. T. (1987). Self-discrepancy: A theory relating self and affect. *Psychological Review, 94,* 319–340.

Hull, J. G. (1981). A self-awareness model of the causes and effects of alcohol consumption. *Journal of Abnormal Psychology, 90,* 586–600.

Hull, J. G., & Young, R. D. (1983). Self-consciousness, self-esteem, and success–failure as determinants of alcohol consumption in male social drinkers. *Journal of Personality and Social Psychology, 44,* 1097–1109.

Hull, J. G., Young, R. D., & Jouriles, E. (1986). Applications of the self-awareness model of alcohol consumption: Predicting patterns of use and abuse. *Journal of Personality and Social Psychology, 51,* 790–796.

Janus, S., Bess, B., & Saltus, C. (1977). *A sexual profile of men in power.* Englewood Cliffs, NJ: Prentice-Hall.

Jones, E. E., & Berglas, S. C. (1978). Control of attributions about the self through self-handicapping strategies: The appeal of alcohol and the role of underachievement. *Personality and Social Psychology Bulletin, 4,* 200–206.

Jones, E. E., & Wortman, C. (1973). *Ingratiation: An attributional approach.* Morristown, NJ: General Learning Press.

Keck, J. N., & Fiebert, M. S. (1986). Avoidance of anxiety and eating disorders. *Psychological Reports, 58,* 432–434.

Krafft-Ebing, R. von. (1922). Psychopathia sexualis (F. S. Klaff, Trans.). In T. Weinberg & G. Kamel (Eds.), *S and M: Studies in sadomasochism* (pp. 25–29). Buffalo, NY: Prometheus, 1983.

Masters, W. H., & Johnson, V. E. (1970). *Human sexual inadequacy*. Boston: Little, Brown.

Monat, A., Averill, J. R., & Lazarus, R. S. (1972). Anticipatory stress and coping reactions under various conditions of uncertainty. *Journal of Personality and Social Psychology, 24,* 237–253.

Polivy, J. (1976). Perception of calories and regulation of intake in restrained and unrestrained subjects. *Addictive Behaviors, 1,* 237–243.

Polivy, J., Heatherton, T. F., & Herman, C. P. (1988). Self-esteem, restraint, and eating behavior. *Journal of Abnormal Psychology, 97,* 354–356.

Sackett, D. L., & Snow, J. C. (1979). The magnitude of compliance and noncompliance. In R. B. Haynes, D. W. Taylor, & D. L. Sackett (Eds.), *Compliance in health care* (pp. 11–22). Baltimore: Johns Hopkins University Press.

Scarry, E. (1985). *The body in pain: The making and unmaking of the world.* New York: Oxford University Press.

Steele, C. M., & Josephs, R. A. (1988). Drinking your troubles away: II. An attention-allocation model of alcohol's effect on psychological stress. *Journal of Abnormal Psychology, 97,* 196–205.

Steenbarger, B. N., & Aderman, D. (1979). Objective self-awareness as a nonaversive state: Effect of anticipating discrepancy reduction. *Journal of Personality, 47,* 330–339.

Tice, D. M. (in press). Esteem protection or enhancement?: Self-handicapping motives differ by trait self-esteem. *Journal of Personality and Social Psychology.*

Vallacher, R. R., & Wegner, D. M. (1985). *A theory of action identification.* Hillsdale, NJ: Erlbaum.

Vallacher, R. R., & Wegner, D. M. (1987). What do people think they're doing: Action identification and human behavior. *Psychological Review, 94,* 3–15.

Wegner, D. M., Schneider, D. J., Carter, S. R., & White, T. L. (1987). Paradoxical effects of thought suppression. *Journal of Personality and Social Psychology, 53,* 5–13.

Weiss, J. M. (1971a). Effects of coping behavior in different warning signal conditions on stress pathology in rats. *Journal of Comparative and Physiological Psychology, 77,* 1–13.

Weiss, J. M. (1971b). Effects of coping behavior with and without a feedback signal on stress pathology in rats. *Journal of Comparative and Physiological Psychology, 77,* 22–30.

CHAPTER THIRTEEN

Social versus Clinical Approaches to Self Psychology: The Self-Evaluation Maintenance Model and Kohutian Object Relations Theory

ABRAHAM TESSER

The self is currently an important construct in experimental social psychology and in clinical psychology. In spite of identical names for the work, "self psychology," the usage and intellectual history of the concept of self in these two behavioral science disciplines is quite different.

The concept of self was very important to William James (1890), one of social psychology's founders. However, what we think of as modern social psychology, with its emphasis on experimental research and mini-theories, really began at about the time of World War II. Except for isolated studies (e.g., Dittes, 1959), experimental[1] social psychology was remarkably bereft of systematic work on the self until the late 1970s. It was at about that time that Wicklund (1975) began publishing his work on objective self-awareness; some people were noticing Aronson's (1969) suggestion that cognitive dissonance may be understood in terms of self-esteem (Greenwald & Ronis, 1978); many of us were arguing about the motivational status of "self-serving biases" (e.g., Ross & Sicoly, 1979; Zuckerman, 1979); and Hazel Markus (1977) was telling us about self-schemas. Now, there are a number of systematic research programs on the self, and many introductory social psychology texts (e.g., Brehm & Kassin, 1990; Worchel, Cooper, & Goethals, 1988) have whole chapters devoted to the "self." (To my knowledge, neither Freud nor the psychoanalytic movement plays an important role in the experimental social-psychological work on self.)

Self psychology in clinical practice, on the other hand, has evolved within a psychoanalytic tradition. Self psychology grew out of the object relations movement and is most closely associated with the name of Heinz

Kohut (1971, 1977, 1984). The object relations movement started in the 1950s (Cashdan, 1988) with the work of Melanie Klein (1948), W. R. D. Fairbairn (1954), and Margaret Mahler (1952). Rather than focusing on sexual or aggressive energy (libido), as in classical psychoanalysis, these theorists emphasized processes of the self (ego) in the context of significant interpersonal (object) relationships. In Kohut's view, not only must the child's more obvious needs be met (e.g., food), but he or she also (1) must be admired for accomplishments by significant others (i.e., "mirroring"), and (2) must have the opportunity to "idealize" significant others.[2] It is the individual's experience of satisfaction or lack of satisfaction of these self-oriented (narcissistic) needs that drives current (inter)personal functioning.

Kohutian theory has some striking similarities (and differences) with some work that I have been doing within the tradition of experimental social psychology. The similarity of basic assumptions about the importance of self-esteem in influencing behavior and the focus on self-esteem in social processes is obvious to anyone who has even passing familiarity with Kohutian theory and the self-evaluation maintenance (SEM) model (Tesser, 1988). Remarkable, however, is the similarity in the *specific* social-psychological (psychosocial) processes assumed to be important (Friedlander, 1986). On the other hand, there are some fundamental differences in the model dynamics, the epistemological foundations of the evidential base, and the clinical implications of each approach. The purpose of this chapter is to explore some of these similarities and differences. Perhaps such an exercise will enrich each approach.

THE BASIC ASSUMPTIONS AND PROCESSES

Both Kohutian theory and the SEM model are predicated on the notion that the satisfaction of the self's needs are part and parcel of normal functioning. Furthermore, both approaches assume that the feelings of competence that affect the self are a result of social processes. Kohut calls these processes "mirroring" and "idealization." In the SEM model, the processes are called "comparison" and "reflection." The Kohutian and SEM processes appear to have some interesting and important parallels.

The SEM Perspective

The notion of "self-evaluation" (i.e., how positive an individual feels about himself or herself) is central to the SEM model. Self-evaluation does not mean the chronic feelings a person has about himself or herself. Rather, this construct taps the dynamic aspect of feelings toward the self (i.e., the variation around some usual or characteristic set of feelings toward the self). Thus, it is not characterized as an individual-difference variable, but rather as a basic psychological process.

Persons feel positive or negative about themselves for a variety of reasons. "Self-evaluation" as used here is a result of real or implied social feedback in performance settings. That is, one can feel and look good by basking in the reflected glory of the better performance of a close other, and/or one can feel and look bad by comparison to the outstanding performance of a close other.

The self-evaluation construct is related to what other investigators term "self-esteem." Indeed, in some earlier work, the term "self-esteem" was used to refer to the self-evaluation construct (Tesser, 1980; Tesser & Campbell, 1980; Tesser & Smith, 1980). However, "self-esteem" has been abandoned because it has too much surplus meaning for present usage. Self-esteem is a relatively general construct. In contrast, self-evaluation has been narrowly and strictly defined in terms of the model components to be described below. There are literally hundreds of studies dealing with self-esteem (Wylie, 1974), and the term is also widely used in a nontechnical way. With that kind of background, the temptation to think of something called self-esteem as real, tangible, and observable is great. On the other hand, self-evaluation is a theoretical construct. Self-esteem is often treated as a chronic, individual-difference variable. In contrast, self-evaluation is presumed to be an interactive function of defined situational influences. It is not fixed; it is dynamic.

Two Antagonistic Processes: Reflection and Comparison

Self-evaluation is assumed to be the result of two separate processes: the reflection process (i.e., the process by which a psychologically close other's good performance can raise self-evaluation) and the comparison process (i.e., the process by which a psychologically close other's good performance can lower self-evaluation). These two processes are, in turn, composed of the constructs of closeness to another and performance of another. Furthermore, the reflection and comparison processes are weighted by the relevance of another's performance to one's own self-definition.

The Reflection Process. According to Cialdini et al. (1976), people are quick to communicate their associations with others who perform well. Since they have not been instrumental in the accomplishments of those others, it appears as if they point out these associations simply to bask in the reflected glory of others' accomplishments; such associations appear to raise the individuals' self-evaluation.

Reflection has two distinct components: closeness and performance. If another person is psychologically distant, then regardless of how good the performance is, one will not be able to bask in his or her reflected glory. As Heider (1958) puts it, "Boasting implies that the person who does the boasting and the object about which he boasts form a unit" (p. 180). Similarly, if another's performance is not particularly good, then regardless of how psychologically close he or she is, one will not gain in reflected glory. In short, the reflection process depends on the interaction of closeness to the other person and the other person's performance. It will produce gains in self-evaluation to the extent that another is psychologically close and the performance is good.

The Comparison Process. While the reflection process suggests that a close association with others who perform well can raise self-evaluation, the opposite expectation is also plausible: Namely, a close association with others who perform well can lower self-evaluation. One's own performance pales in comparison to that of someone who performs better. Comparison, like reflection, has two components. If another is psychologically close, comparison processes are more likely to be engaged; therefore, the effects of the other's performance on one's self-evaluation will be more pronounced than if the other is distant. A performance that is better than an individual's own will be a greater blow to the individual's self-evaluation if the other is psychologically close.[3] Also, if another's performance is mediocre, the individual's self-evaluation will not be affected very much, regardless of how close or distant the other person is. As in the case of reflection, closeness and performance appear to combine multiplicatively in determining comparison.

Elements of the Reflection and Comparison Processes

Social-Psychological Closeness. Reflection and comparison processes depend on social-psychological closeness and performance. "Closeness" refers to the psychological proximity between a person and another from the perspective of the self. The definition of closeness draws heavily on Heider's (1958) notion of "unit relation" as it is applied to the relationship between persons. In general, to the extent that there is a unit relation between two persons, they are close. Following Heider (1958), the SEM model posits a number of factors that should increase closeness. For example, proximity in space; similarity in attitudes, values, age, or personality; and common origins, nationality, religion, or familial background tend to increase closeness. Friends are likely to be closer than strangers.

Again, much as in Heider's (1958) notion of unit relation, the closeness of two individuals is not fixed but varies with context. Two persons from Brooklyn, New York will be closer if they are in Athens, Georgia than if they are in Brooklyn, New York. The addition of a third person to a pair will change the closeness of the pair. If a third person is more similar to a member of the original pair than is the other original member, the original pair will become less close. If the third member is less similar to the original pair members than the pair members are to each other, the pair will seem closer. Miller, Turnbull, and McFarland (1988) have completed an integrated series of studies showing that closeness increases when persons share distinctive attributes. Finally, the situation can make different aspects of the members of a pair salient and thus change closeness in that way. Heider (1958) gives Ichheiser's (1949) example of "two people who are thought of as doctor and patient when seen in the physician's office, as radical and conservative when seen at a political rally and as two Englishmen should they meet in Italy" (Heider, 1958, p. 179).

Performance. "Performance" refers to the relative quality of another's performance in a particular domain.[4] If is assumed that one's own performance serves as an anchor or point of comparison in judging the performance of others. Another's performance is good to the extent that it is better than one's own. Performance, like the other variables, is taken from the perspective of the actor. Like changes in closeness and relevance, changes in performance may represent changes in perception as well as objective changes in actual levels of performance. Furthermore, since performance is defined relatively, it can be affected by both the actor's and the other's perceived level of performance. Thus, the relative performance of another can be increased by improving the other's performance or by decreasing one's own level of performance. The relative performance of another can be decreased by improving one's own performance or by decreasing or interfering with the other's performance.

Weighting the Reflection and Comparison Processes: Relevance

The reflection and comparison processes are antagonistic. When another's closeness and performance are both high, one's self-evaluation should be raised—by reflection. At the same time, however, self-evaluation should be threatened—by comparison. How are we to reconcile this apparent contradiction? The model asserts that reflection and comparison processes are now always equally important. The relevance of the other's performance to one's self-definition is presumed to determine the relative weights of these two processes.

"Relevance" refers to the extent to which another's performance is on a dimension that is self-defining for a person. We all recognize and value good performance on any number of dimensions (marathon running, violin playing, etc.). Our own aspirations, however, exist only with respect to a small subset of these. Another's performance, then, is relevant to the extent that it is on one of these few dimensions that are self-defining for us. Thus, if one aspires to be a good surfer but does not play the piano, then another's surfing performance is high in relevance but his or her piano performance is not. The model (following Festinger, 1954) also asserts that if another's performance is too much better or too much worse, thereby rendering comparison difficult, then it will also be low in relevance even if it is on a self-defining dimension.

The relevance of another's performance increases the importance of the comparison process, relative to the reflection process. When relevance is high, the comparison process is more important than the reflection process. A good performance by another is threatening to self-evaluation, and the closeness of that other increases the threat. When relevance is low, the reflection process is relatively more important. Another's good performance will bolster one's self-evaluation, especially when that other is close. For example, if John aspires to be a good baseball player and his brother (high closeness) hits a grand slam in a game in which John goes hitless, his self-evaluation will suffer by comparison. If, on the other hand, John has no musical aspirations and his brother gets rave notices for a violin recital, John's self-evaluation will be raised—by the process of reflection.

Self-Enhancement: The Core Assumption

The assumption that makes the SEM model work is as follows: *Persons behave so as to maximize their self-evaluation (or minimize loss in self-evaluation).* That is, they will regulate their behavior in order to maintain a positive self-regard. On the surface, this assumption seems noncontroversial. However, there is a literature suggesting that some persons do not regulate their behavior to produce positive self-outcomes. For example, if people prefer consistent feedback, then people low in self-esteem may behave in ways to maintain that low self-esteem (e.g., Lecky, 1945; Swann, 1983). There are now several studies (e.g., McFarlin & Blascovich 1981; Moreland & Sweeney, 1984; Swann, Griffin, Predmore, & Gaines, 1987) and reviews (e.g., Jones, 1973; Shrauger, 1975) that address this question. They suggest that cognitive and affective responses to performance feedback should be distinguished. Affective responses seem to follow a self-enhancement rule: Even persons low in self-esteem or persons who are depressed show positive affective responses to situations that enhance their self-esteem or self-evaluation, and negative affect to situations that threaten their self-esteem. On the other hand, their expectations (i.e., cognitive responses) concerning feedback about their behavior tend to be consistent with their self-esteem. Thus, there appears to be some independence between the cognitive and affective systems. Since the core assumption of the model concerns the affective system, it remains plausible.

The Kohutian Perspective

Kohut's ideas about the self grew out of his clinical practice. In this practice, he encountered a greater incidence of narcissistic personality disorders and behavior disorders than he would have expected on the basis of previous literature in the psychoanalytic domain. Perhaps societal changes were producing narcissistic symptoms (Lasch, 1978). The traditional view of narcissism or self-love from the psychoanalytic perspective was pessimistic (Reich, 1960), but not so for Kohut (Chessick, 1985). Indeed, "Kohut (1977) contends that narcissism is the normal and central trend in personality development. The development of the self is therefore, the transformation of narcissism" (Patton, Connor, & Scott, 1982, p. 271).

For Kohut, the person's inner self is crucial. "The therapist learns about this through empathy or vicarious introspection and attempts to understand the rising and falling of self-esteem in relation to the person's largely unconscious ambitions, on the one hand, and largely unconscious ideals on the other" (Chessick, 1985, p. 82). These ambitions and ideals have their genesis in the "grandiose self," an infantile organization of self (at about 2 years of age) in which one's natural needs for exhibitionism and idealizing are strongly felt. Empathic parents will recognize, echo, reflect, admire, and approve the child. This process, called "mirroring," satisfies the child's exhibitionistic needs. At the same time, the empathic parent will be an accepting target of the child's idealization needs.

The repeated use of the term "empathic" is deliberate. Unconditional approval or inappropriate approval from the child's point of view will not produce effective mirroring. The parent must empathize with the child (i.e., put himself or herself in the place of the child) to understand what it is the child is exhibiting or "holding up" for reflection, in order to produce effective mirroring. It is the echoing of the child's own agenda that leads to effective mirroring. Presumably, the parent must also empathize with the child to serve as an effective target for idealization. Empathic responding allows the child to feel as if he or she were the center of the universe (via mirroring) and at the same time one with the perfect and omnipotent parents (via idealizing). This sets the stage for the development of a mature, cohesive, bipolar self with a healthy level of self-esteem (Patton et al., 1982).

Healthy development, however, is not simply the result of the satisfaction of all the child's exhibitionistic needs and needs for idealization.

Inevitable failures in empathy or availability of the parent (selfobject) leads to frustration. If the frequency and timing of these episodes are optimal, the child himself or herself gradually learns to take over the mirroring and idealizing functions performed by the selfobject. This process is called "transmuting internalization." "Thus, outer signs of approval become internalized as self-esteem and feelings of vitality, while exhibitionism and grandiosity mature into healthy self-assertive behavior and the pursuit of ambitions" (Kahn, 1985, p. 897). On the other hand, optimal frustration of idealization leads the child gradually to acquire his or her own self-soothing ability, and, later in childhood, to internalize the values and ideal of the idealized selfobject. These internalized values and ideals manifest themselves as goals in adulthood.

It is noteworthy that selfobjects are not unimportant to the healthy adult self. The adult continues to depend on others to satisfy mirroring and idealization needs. A mature relationship is one in which each can assert his or her own (exhibitionistic) needs and for which there is "empathic resonance" on the part of each partner. It is also a relationship in which partners do not idealize each other, but have respect for each other's realistic qualities.

In sum, Kohutian theory gives prominence to two psychosocial processes for the self's functioning. The mirroring process is one in which the self's accomplishments are recognized and applauded by important selfobjects. The idealization process is one in which important selfobjects are held up for admiration.

Comparing the Basic Assumptions and Processes

This short description of the SEM model and Kohutian theory makes clear a number of similarities. For each, self-esteem is crucial and the self's needs drive much of behavior. Both approaches emphasize performance and are concerned with competence, achievement, and so on as being crucial to positive feelings about the self. Both are concerned with the closeness of others/selfobjects. Moreover, the specific psychosocial processes of mirroring and idealizing seem to have a rough correspondence to the social-psychological processes of comparison and reflection.[5] Even within these broad similarities, though, the SEM model and the Kohutian model differ somewhat in the basic constituents of their processes.

Comparing the Comparison and Mirroring Processes

Both models put emphasis on the mixture of the self's own accomplishments and the social context of those accomplishments. However, the

TABLE 13.1. Comparison of Basic Processes

	SEM model	Kohutian model
Dimension	Comparison process	Mirroring process
Focus of process	Self-glorification	Self-glorification
Locus of action	Self	Selfobject
Interpersonal relationship	Social-psychological closeness	Psychosocial closeness
Motive	Self-protection	Self-enhancement
Performance domain	High self-relevance	High self-relevance
	Reflection process	Idealization process
Focus of process	Glorification of other	Glorification of other
Locus of action	Self	Self–selfobject
Interpersonal relationship	Social-psychological closeness	Psychosocial closeness
Motive	Self-enhancement	Self-protection
Performance domain	Low self-relevance	Unspecified

details by which these accomplishments affect the self are quite different. As can be seen in Table 13.1, the theories can be compared on five dimensions.

Both the comparison process and the mirroring process are social. Each requires the self and another. Furthermore, both are concerned with self-glorification. The comparison process is predicated on the idea that being outdone by another can be threatening, and the mirroring process points to the need for others to recognize the self's accomplishments. Notice, however, that they differ in the extent to which the self is the active agent. Mirroring depends on the *other's*, the selfobject's, taking the active role in admiring, recognizing and validating the accomplishments of the self. Although the impact of mirroring is on the self, it is the other who takes the active role. From the perspective of the SEM model, on the other hand, the comparison process will unfold even with a passive other, one who may even be unaware of the implications of his or her performance for the self. Although the good performance of a close other is involved in the comparison process, the action in this process is intrapsychic (i.e., with the self).[6] Theoretically, the self is the active agent in controlling/perceiving one's own and the other's relative performance, for example.

Both the comparison process and the mirroring process depend on the self's relationship to another. The threat of comparison increases with the *social-psychological closeness* of the other. As spelled out earlier, "social-psychological closeness" refers to unit relatedness in the Heiderian (1958) sense (e.g., similarity of background, contiguity). The appropriate self-object for mirroring presumably must be a significant other in the self's life (i.e., someone who is *psychosocially close*). At first, it is the primary caretaker. But in adult life it could be the therapist who, through transference processes, takes on the role of the primary caretaker. Presumably, it could also be a spouse or a close friend. Although in both cases the other must have some special significance to the self, the parameters bounding the relationship for the comparison process and the mirroring process are quite different. However, in neither theory are these boundaries well articulated.

Both the SEM model and Kohutian theory are clearly motivational. However, the characterization of the motivational underpinnings of the comparison and mirroring processes are quite different. The mirroring process directly satisfies the derivative of infantile needs for grandiosity and exhibitionism. The comparison process, on the other hand, is motivated by *threat avoidance*. Being outperformed by a close other in a self-relevant domain is assumed to be threatening, and therefore the individual is motivated to avoid it. Thus, mirroring is positive (i.e., the validation of one's achievements), whereas comparison is negative, implying a threat to one's sense of accomplishment.

The SEM model suggests that the comparison process only becomes important when a self-relevant performance domain is in question. (When relevance is low, the reflection process will be more important.) According to Kohut, the individual has natural skills and talents. If all goes well, these skills and talents are developed. Although Kohut does not distinguish areas of self-relevance as does the SEM model, Kohut's emphasis on *empathy* leads me to infer that the models are similar with respect to this dimension. For mirroring to work, the selfobject must empathize with the self; that is, the selfobject must understand what it is that the self is offering for mirroring. If the selfobject is not empathic and mirrors the wrong thing, then the process will not play itself out appropriately. What is it that the self offers up for mirroring? Presumably, the accomplishments that are important (i.e., relevant) to the self.

In sum, the comparison process of the SEM model and the mirroring process of Kohutian theory point to the individual's need to feel *self-competent* with respect to personally important dimensions and the importance of close others in generating these feelings. However, they differ in their definitions of closeness, the precise motivational underpinnings of the process, and the agentic roles of self and other.

Comparing the Reflection and Idealization Processes[7]

Central to both the SEM model and Kohut's model is the idea that the perception of the outstanding performance of a close other can be beneficial to the self. In the case of both reflection and idealization, it is the self who takes the active role. The other need only be available for this to happen, although Kohut suggests that the other must allow this to happen. Also, both the reflection and idealization processes depend on the target other's being close. But as with the comparison and mirroring process, the nature of closeness differs.

The major differences between the reflection and idealization processes concern the underlying motives and the performance domain. From the perspective of the SEM model, it is simply assumed that being associated with a "winner" reflects positively on the self (e.g., Cialdini et al., 1976; Sigall & Landy, 1973). This tendency is presumed to derive from primitive empathic mechanisms in which the infant tends to "catch" the emotions of those around him or her (Tesser, 1984). Reflection leads to self-enhancement and is a positive thing. For Kohut, the infant wishes to identify with an omnipotent other for security. It is through merging with powerful others that the individual learns to control anxiety and soothe the self. Thus, idealization is a self-protective rather than a self-enhancing motive.

Kohut does not delineate the spheres of performance within which we can expect to find idealization. Since the motive for idealization is security, and since empathy is important, perhaps we can infer that idealization takes place on dimensions along which the individual feels threatened or incapable of self-coping. On the other hand, the SEM model assumes that the individual will bask in the reflected glory of a close other's good performance as long as that performance is not threatening via comparison (i.e., as long as it is low in self-relevance).

Conclusion

This review of the processes associated with the SEM model and the Kohutian model points up a number of similarities and differences. Both models have a process that emphasizes enhancement of the self, and both models have a process that emphasizes threat to the self. Given the juxtaposition of these motives in Table 13.1, each model might learn a lesson from the other. The comparison process maps onto the mirroring process, and thus there may be a role for self-enhancement in the comparison process and a role for self-protection or threat in the mirroring process. For example, Beach and I (Tesser & Beach, 1989; Beach, in press) have begun to explore the possibility of self-enhancement through outperforming a close other on a highly relevant dimension (i.e., the comparison process). In a similar vein, Kohutian theory might be enriched by recognizing that aspects of the mirroring process have the potential for threat. Telling another individual that he or she is good in an area that is self-relevant implies that the selfobject thinks he or she is in a position to judge and perhaps is superior. Similarly, since the reflection and idealization processes map onto each other, there may be a role for self-protection in the reflection process and a role for self-enhancement in the idealization process.

The SEM model puts a great deal of emphasis on locating the action in the self, whereas Kohutian theory puts the "action" in the selfobject. Each perspective might be improved by trying to accommodate the point of view of the other. The SEM model might be developed to look at the functions of the self object or other person in the situation, and the Kohutian model could put a greater emphasis on the initiation of action in the self. For example, the SEM model could be expanded to reorganize the importance of interpretive feedback from others. The presence of a "mirroring" other could make what feels like a failure, relative to another person, into a success. Kohutian theory could put more of the action into the self. It seems plausible that the individual may be able to seek out circumstances that will allow for good performance and self-glorification without the initiation of the selfobject.

Finally, a fine-grained analysis of interpersonal relationships would be helpful from both perspectives. I think Kohutian theory could be made richer by making discriminations in domains of the self as the SEM model has done. Clearly, the possibility that the SEM and Kohutian perspectives will enrich each others seems to be present.

DYNAMICS

The SEM model and the Kohutian model seem to have some overlap and some differences in the constituents of their processes. Now, I turn to the macro- and microdynamics of the processes. From a global or macro perspective, the Kohutian processes appear to function independently, where the SEM model processes function systemically; Kohutian dynamics are based on the individual's developmental history, whereas SEM dynamics are based on the present situation. On the microdynamic level, emotions play a role in the unfolding of specific behaviors in both models, but the role is not identical. According to the SEM model, emotion is a marker, an experience, and a mediator of behavioral change; for Kohutian theory, it is a symptom.

Macrodynamics

Kohut's description of the mirroring and idealization process suggests that their functioning is relatively additive/independent. As can be seen in

Figure 13.1, Patton et al. (1982) picture Kohutian development as taking place in parallel. Indeed, although there is some overlap, problems with mirroring result in one set of symptoms, while problems with idealization can result in a qualitatively different set of symptoms. For example, frustration of mirroring needs produces a "mirror-hungry personality," a person constantly on display, moving from relationship to relationship with an insatiable desire for attention. Frustration of idealization needs can produce the "ideal-hungry personality," a person who is "forever in search of

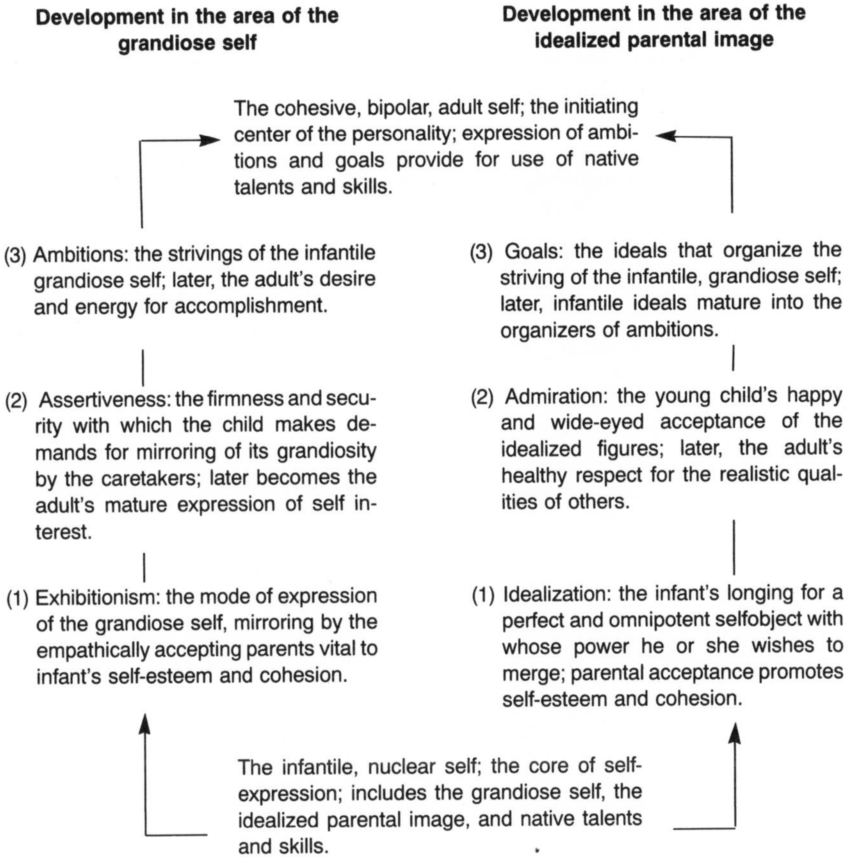

Development in the area of the
grandiose self

Development in the area of the
idealized parental image

The cohesive, bipolar, adult self; the initiating center of the personality; expression of ambitions and goals provide for use of native talents and skills.

(3) Ambitions: the strivings of the infantile grandiose self; later, the adult's desire and energy for accomplishment.

(3) Goals: the ideals that organize the striving of the infantile, grandiose self; later, infantile ideals mature into the organizers of ambitions.

(2) Assertiveness: the firmness and security with which the child makes demands for mirroring of its grandiosity by the caretakers; later becomes the adult's mature expression of self interest.

(2) Admiration: the young child's happy and wide-eyed acceptance of the idealized figures; later, the adult's healthy respect for the realistic qualities of others.

(1) Exhibitionism: the mode of expression of the grandiose self, mirroring by the empathically accepting parents vital to infant's self-esteem and cohesion.

(1) Idealization: the infant's longing for a perfect and omnipotent selfobject with whose power he or she wishes to merge; parental acceptance promotes self-esteem and cohesion.

The infantile, nuclear self; the core of self-expression; includes the grandiose self, the idealized parental image, and native talents and skills.

FIGURE 13.1. The parallel lines of development of the self. From "Kohut's Psychology of the Self: Theory and Measures of Counseling Outcome" by M. J. Patton, G. E. Connor, and K. J. Scott, 1982, *Journal of Counseling Psychology, 29,* 268–282. Copyright 1982 by the American Psychological Association. Reprinted by permission.

others whom [he or she] can admire for their prestige, power, beauty, intelligence or moral stature" (Maddi, 1989, p. 303). Depending on the client's symptoms, the therapist can either mirror the client or work with the client's idealization needs.

In contrast, the SEM model is *systemic* (Carver & Scheier, 1981; Powers, 1973). The model predicts that persons will regulate their behavior so as to maintain a positive self-evaluation. In doing so, they may alter interpersonal closeness, relative performance, or their own self-definition (relevance). Since these variables are in a *systemic* relationship to one another, each is at once both a cause and a consequence of the other two. A useful metaphor is the way in which Boyle's law of gases relates heat, volume, and pressure to one another. The systemic aspect of the model is presented schematically in Figure 13.2. Circles represent the variables of performance, closeness, and relevance; the arrows represent the direction of flow in causal influence; and the open ellipses represent variables that interact with a particular cause. Thus, performance, in interaction with

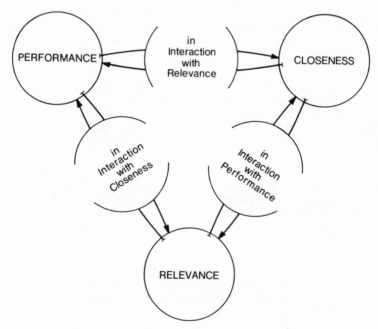

FIGURE 13.2. The systemic character of the SEM model. From "Toward a Self-Evaluation Maintenance Model of Social Behavior" by A. Tesser, 1988, in L. Berkowitz (Ed.), *Advances in Experimental Social Psychology* (Vol. 21, pp. 181–227), New York: Academic Press. Copyright 1988 by Academic Press, Inc. Reprinted by permission.

relevance, will affect closeness; closeness, in interaction with performance, will affect relevance; and relevance, in interaction with closeness, will affect performance. Given the systemic nature of the processes, change processes are not independent.

Historical perspective represents another difference in the macrodynamics of the Kohutian and SEM approaches. From the point of view of Kohut's clinical theory, the dynamics of everyday functioning are largely determined by the individual's past. If early exhibitionist and idealizing needs were met and periodically (optimally) frustrated, the individual will develop a mature, coherent self capable of self-assertion, with realistic admiration for others, and a healthy set of goals and ambitions. On the other hand, if the individual does not have this optimal developmental history, he or she will have problems in some of these areas. Since the problems are rooted in the past, the way to deal with them is for a therapist to provide the kind of experiences the individual should have had at an earlier stage. In short, the past is crucial to present functioning.

The focus of the SEM model is on the present. Obviously, there are individual differences: People have different developmental histories, and these histories will leave their imprint on present functioning. However, present functioning is largely determined by the individual's perceptions of his or her own current circumstances. To the extent that he or she is presently being outperformed by a close other on a relevant dimension of self, the individual will suffer by comparison. Regardless of past history, the individual will be motivated to reduce closeness, change relevance, or alter the relative performance difference. The reflection process is similarly highly dependent on the perception of the present situation.

Microdynamics

Microdynamics focus on the most immediate correlates of behavioral change. For the SEM model, these correlates are emotional. Emotion serves as a marker of the operation of SEM processes, as a subjective experience accompanying the operation of the processes, and as a mediator of the observed behavioral changes.

According to the SEM model, people change their behavior so as to control their own self-evaluation. If people strive for positive changes and avoid negative changes in self-evaluation, then circumstances under which the model anticipates positive changes in self-evaluation ought to produce positive emotional responses, and circumstances under which the model anticipates negative changes in self-evaluation ought to produce negative changes in emotion. My colleagues and I have looked at two aspects of emotional responding as markers of SEM functioning: arousal (intensity) and affect (positive vs. negative tone). We have relied on these aspects because they are labile enough to register fast changes; their measurement does not have to rely on self-report; and the subject does not have to be aware of his or her feelings for these aspects to manifest themselves. One set of studies (Tesser, Millar, & Moore, 1988) revealed that emotion does *mark* the SEM processes. That is, behavioral measures of arousal (performance on complex and simple tasks) and measures of facial affect covaried with the comparison and reflection processes as predicted. Being outperformed by a close other produced arousal. When relevance was high, being outperformed by a close other produced negative affect; when relevance was low, it produced positive affect.

The aspects of emotion—arousal and affect—that we have used as markers of the operation of the reflection and comparison processes are useful, in that they do not depend on conscious representation or self-reports to be detected. On the other hand, they lack the richness of and do not convey the *subjective emotional experiences* that accompany the SEM processes. For example, the threat associated with comparison ought to be experienced as jealousy or envy (e.g., Salovey & Rodin, 1984). When there is the potential to be outperformed by a close other on a relevant dimension and the threat is not realized (i.e., when self outperforms other), the emotion of pride ought to be experienced. Thus, at least part of the experience of high and low levels of comparison ought to be manifested in feelings of jealousy/envy and pride, respectively. The experience of reflection is more difficult. I know of no single word in English that describes the feeling of "pride in other," although there are such words in other languages (e.g., *kvell* and *nachas* [transliterations] in Yiddish, *orgullo* in Spanish). However, it is a pride in the other that we expect to covary with the reflection process. We (Tesser & Collins, 1988) asked subjects to recall personal situations that varied with respect to relevance, performance, and closeness. Although closeness did not have as much impact as we expected, subjects' ratings of their own emotions in those situations roughly paralleled our expectations.

The SEM processes are marked by emotion and accompanied by subjective emotional experiences. We also believe that emotion *mediates* SEM behavior. One possibility is that there is a two-step causal sequence. A change in external circumstances triggers the SEM processes that result in arousal. Increased arousal leads to a cognitive search (e.g., Berscheid, 1983; Mandler, 1975), resulting in a change of behavior in order to eliminate or reduce the potential pain of comparison or to maintain or increase the potential pleasure of reflection. If this line of reasoning is correct, then the SEM pattern of behavior should covary with emotional arousal. The SEM pattern should be clear when arousal is high and become fuzzy or disappear when arousal is low. The SEM pattern should also dissolve if the arousal that is present is misattributed to some irrelevant source. Both of these sets of predictions were recently confirmed (Tesser, Pilkington, & McIntosh, 1989; Tesser, Achee, & Pilkington, 1990). Thus, emotion appears to play a key mediational role in SEM processes.

Although emotion plays a role in behavior from the Kohutian perspective, its role appears to be that of a symptom of self-fragmentation rather than as a mediator of change. Thus, small interpersonal slights can result in withdrawal or episodes of rage. "Feelings of inner emptiness or depression, caused by the chronic self-object failures, are defended against by compulsive attempts to stimulate or soothe the self via sexual excitement, aggressive attacks, the intake of drugs or food, or by other means" (Kahn, 1985, p. 899).

Actually, the microdynamics of behavior change are not well articulated by Kohutian theory. Kohut (e.g., 1979) gives examples of behavior and behavior change, but the examples are exemplars of patterns of behavior that are relatively distally controlled by underlying self-issues. It is not a concern with predicting behavior that drives the enterprise. Rather, it is the understanding or interpretation of behavior that is really at issue. If there is an underlying microdynamic associated with behavior, it is frustration. If the individual experiences a lapse in the satisfaction of the self's needs with which he or she is unprepared to deal, the result will be rage, or depression, or sexual perversity, or the like. If there is frustration of the self's needs under optimal circumstances—that is, when there is a satisfactory relationship between self and other (e.g., a therapist) and the other fails to provide for the self's needs—the self will respond with changes in the direction of growth. The self will become better able to deal with its own needs.

THE AWARENESS ISSUE

Kohut's theory of the self is derived from psychoanalytic theory. In traditional psychoanalysis, one of the major goals of therapy is the widening of consciousness. In contrast, although drives are not open to introspection (Kohut, 1982), the primary goal of Kohutian therapy is not "insight," but rather the establishment of empathic "in-tuneness" in order to strengthen the structure of self (Kahn, 1985).

The SEM model emerges from a social-psychological tradition in which phenomenological self-reports are the usual stock in trade. Research experience with the model, however, suggests that people are often unaware of the extent to which their behavior conforms to the model. There are a number of examples. In one study (Tesser & Campbell, 1982), subjects indicated on a computer how well a friend or a stranger performed on tasks that were either relevant or irrelevant to their (the subjects') own self-definition. In another study (Tesser & Smith, 1980), subjects were given the opportunity to affect the performance of either a friend or a stranger on a task that was either high or low in self-relevance. In both cases, subjects' behavior conformed to the model, while subsequent self-reports about their behavior did not. The self-reports indicated that they were kinder to the friend than they actually were. Similarly, we (Tesser et al., 1988) tracked the pleasantness of expression on people's faces when they were confronted with information about their performance on either a high- or low-relevance task relative to a friend or a stranger. Facial expressions were predicted by the SEM model, but subjects' self-reports of mood were not.

In each such case, there is a discrepancy between the actual behavior and the individual's self-report. Perhaps the individual is quite aware of his or her behavior, but simply provides a self-report intended to make him or her look good to the experimenter. This seems unlikely, because the subject knows that the experimenter has access to the previous behavior. (Indeed, in some cases the behavior was recorded by computer or by video camera.) If anything, a "lie" about previous behavior could make the individual look worse. Therefore, it appears that at least some of the changes associated with the SEM model are made without awareness.

In sum, although Kohut's theory and the SEM model come from intellectual traditions that take diametrically opposed stands on the awareness issue, they are remarkably similar. Both agree that much of what happens in the service of the self is not available to self-awareness, but for neither is awareness the important issue.

QUESTIONS OF EPISTEMOLOGY

Psychoanalytically derived theories and social-psychological theories also differ with respect to how they learn about the world. The answers to such questions as "What are the populations of interest?", "Where are the important theoretical invariances to be found?", and "What constitutes good data for validating knowledge?" all differ fundamentally.

For Kohut's clinical theory of the self, the population that is available for observation consists of clients presenting themselves for therapy. For the SEM model, the population consists of normal adults; to be more specific, since most of the research takes place in an academic setting, the population consists mainly of young adults taking introductory psychology courses. Persons interested in therapy are focused on their problems, what is intolerable in their lives, and their need for change. The relationship they enter into with the therapist is likely to be long-term and intimate—a relationship in which it will be difficult to keep from revealing very much. The unselected college student is less likely to be short-term and specifically focused. Rather than being preoccupied with problems, the student is likely to be trying to put his or her best foot forward. Clearly, what is available for observation in these two populations is not the same.

Theory development involves a construction of invariances or rules that govern phenomena of interest. The theorist's metatheory about behavior will have a profound impact on the kind of invariances he or she is likely to develop. Psychoanalysts and social psychologists have fundamentally different metatheories of behavior. Thus, it is not surprising to discover that the kinds of invariances associated with Kohut's theory involve early interactions between child and caretaker. The invariances associated with the SEM model, in contrast, concern the dynamics of one's present, changing circumstances.

An epistemology also must have rules for gathering data and criteria for how such data can be used to validate inferences or hypotheses. Again, the psychoanalytic and social-psychological approaches diverge. Kohut (1978) is quite clear on how one learns about the psychological world as distinct from the physical or biological world: "The inner world cannot be observed with the aid of our sense organs. [However,] our thoughts, wishes, feelings, and fantasies . . . are real, and we can observe them as they occur in time: through introspection in our selves, and through empathy (i.e., vicarious introspection) in others" (pp. 205–206). Although other methods may be used and amalgamated for Kohut "the final and decisive observational act, however, is introspective or empathic" (pp. 209–210). For example, we may use a yardstick to show that an individual is very tall, but it is only through empathy that we can understand the psychological significance of this height.

Kohut's insistence on empathy and "near experiences" as a vehicle for knowing precludes the use of contemporary social psychology's *modus operandi*, the systematic testing of hypotheses using operational definitions of variables and statistical tests of observations. In contrast to Kohutian theory, the insights from the SEM model have been subjected to laboratory experiments and field studies which focus on perceptions, behaviors and feelings. (Summaries of this work are available in Tesser, 1986, 1988, and in press.) The goal here is also understanding, but the understanding is achieved through prediction and control rather than empathy.

CLINICAL IMPLICATIONS

The self psychology of Kohut was developed in the context of a psychoanalytic clinical practice. Thus, it tenets for what to do in this setting are rich, well developed, and rather fully articulated and commented upon. On the other hand, the implications of the SEM model for clinical practice are not well developed. The theory was not developed for this purpose and until only recently did not have the attention of clinical practitioners. Thus, the implications to be drawn are still quite tentative and have not undergone the test of repeated use in a clinical setting.

For both approaches, clinical practice follows from the processes they have identified as important: Both seek to maximize self-esteem through the use of social relationships. But there are some fundamental differences in the techniques to accomplish this. In principle, change agents can be anyone to whom the client is close. However, Kohutian therapy is crucially dependent on transference phenomena and trained empathic responding. The therapist must optimally time the presentation and withdrawal of the mirroring and the idealization process; thus, therapy tends to be individual. The SEM model, on the other hand, is making its first foray into clinical practice in terms of marital therapy (e.g., Beach, in press; Tesser & Beach, 1989). Perhaps because we have observed behavior change as a result of relatively minor laboratory manipulations, we are optimistic that marital partners can help each other change the construals of circumstances that lead to unproductive interpersonal feelings and behavior.

The focus of change in Kohutian therapy is the person rather than the environment. Problems are seen as being in the client, who has a narcissistic personality, a fragmented self, or the like. Therefore, therapy must change the structure of the individual's self. Furthermore, since these problems are seen to arise from faulty development, the temporal focus of the therapy is on the past. Transference is important because it allows the therapist to take over the role of early caretakers and to provide the psychological sustenance and challenge that those early caretakers did not. The SEM model, on the other hand, assumes that problems do not necessarily arise from a faulty self or a faulty development. Problems may result from the structure of the environment or from an individual's perception of the environment. Thus, significant beneficial changes can come from changing the environment or the client's perception of the environment. For example, to reduce the pain of comparison, clients can be encouraged to seek out environments where their own performance is among the best; or they can be encouraged to limit the breadth of areas that are relevant to their self-definition.

A CONCLUDING OBSERVATION

There is an overriding difference between Kohutian theory and the SEM model—a difference so large that most of the details seem to be implications of it. It is that Kohutian theory is driven by clinical concerns and the SEM model by more general, basic science concerns. Perhaps what is most remarkable in the face of this difference is that each approach sees human behavior as unfolding according to very similar social-psychological processes. It is in this commonality that we begin to discern a more universal way of thinking about behavior, and it is the complementary—or perhaps I should say mirrored/reflected—differences that provide the potential for the growth of each perspective. For example, a broader SEM model that includes self-generated rehearsal of one's own achievements and self-generated rehearsal of achievements of close others as potential responses to frustration and perceived failure is entirely consistent with the current SEM model, yet goes beyond its current bounds. Thus, it might be posited that in addition to changing closeness, or relative performance on a task when outperformed by a close other, a person could also rehearse *previous* good performances by the self on relevant tasks or previous good performances by others on tasks low in relevance. This self-soothing activity has the form of a Kohutian response to frustration, but is couched in SEM terminology. Perhaps similar implications of the SEM model for developments in Kohutian theory may also be forthcoming.

ACKNOWLEDGMENTS

I am grateful to Winter Giddings, who first introduced me to Kohut's ideas, and to Steven Beach, Carmen McClendon, and Janet Moore, who made helpful comments on a draft of this chapter. I also wish to acknowledge the support of the National Institute of Mental Health, Grant No. 1R01MH41487-01.

NOTES

1. During this time a number of investigators were doing *individual-difference* work on self-related constructs, such as internal–external locus of control (e.g., Rotter, 1966) and self-esteem (Wylie, 1974).

2. Kohut (1984) outlined a third aspect of the self's functioning, having to do with "twinship" needs, or the need simply to be close to someone who is similar to the self. It is through such closeness that talents and skills are optimally developed. This aspect of the self's functioning has not been fleshed out or developed theoretically to the extent that mirroring and idealization have (Kahn, 1985). In the self-evaluation maintenance (SEM) model, there is no need for a close other, per se. In the SEM model, close others potentiate the effects of relevance and performance: The closer the other, the greater the impact on the self. Therefore, although I refer to closeness needs throughout the rest of this chapter, I focus primarily on Kohut's bipolar self (i.e., the needs for mirroring and idealization).

3. There is a kind of paradox here: As closeness increases, so do the possibilities

for comparison. However, one can imagine situations in which two persons are so close that the unit is the pair rather than the individual. Under these conditions, the question of comparison is not relevant; that is, one person's actions are totally substitutable for the other's. However, I suspect that such situations are rare.

4. Performance and relevance are not completely independent. When another's performance is particularly discrepant from one's own, comparison becomes difficult and relevance decreases.

5. It appears as if mirrors are an obvious analogy for thinking about the inherent reflexiveness in the concept of self. Both Kohut and the SEM model make use of a mirror analogy in labeling the processes of interest. When the processes from one theory are mapped onto the processes of the other, the mirror analogy labels are appended to different processes. Thus, the SEM's comparison process maps onto Kohut's mirroring process, and Kohut's idealizing process maps onto the SEM reflection process.

6. The bulk of work on the SEM model focuses on intrapsychic processes. However, it also appears likely that self-presentation concerns may be at work. See Tesser and Moore (1986) and Tesser and Paulhus (1983) for more complete discussions of this issue.

7. From my perspective, the comparison process from the SEM model maps most easily onto the mirroring process of Kohut. Robert Stolorow, an expert on Kohutian theory (e.g., Stolorow, Brandchaft, & Atwood, 1987), suggests (personal communication, March 24, 1990) that it is possible to map the comparison process onto the Kohutian category of "twinship." "The performing other is experienced as a replica or twin of the subject's *self-ideal*, and the subject experiences a painful discrepancy between his perception of his actual self and self-ideal, evoking shame and envy. This is very different from the reflection situation, in which the performing other is experienced as an idealized object in whose glory one can participate."

REFERENCES

Aronson, E. (1969). The theory of cognitive dissonance: A current perspective. In L. Bekowitz (Ed.), *Advances in experimental social psychology* (Vol. 4, pp. 2–32). New York: Academic Press.

Beach, S. R. H. (in press). Social cognition and the relationship repair process: Toward better outcomes in marital therapy. In G. Fletcher & F. Fincham (Eds.), *Cognition in close relationships*. New York: Guilford Press.

Berscheid, E. (1983). Emotion. In H. H. Kelley, E. Berscheid, A. Christensen, J. Harvey, T. L. Huston, G. Levinger, E. McClintock, A. Peplau, & D. R. Peterson, *Close relationships* (pp. 110–168.) San Francisco: W. H. Freeman.

Brehm, S. S., & Kassin, S. M. (1990). *Social psychology*. Boston: Houghton-Mifflin.

Carver, C. S., & Scheier, M. F. (1981). *Attention and self-regulation: A control-theory approach to human behavior*. New York: Springer-Verlag.

Cashdan, S. (1988). *Object relations therapy*. New York: Norton.

Chessick, R. D. (1985). *Psychology of the self and the treatment of narcissism*. Northvale, NJ: Jason Aronson.

Cialdini, R. B., Borden, R. J., Thorne, A., Walker, M. R., Freeman, S., & Sloan, L. R. (1976). Basking in reflected glory: Three (football) field studies. *Journal of Personality and Social Psychology, 34*, 366–375.

Dittes, J. (1959). Attractiveness of group as a function of self-esteem and acceptance by group. *Journal of Abnormal and Social Psychology, 59*, 77–82.

Fairbairn, W. R. D. (1954). *An object relations theory of personality*. New York: Basic Books.

Festinger, L. (1954). A theory of social comparison processes. *Human Relations, 7*, 117–140.

Friedlander, M. (1986). *The phenomenal self, strategic self-presentation, and Kohut's self psychology*. Paper presented at the annual convention of the American Psychological Association, Washington, DC.

Greenwald, A. G., & Ronis, D. L. (1978). Twenty years of cognitive dissonance: Case study of the evolution of a theory. *Psychological Review, 85*, 53–57.

Heider, F. (1958). *The psychology of interpersonal relations*. New York: Wiley.

Ichheiser, G. (1949). Misunderstandings in human relations. *American Journal of Sociology, 55*(2), Part 2.

James, W. (1890). *The principles of psychology* (Vol. 1). New York: Henry Holt.

Jones, S. C. (1973). Self and interpersonal evaluations: Esteem theories versus consistency theories. *Psychological Bulletin, 79*, 185–199.

Kahn, E. (1985). Heinz Kohut and Carl Rogers: A timely comparison. *American Psychologist, 40*, 893–904.

Klein, M. (1948). *Contributions to psychoanalysis*. London: Hogarth Press.

Kohut, H. (1971). *The analysis of the self*. New York: International Universities Press.

Kohut, H. (1977). *The restoration of the self*. New York: International Universities Press.

Kohut, H. (1978). Introspection, empathy, and psychoanalysis: An examination of the relationship between mode of observation and theory. In P. Ornstein (Ed.), *The search for the self* (Vol. 1, pp. 205–232). New York: International Universities Press.

Kohut, H. (1979). The two analyses of Mr. Z. *International Journal of Psycho-Analysis, 60*, 3–27.

Kohut, H. (1982). Introspection, empathy, and the semi-circle of mental health. *International Journal of Psycho-Analysis, 63*, 395–407.

Kohut, H. (1984). *How does analysis cure?* (A. Goldberg & P. E. Stepansky, Eds.). Chicago: University of Chicago Press.

Lasch, C. (1978). *The culture of narcissism*. New York: Norton.

Lecky, P. (1945). *Self-consistency: A theory of personality*. New York: Island Press.

Maddi, S. R. (1989). *Personality theories: A comparative analysis* (5th ed.). Homewood, IL: Dorsey Press.

Mahler, M. S. (1952). On child psychosis and schizophrenia: Autistic and symbiotic infantile psychoses. *Psychoanalytic Study of the Child, 7*, 286–305.

Mandler, G. (1975). *Mind and emotion*. New York: Wiley.

Markus, H. (1977). Self-schemata and processing information about the self. *Journal of Personality and Social Psychology, 35,* 63–78.

McFarlin, D. B., & Blascovich, J. (1981). Effects of self-esteem and performance on future affective preferences and cognitive expectations. *Journal of Personality and Social Psychology, 40,* 521–531.

Miller, D. T., Turnbull, W., & McFarland, C. (1988). Particularistic and universalistic evaluation in the social comparison process. *Journal of Personality and Social Psychology, 55,* 908–917.

Moreland, R. L., & Sweeney, P. D. (1984). Self-expectancies and reactions to evaluations of personal performance. *Journal of Personality, 52,* 156–176.

Patton, M. J., Connor, G. E., & Scott, K. J. (1982). Kohut's psychology of the self: Theory and measures of counseling outcome. *Journal of Counseling Psychology, 29,* 268–282.

Powers, W. T. (1973). *Behavior: The control of perception.* Chicago: Aldine.

Reich, A. (1960). Pathological forms of self-esteem regulation. *Psychoanalytic Study of the Child, 15,* 215–232.

Ross, M., & Sicoly, F. (1979). Egocentric biases in availability and attribution. *Journal of Personality and Social Psychology, 37,* 322–336.

Rotter, J. B. (1966). Generalized expectancies for internal versus external control of reinforcement. *Psychological Monographs, 80*(1, Whole No. 609).

Salovey, P., & Rodin, J. (1984). Some antecedents and consequences of social-comparison jealousy. *Journal of Personality and Social Psychology, 47,* 780–792.

Shrauger, J. S. (1975). Responses to evaluation as a function of initial self-perceptions. *Psychological Bulletin, 82,* 581–596.

Sigall, H., & Landy, D. (1973). Radiating beauty: Effects of attractive partner on person perception. *Journal of Social Psychology, 28,* 218–224.

Stolorow, R., Brandchaft, B., & Atwood, G. (1987). *Psychoanalytic treatment: An intersubjective approach.* Hillsdale, NJ: Erlbaum.

Swann, W. B., Jr. (1983). Self-verification: Bringing social reality into harmony with the self. In J. Suls & A. G. Greenwald (Eds.), *Psychological perspectives on the self* (Vol. 2, pp. 33–66). Hillsdale, NJ: Erlbaum.

Swann, W. B., Jr., Griffin, J. J., Predmore, S. C., & Gaines, B. (1987). The cognitive–affective crossfire: When self-consistency confronts self enhancement. *Journal of Personality and Social Psychology, 52,* 881–889.

Tesser, A. (1980). Self-esteem maintenance in family dynamics. *Journal of Personality and Social Psychology, 39,* 77–91.

Tesser, A. (1984). Self-evaluation maintenance processes: Implications for relationships and development. In J. C. Masters & K. L. Yarkin (Eds.), *Boundary areas in psychology: Social and Developmental psychology* (pp. 271–299). New York: Academic Press.

Tesser, A. (1986). Some effects of self-evaluation maintenance on cognition and action. In R. M. Sorrentino & E. T. Higgins (Eds.), *Handbook of motivation and cognition: Foundations of social behavior* (Vol. 1, pp. 435–464). New York: Guilford Press.

Tesser, A. (1988). Toward a self-evaluation maintenance model of social behavior. In L. Berkowitz (Ed.), *Advances in experimental social psychology* (Vol. 21, pp. 181–227). New York: Academic Press.

Tesser, A. (in press). Emotion in social comparison and reflection processes. In J. Suls & T. A. Wills (Eds.), *Social comparison: Contemporary theory and research.* Hillsdale, NJ: Erlbaum.

Tesser, A., Achee, J., & Pilkington, C. (1990). *On the role of arousal in self-evaluation maintenance processes.* Unpublished manuscript, University of Georgia.

Tesser, A., & Beach, S. (1989). *Emotion in marriage: The role of social reflection and comparison.* Unpublished research proposal, University of Georgia.

Tesser, A., & Campbell, J. (1982). Self-evaluation maintenance and the perception of friends and strangers. *Journal of Personality, 50,* 261–279.

Tesser, A., & Collins, J. (1988). Emotion in social reflection and comparison situations: Intuitive, systematic, and exploratory approaches. *Journal of Personality and Social Psychology, 55,* 695–709.

Tesser, A., Millar, M., & Moore, J. (1988). Some affective consequences of social comparison and reflection processes: The pain and pleasure of being close. *Journal of Personality and Social Psychology, 54,* 49–61.

Tesser, A., & Moore, J. (1986). On the convergence of public and private aspects of self. In R. Baumeister (Ed.), *Public self and private self* (pp. 99–116). New York: Springer-Verlag.

Tesser, A., & Paulhus, D. (1983). The definition of self: Private and public self-evaluation maintenance strategies. *Journal of Personality and Social Psychology, 44,* 672–682.

Tesser, A., Pilkington, C., & McIntosh, W. (1989). Self-evaluation maintenance and the mediational role of emotion: The perception of friends and strangers. *Journal of Personality and Social Psychology, 57,* 442–456.

Tesser, A., & Smith, J. (1980). Some effects of friendship and task relevance on helping: You don't always help the one you like. *Journal of Experimental Social Psychology, 16,* 582–590.

Wicklund, R. D. (1975). Objective self-awareness. In L. Berkowitz (Ed.), *Advances in experimental social psychology* (Vol. 8, pp. 233–275). New York: Academic Press.

Worchel, S., Cooper, J., & Goethals, G. R. (1988). *Understanding social psychology* (4th ed.). Homewood, IL: Dorsey Press.

Wylie, R. C. (1974). *The self-concept* (rev. ed., Vol. 1). Lincoln: University of Nebraska Press.

Zuckerman, M. (1979). Attribution of success and failure revisited, or: The motivational bias is alive and well in attribution theory. *Journal of Personality, 47,* 245–287.

CHAPTER FOURTEEN

Self-with-Other Representation as a Unit of Analysis in Self-Concept Research

DANIEL M. OGILVIE
RICHARD D. ASHMORE

INTRODUCTION

This chapter deals with a decision we made concerning what information about the "social self" would be most useful to collect in the context of a research project titled "Gender Identity, Sex Stereotypes, and Social Action" (Ashmore & Ogilvie, 1989). Eventually, we will piece together a vast array of information related to the causes, contents, and consequences of gender-related beliefs about the self and others. In addition to obtaining information about research participants' interests and abilities, goals and actions, personality traits and characteristic feelings, perceptions of their own and others' physical appearances, and so on, we wished also to gather something crucial concerning their social self-concepts. Specifically, our aim was to assess what aspects of the self are brought out in participants' primary relationships with specific other people in their lives and to represent how these self-with-other experiences are organized.[1]

Although our two careers in psychology are vastly different, we converged at the same intersection regarding the importance of interactions with others as critical to understanding the formation, maintenance, and transformation of the self-concept. Within this general perspective, we give special scrutiny to the individual's construction of internal representations of interactions with specific people, and this focus has led to the creation of a unit of analysis that is unique in social-psychological investigations of the self. This unit of analysis, "self-with-other," is the primary focus of the remainder of this chapter.

Prior to elaborating on our "self-with-other" construct, we look first at the research of others and discuss variables commonly used in various designs. We do this for the purpose of showing how our approach is similar to and yet different from extant models. Our views of the self as a multiplicity, its hierarchical organization, its cognitive representation, and the like grow in many ways from the work of other researchers in the field. Indeed, the supportive links and invigorating areas of overlap between our work and the advancements made by others make it mandatory that we acknowledge our indebtedness. In doing so, we also create a context for making some distinctions we wish to preserve.

AN OVERVIEW OF MODERN RESEARCH ON THE SELF

Most research investigations related to the "self" focus either on individuals' perceptions of themselves *or* on their perceptions of others. The following partial survey of the literature reflects that division.

Self-Perception

Wylie (1974) has provided a compendium of thousands of studies that view the self as a single entity. A shared notion of much of this research is that the "self" is a concept that can be brought to mind and objectified for the purpose of evaluation.[2] In effect, the self is treated as an idea or "thing" (albeit a very important thing) that can be described, rated, and assessed using the same processes that one might use in evaluating other objects.

A more recent view taken in self-concept research is that the self can be decomposed into a confederacy or multiplicity of "selves." The theoretical precedence for this distinction runs deep. From James's (1890) argument that we have as many selves as there are persons with whom we are socially engaged, to Mead's (1934) theory of complexity of the self as a result of individuals' interactions with others in a structured society, the stage had been set for a multifaceted view of the self many years before research from this perspective began in earnest. The Twenty Statements Test developed by Kuhn and McPartland (1954) was among the first instruments created to elicit multiple domains of self-definition. This open-ended method requires respondents to answer the question "Who am I?" 20 times. The Twenty Statements Test was used by numerous researchers, especially in the 1960s and early 1970s, who categorized responses using several different content analysis systems. (See Zurcher, 1977, for a review of this work, and McGuire & McGuire, 1988, for an example of an alternative approach to open-endedly gathering self-descriptive information.)

New conceptualizations of the self as a multiplicity and methods relating to these theories were developed in the 1980s. Much of this work is reviewed by Markus and Wurf (1987). Here, we are more interested in the procedures and units of analysis selected for research than in the theoretical substance behind the investigations. In some studies, respondents are asked to assess themselves in terms of experimenter-generated self-concept categories. For example, Higgins and his coinvestigators (Higgins, Klein, & Strauman, 1985; Higgins, Bond, Klein, & Strauman, 1986) divide the self in to "real," "ideal," and "ought" components and ask respondents to describe each component using 10 features. Scores representing discrepancies between the real and ideal selves, and between the real and ought selves are derived from these descriptions and are shown to be variously related to the mood states of depression and anxiety. A different strategy is used by Linville (1985) in her work on self-complexity. Linville provides her respondents with 33 traits and asks them to sort them into self-descriptive piles. Each pile is assumed to reflect a unit or aspect of the self.

Other investigators are concerned with the structure of multiple identities. Stryker and Serpe (1982) approach the problem from a symbolic interactionist perspective and argue that commitment to an identity leads to its salience, and that salience, in turn, affects role-related behavioral choices. Thus, the location of an identity in the overall structure of identities is a function of the individual's commitment to it. The identities about which respondents make judgments are predetermined by Stryker and Serpe. By contrast, Rosenberg and Gara (1985) and Ogilvie (1987a) rely on respondents to generate their own identities *and* their own vocabulary for describing these identities. After identities and features are determined, respondents rate every identity on all features. The resulting matrix is then analyzed in a manner that represents identity structure in terms of identity equivalence, disjunctiveness, and subset–superset relations. We have a great deal more to say about this method of analysis later on. For now, the primary point we wish to make is that a common denominator of self-perception research is this: Participants are asked to bring to mind identities or aspects of themselves and to describe, either in their own terms or in terms provided by investigators, how they are or how they feel about themselves in any particular identity.

Another approach to self-perception research is being taken by cognitive–social psychologists. The focus of this work is primarily on the question of how self-knowledge is mentally organized and processed. In general, the self is envisioned as a node in an associative memory network (Cantor & Kihlstrom, 1987; Kihlstrom et al., 1988). This node is linked to other nodes representing semantic information (e.g., traits and characteristics) and other nodes representing episodic information (e.g., specific actions). The researcher's task is to activate a self node and, through various reaction time designs, begin to plot the structure of the associative network. Using this strategy, hypotheses regarding the effects of self-schematic and self-aschematic knowledge on the speed of information processing can be tested (e.g., Markus, 1977, 1983). It is important to note that most researchers in this arena are more concerned with locating general rules for processing self-related information than they are with the issue of individual differences regarding structure of the self.

Perceptions of Others

Most studies in the area of person perception are designed to uncover and describe implicit dimensions individuals use to organize their perceptions of others. Generally, these studies are nomothetic and, given researchers' normative intentions, the self is seldom implicated. However, a large body of literature spawned by George Kelly's (1955) work on construct systems is relevant to the present discussion. Kelly argued that an individual's personality *is* his or her construct system. As lay scientists, human beings create theories about what other people are like and how they are predisposed to behave. The basic elements of lay theories are individually held constructs. Constructs are uncovered by asking respondents to compare three people in their lives, showing how two of them are alike and the third is different. A result may be that two people are construed as alike in that they are both friendly (the construct pole) and the third person is different because he or she is critical of others (the contrast pole). By sorting and labeling numerous triads of people in this manner, the participant reveals the primary constructs he or she uses in organizing perceptions of others.

After personal constructs have been obtained, Kelly and his followers make a noteworthy inference. That is, the constructs individuals use to construe other people, and the manner in which these constructs are hierarchically arranged, say something vital about the respondent's own personality. In other words, it is assumed that the constructs applied to others are also central items of self-evaluation. By obtaining information about the constructs individuals use for organizing their perceptions of *others*, one becomes informed about the beholders' personalities.

In summary, most research on the self as a multiplicity asks respondents to think about themselves or aspects of themselves as objects of investigation. Other researchers (notably Kelly and his followers) obtain information about personality structure by having respondents bring to mind other people as objects of comparison. Although it might appear that our focus of investigation alternates between perceptions of the self *and* the other, in fact our unit of analysis captures something quite different. Self-with-other units are mental representations of self–other *interactions*. It is now essential that we describe this unit and its theoretical underpinnings in sufficient detail to demonstrate how it is an altogether new unit for a social psychological approach to the analysis of the self. The next two sections are written for that purpose.

SELF-WITH-OTHER AS A UNIT OF ANALYSIS

We concur with others (see the preceding review) that an essential aspect of human existence is the formation and reformation of cognitive representations of one's self. Much of this activity occurs in the context of real or imagined interactions with an audience. People recall how they were in various situations, and this forms a basis for self-knowledge. Self-images are also formed from notions of "how I would ideally like to be," "how I ought to be" (Higgins et al., 1985), and "me at my worst" (Ogilvie, 1987b), as well as from ideas of what may be possible in the future (Markus & Nurius, 1986). These self-images are internalized and serve as guides to ongoing and future behavior. Fortunately for researchers, they can also be called to mind and objectified for the purpose of description and evaluation. We also internalize and mentally arrange images of other people, partly for the purpose of simplifying a complex world. Like images of the self, images of others can be brought to consciousness and manipulated for a variety of purposes. Our model goes beyond these two domains of affective and cognitive encoding, the self and the other, and declares that we also internalize the whole of our relationships. That is, we not only internalize and mentally represent our selves and others; *we also form images of what we are like and how we feel when we are with specific other people in our lives.*

There are several areas of overlap between our self-with-other representational unit and the theoretical work of others. For example, we suspect that it captures a central aspect of what Tomkins (1987) means by "scenes" in his script theory. A scene represents a "happening" that minimally includes one affect and one object of that affect. In most instances, a scene is a composite image extracted from a pattern of multiply recurring events involving the self, an affect (or a particular blending of affects), and an object (i.e., another person). Thus, a scene is formed from an average of repeated self-with-specific-other experiences; as a consequence, it can portray a self-with-other relationship that never happened, precisely as the generalized scene depicts it.

Most scenes, or self-with-other units, rest beneath everyday consciousness. Despite their nonconscious status (or perhaps *because* they are not conscious), they are powerful motivators of behavior. According to Tomkins (1987) and Carlson (1988), we strive to magnify a family of safety-related scenes by seeking ways to re-enact them. We embellish thrilling scenes in order to enhance experiences of excitement. We are also motivated to avoid recreating anxiety-related scenes—scenes wherein we have experienced discomfort or insecurity. Important elements of scenes are "scripts," which contain rules for enhancing, creating, interpreting, defending against, or modifying external reality (or our construal of reality) in accordance with families of internalized scenes. Thus, the activation of a scene leads to a simultaneous activation of scripted behaviors pertaining to that scene.

Psychoanalytic theorists have worked with concepts similar to Tomkins's "scenes" and "scripts" ever since Freud (1914) addressed himself to the phenomenon of transference in the patient–therapist relationship. Rather than dismissing seemingly uncalled-for outbursts of anger or undue expressions of love and affection for the therapist by a client as further evidence of pathology, Freud came to view such episodes as vital ingredients of successful therapy. In effect, as therapy progresses, repressed "scenes" seek new avenues for expression. Since some affect-laden scenes are shielded from memory, the patient cannot form conscious representations of them. Instead, the patient re-enacts aspects of a repressed relationship (an unconscious "scene") in his or her here-and-now relationship with the therapist. In effect, transference was viewed as a conflict-driven symptom to be unraveled and explored. It became a tool for inspecting patterns of troubled and incomplete past relationships.

Transference continues to be a topic of interest among modern-day object relations theorists. For example, Kernberg (1976), in addressing character pathology, writes:

> The more rigid and neurotic the character traits are, the more they reveal that a past pathogenic internalized object (representing a particular conflict) has become "frozen" into a character pattern. Psychoanalytic exploration and resolution of character traits as they become transformed into active transference dispositions consistently reveal the activation of *units of self- and object-representations linked by a particular affect disposition*. (p. 79, emphasis ours)

Thus, Kernberg's basic unit is comprised of the self, an object (another person), and an "affect disposition."

Further evidence of the significance granted something like our "self-with-other" units of analysis in the field of psychoanalytic self psychology is the now-standard practice of combining the words "self" and "object" into one word, "selfobject." Kohut (1977) elaborates the self object into a "self/self-object unit" (p. 86). Other concepts that highlight the clinical importance of the self in interaction with others include Mitchell's (1988) "relational model," Beebe and Lachmann's (1988) "influence structures," Modell's (1984) "two-person psychology," and Atwood and Stolorow's (1984) notion of "intersubjective contexts." Stolorow (Chapter Two, this volume) considers Mitchell to have captured the essence of "relational-model" theories in the following passage:

> In this vision the basic unit of study is not the individual as a separate entity whose desires clash with an external reality, but an interactional field within which the individual arises and struggles to make contact and to articulate himself. *Desire* is experienced always *in the context of relatedness*, and it is that context which defines its meaning. Mind is composed of relational configurations. . . . Experience is understood as structured through interactions. . . . (Mitchell, 1988, pp. 3–4, emphasis in original)

Stolorow expresses his own views regarding relational models when he writes, "To my mind, the most important development in psychoanalysis over the past decade has been the growing recognition that intrapsychic phenomena must be understood in the context of the larger interactional systems in which they take form" (Stolorow, Chapter Two, this volume).

Lastly, Stern (1985) discusses his own relational model in terms of internal "representations of interactions that have become generalized," abbreviated as "RIGs." RIGs are representations in the minds of infants of repeated episodes of interactive experience with a "self-regulating other" (usually the primary caregiver). A RIG is a composite, usually nonconscious, image of past self-with-other experiences that represents an average of these experiences. A RIG is similar to Sullivan's concept of "dynamism," an energy unit formed from a pattern of "insignificant particular differences" (Sullivan, 1953, p. 104). It is through the development of RIGs or interactive dynamisms that the infant comes to know its interpersonal world and know how to behave within it. When a RIG is triggered, or a dynamism is activated, by the infant or another person, "it packs the same wallop of the original lived experience" (Stern, 1985, p. 110).

In summary, what we refer to as "self-with-other" representational units can be viewed as yet a new name attached to mental activity that has a long history of theoretical investigation in psychoanalytic psychology, culminating in a recent surge of theoretical interest. Clinical ideas seldom penetrate research-oriented personality and social psychology. To a very great degree, these two domains of psychology exist worlds apart. However, research methods are now available for some bridge building. Retrospectively, our own research can be viewed as an attempt to transport ideas generated by clinically formulated relational models into a social–personality–cognitive model of self-perception. This characterizes Ogilvie's entry point into this research more than it does Ashmore's, whose cognitive–social-psychological model (see Ashmore & Del Boca, 1986) was developed completely outside any clinical considerations and well before it became apparent how directly our model bears on present-day psychoanalytic theory.

Finally, in order not to be buried in a web of overlapping considerations, we need to bear in mind one important difference between our framework and clinically derived conceptualizations. Most clinical models were developed to provide greater understanding of therapist–patient interactions. The intersubjective, relational worlds referred to in clinical self psychology come up most frequently in the context of investigating the intersubjective transactions (transference and countertransference) that occur in clinical settings. Our self-with-other unit refers to the internalization of past and present interactions that are fully contained in the minds of individuals. They form the foundation of our being in the world of others and provide us with a sense of continuity between past and present interactive experiences. Before describing how our unit of analysis is operationalized, we offer the following brief summary of our guiding theoretical notions.

TOWARD A THEORY OF SELF-WITH-OTHER REPRESENTATIONS

In line with the views of several theorists mentioned in the preceding section, we begin with the notion that critical elements of important self-with-other experiences are mentally encoded. These mentally recorded, affectively toned events enable individuals to identify ongoing interpersonal interactions as similar to or different from previous patterns of self-with-other interactions.

The most important self-with-other sets of experiences in infancy are the child's self-with-mother (or self-with-primary-caretaker) experiences. We concur with clinical theory that more than one internal representation of self-with-Mom can be created. For example, a child may form a self-with-Mom-when-she-is-in-a-good-mood representation of interactions and another self-with-Mom-when-she-is-upset encoding. This kind of mental activity is a vital ingredient of self–selfobject splitting often referred to in clinical literature, and is probably a normal aspect of development in the preverbal child.

As the infant develops and other relationships are formed, new self-with-other interactions take shape. New "others" include Dad, brothers and sisters, and various extended family members who are actively involved in the child's life.

Internalized self-with-other representations created and organized in childhood from nonconscious building blocks for later self-with-other experiences. They inform us about how to interpret events, what to *feel* during different interactions, and how to behave in various self-with-other episodes. Although we consider self-with-other representations formed in childhood to be very important, we do not wish to overplay the impact they have on later interpersonal development. We grant that profoundly disturbed early object relations can have an overbearing effect on subsequent relationships, but we view such disturbances as exceptions, not the rule. Psychologically healthy individuals do not simply graft new relationships onto pre-existing primary internal representations formed from earlier self-with-other constellations of experience. Stasis is a condition of assimilating new interpersonal experiences into fixed and unchanging internal representations of previously encoded self-with-other experiences. Growth, however, involves updating, modifying, regrouping, and even transforming earlier representations in a manner that brings them more in line with present-day interactive experiences. The self is not a static object; it is a process. Likewise, internalized self-with-other representations in the healthy individual are not static entities. They are responsive to new relationships and are capable of accommodating themselves to the here-and-now "realities" of interpersonal relationships.

Propositional Summary

Although it is premature to cast our thinking about the self-with-other unit as a formal theory, we can summarize our working framework in terms of the following series of seven propositions:

1. The self-concept comprises multiple components.

2. One particularly important constituent is the social or interpersonal self.

3. A crucial, yet to date neglected, unit of analysis in investigating the social self is "self-with-other." The "self-with-other" variable is a hypothetical construct. It is provisionally defined as a mental representation that includes the set of personal qualities (traits, feelings, and the like) that an individual believes characterizes his or her self when with a particular other person.

4. Although each self-with-important-other internal representation is unique, the individual develops groupings of similar self-with-other representations. As an individual experiences self similarly in relationships with multiple specific others, a self-with-other family or constellation develops; for example, a preschool boy experiences himself as competent and comfortable with Mom, with Judy (a teenage babysitter), and with Grandpa.

5. Constellations of self-with-others are, in turn, mentally organized into an overall self-with-others structure. The exact nature of this structure

is impossible to specify at this time, and it is likely to vary considerably from person to person. At the same time, however, it is useful as a starting point to construe self-with-others groupings to be hierarchically arranged. This assumption is congruent with most current models of long-term memory and allows for the identification of self-with-others that vary in specificity versus generality.

6. Individually and as an overall structure, the mental representations of self-with-others are assumed to serve a variety of important functions for the individual. These include (a) summarizing past experience; (b) guiding present actions, especially interpersonal behavior; and (c) interpreting own and others' (especially interaction partners') behavior.

7. Although self-with-other representations are dynamic rather than static, they are, for most adults most of the time, sufficiently stable to allow reliable measurement.

We now turn to the issue of assessment.

Preview of Methods and Procedures

Our general research strategy seeks to integrate idiographic and nomothetic principles. That is, our aim is to describe each individual as fully and accurately as possible and, at the same time, to identify and quantify cross-person variables from each individual's data. In terms of specifics, the initial foray into assessing the self-with-other unit entails four separate data-gathering sessions: (1) By means of a face-to-face interview, we determine each participant's set of important others and personal vocabulary for thinking about others and self-with-others; (2) and (3) using an interactive computer procedure, the participant describes each other person and self-with-each-individual; (4) the results of multivariate structural analyses of these data are presented to and discussed with the participant. We now describe these sessions in depth, present the results for two individuals, and discuss strategies for making nomothetic comparisons.

METHODS AND PROCEDURES

At the time of this writing, we have conducted 6 of 11 sessions with 71 young adult participants in a 2-year study of the multiple components of gender identity (Ashmore & Ogilvie, 1989; Ashmore, 1990). The first four of these sessions pertain directly to our present topic, and the procedures used therein are now our focus. You, the reader, are invited to imagine having agreed to serve as a paid participant in this study, which was described as aimed at assessing the various aspects of self-concept. The following is a session-by-session review of what you and the investigators accomplished in four 80-minute sessions during the first 3 months of the study.

Session 1

In a letter mailed to you prior to your first session, you were asked to create a list of past and present "important people in your life." This list was to include parents, relatives, friends, enemies, and other acquaintances who have had a strong influence on you in negative as well as positive ways. In accord with the average number of names generated by the other participants, you created a list of 29 important people and brought this list with you to your session.

Your interviewer informed you that the purpose of this session was to develop a list of words and phrases that you typically use to describe other people and yourself when you interact with others who are prominent in your life. Your interviewer began this process by asking you to look over your "important people" list and find a person who was easy for you to describe. You selected a male colleague whom you consider to be ambitious, obnoxious, insensitive to others' feelings, pushy, and untrustworthy. "Angry" and "upset" were the two words you used when you were asked whether this individual made you feel any particular way when you were with him. As you spoke, the interviewer wrote down some key information about your colleague on a 3 × 5 card and, on a separate sheet of paper, began your list of descriptors (i.e., "ambitious," "obnoxious," "upset," etc.). Henceforth, we refer to descriptors as "features."

As you described the people on your list, you came across two instances where you found the task particularly difficult. In both cases, the problem had to do with a dramatic change that had occurred in your relationships with these two individuals. There had been a critical turning point in the quality of your interactions with them. In both instances, your interviewer suggested that you make Time 1–Time 2 distinctions, allowing you to create two individuals from one (e.g., "my colleague when we used to collaborate," "my colleague after we ceased to collaborate"). You accepted that option and understood that a consequence of the two divisions you made was that each individual you split in that manner would henceforth be treated as two different interactive partners.

It took 70 minute to create your features list. In the time remaining, your interviewer asked for your assistance in reducing your list of people to a total of 25. That total included the two individuals for whom you had made Time1–Time 2 distinctions. You were now operating with a total of 31 people, and 6 of these individuals had to be deleted. Strong candidates for deletion had already occurred to you during the interview, as you had realized that some individuals you had included on your original list were little more than distant memories.[3] For you, then, as for most other participants, the limit of 25 others that we imposed on you gave you sufficient opportunity to cover a wide range of the various sorts of people who are, or have been, interpersonally important to you.

After you departed, your interviewer counted the number of features you had produced. The resulting number, 68, had to be reduced to a total of 42 with a list of 8 backup words. This was accomplished by crossing out duplicates, reducing synonyms into exemplar words, and giving some preference for retaining "negative" words over "positive" ones. The third guideline was followed because your "positive" descriptors had outnumbered "negative" ones (which is the rule in research involving open-ended descriptions of self and others), and we wished to preserve the widest possible range of words in your descriptive vocabulary.

In preparation for Session 2, the 42 words from your personal vocabulary were entered into a computer. These terms were combined with a list of 18 words from the project's "consensual vocabulary." This inclusion of project-generated items is one of the few exceptions to our standard practice of working primarily with participants' descriptions in their own words of their thoughts and feelings. This particular exception was made in order to further our interests in comparing our results regarding the effects of gender on self-perception with the work performed by others on this topic. To this end, the consensual list contained words drawn from the results of Williams and Best's (1982) work using Gough's Adjective Checklist to assess sex stereotypes. Eight words were high-consensus male stereotype words, and eight others were high-consensus female stereotype words. These were further subdivided into positive and negative evaluations. Male/positive words were "active," "confident," "independent," and "strong." Female/positive words were "affectionate," "gentle," "sympathetic," and "warm." Male/negative words included "boastful," "coarse," "egotistical," and "hardhearted." Female/negatives were "fussy," "nagging," "weak," and "whiny." Two more words, "feminine" and "masculine," were added to this list. Four of your personal vocabulary words matched words contained in the consensual vocabulary. In order to maintain a list of 60 words, the 4 remaining words were obtained from your backup list.

Finally, the names of your 25 important people were entered into the computer. With this and the already entered features, as well as the specially written computer program to allow you to use these to describe others and self-with-others, the project was prepared for your next visit.

Session 2

When you arrived for the second session, you were escorted to a private room and seated in front of a computer screen; an assistant instructed you how to interact with the computer as follows. Your training consisted of a couple of practice examples wherein the name of a well-known individual appeared near the top of the screen. A feature (e.g., "friendly") then appeared in the middle of the screen, and your task was to rate the individual in terms of how friendly you considered him or her to be. You were given three options. If you considered "friendly" as not a relevant descriptor for this individual, you entered a "0." A "1" indicated that you viewed "friendly" as somewhat descriptive of the individual, and a "2" indicated that "friendly" described the individual quite well.

After you rated the practice target on the first word and had pressed the "enter" key, a new descriptor replaced "friendly" on the screen. After eight descriptors were used in this fashion, a tone sounded indicating that you had completed your ratings of the first practice target, and a second target name (another famous person) replaced the first at the top of the screen. By the end of this trial run, you were now proficient with the task and were ready to begin.

Instead of rating famous people, your task now was to rate the 25 important people in your life that you had worked with in Session 1. In alphabetical order, the first name on your list appeared on the screen. This was followed by the appearance of one of 60 features, also arranged alphabetically. Your task was to form an image of your target person and rate him or her on all 60 features. That is, you were instructed to judge the degree to which each feature was descriptive of the individual you were rating. After you had completed your ratings of the first target, a "beep" alerted you to the fact that a new target name had replaced the old one on the screen. After you had rated 13 targets, a message appeared on the screen encouraging you to take a break and inviting you to partake of refreshments. You did so, returned 5 minutes later, and completed the remaining 12 ratings. The entire session lasted 75 minutes.

Session 3

Session 3 occurred a few weeks later. The computer-interactive format of this session was the same one used in Session 2 with one very critical exception. This time, instead of rating other people using your features list, your task was to rate *yourself* as you perceive yourself to be (or to have been) when you are (or were) *with* the targets on your list. You were instructed to bring to mind an image, memory, or scene of yourself as a partner *in a relationship with* each of your 25 targets, and to rate your experiences of yourself as an interactive participant in this dyad. In this exercise, the features were the same ones used in Session 2. The target names also remained unchanged. However, three additional targets had been added to the target list. They were "Me, as I Would Like to Be," "Me, at My Worst," and "Me, as I Usually Am." One or another of these new entries appeared after a quarter, and half, and three-quarters of the target names had been rated. You had been forewarned that these additions had been made, and were instructed to rate these selves directly instead of in a self-with-other context. Session 3 was concluded after you had completed all "me-with-others" ratings, as well as having made your "ideal," "at-worst," and "as usual" judgments.

Session 4

Session 4 was a feedback session. A letter, mailed to you prior to this session, invited you to bring with you any questions you might have about yourself and your relationships with various people in your life. No particular questions occurred to you—nor did they occur to most other participants. (Questions that were brought in by participants were acknowledged by the interviewer and were discussed, where appropriate, during the sessions.) The first 10 minutes were taken up by your performing some paper-and-pencil ratings of your targets and yourself on four preselected dimensions. (These ratings, though important to our investigative design, are not relevant to the present discussion.) After you completed your ratings, your interviewer informed you that the remainder of the session would be devoted to going over some of the results of your work in the previous three sessions.

You were reminded that the preceding three sessions were directed toward obtaining information about your perceptions of other people and your perceptions of yourself-with-other-people. A goal of the project was to be able to summarize and recover the ratings you had made in Sessions 2 and 3 in a manner that permitted them to be displayed in a clear, concise, and (ideally) personally meaningful fashion. Two computer programs had been written specifically for that purpose. Your interviewer told you that he or she had some technical knowledge of how the displays were computed, but had limited knowledge (hunches at best) about what the figures you were about to review meant. In other words, *you* (not your interviewer) were the specialist on your life, and it was up to you to discover whether the displays contained meaningful information.

At this point, you were shown two diagrams. One displayed the results of Session 2 ratings (perceptions of others), and the second was a figure representing your Session 3 ratings (perceptions of self-with-others). Rather than simply presenting the figures to you for your comment, your interviewer followed a predesigned format that first drew your attention to certain structural features of the figure pertaining to your self-with-others ratings. Your interviewer had you focus on various portions of the structural configuration of your self-with-others ratings, and as he or she did that, you were invited to comment on each segment of the display. During the course of this interaction, you realized that your interviewer was serious about leaving the task of making meanings in your hands. Genuine interest was shown in your comments, associations, discoveries, *and reservations* about your "self-with-others" structure, as witnessed by the notations being made by your interviewer (both on the figure itself and on a separate pad). After reviewing the "self-with-others" display, your interviewer guided you through the figure containing a representation of your perceptions of others. Near the end of the session, after you had become proficient at "reading" the displays, you were able to compare the two figures and identify several structural differences between them.

PURPOSES BEHIND SESSIONS 1 THROUGH 4

In this section, we briefly review some distinctive aspects of the four sessions.

Session 1

Our procedure for obtaining lists of "important people" is a variant of strategies used by others. For example, Kelly (1955) required subjects to fill in the names of people who fit the slots in his Role List prior to completing the Role Construct Repertory (REP) Test. Rosenberg (1977) has had research participants name as many people as come to mind, including individuals known personally and individuals known by reputation only. Although participants in our research are given some guidelines (e.g., immediate family, important relatives, friends, enemies), they are given considerable freedom for identifying people who are now (or have been in the past) influential.

Participants' final list is restricted to *important* people known personally by them, and the list may contain no more than 25 names. As yet, no research has been conducted that enables anyone to declare what an optimal number of targets is. Our own experience in this regard is that 25 names presses the limits for some individuals, and for others it is close to the mark. The average number of names spontaneously generated by our participants was 29. An additional consideration that went into our decision to limit the number of rating targets to 25 and features to 60 come from pilot work showing that a 25 × 60 rating matrix could be completed within our 80-minute time frame. Any increase in those dimensions would require more of the participants' time and would undoubtedly exceed participants' patience with such a repetitive exercise.

Session 2

The task of rating others on a list of attributes is a standard procedure in person perception research. Up to the late 1970s, feature lists were almost always experimenter-generated. Gradually, the statistical advantage of such uniformity began to crack under the pressure of realizing that many of the attributes experimenters were interested in had no particular bearing on the meaning structure in individuals' minds. As a consequence, free-response procedures were developed; in time, methods for comparing idiographic data of this sort were created (see especially Rosenberg, 1977). In our research, over two-thirds (42 words or phrases) of a participant's features list is self-generated. The remaining 18 words are supplied by us. As previously mentioned, these "gender-related" words are critical ingredients to the final fulfillment of the goals of our longitudinal investigation of gender identity.

Eventually, a full explication of the results of our research will enable us to discuss various configurations of our participants' perceptions of others. For now, however, this aspect of our study must be underplayed in order for us to concentrate on self-with-other representations. Thus, we make only comments "in passing" about the person perception aspects of our research in the ensuing discussion.

Session 3

It is in Session 3 that our "self-with-other" unit of analysis is operationalized. Respondents are asked to create images of themselves in interaction with specific people in their lives and to rate how they experience themselves in the context of each of these important relationships. This is one of the few times in research of this nature that the "self-with-other" unit of analysis has been isolated from other sorts of ratings.[4] Other research has approximated this variable by having respondents rate their identities. For example, Ogilvie (1987a), in a study of identity structure in later life, asked research participants to self-generate a list of their own identities. These identities were then treated as targets for feature ratings. In order to rate some identities, such as "mother," "caretaker for aunt," and "wife," respondents probably brought to mind specific instances of when they enacted a target identity (e.g., "wife" = "me-with-my-husband"). Such specificity was less likely to occur with other identities. For example, "mother" would entail thinking of "me as a mother, generalized" for women with more than one child. And other identities, such as "former supervisor," "Orthodox Jew," and "retired person," were likely to be rated outside the context of thinking about the self in relationship with a specific person. Robey, Cohen, and Gara (1989) used a self-with-other unit (e.g., "me-with-mother") in their research, but these units were analyzed in a space also occupied by generalized identities (e.g., "artist," "golfer," and "American"), which are units that are less interpersonally specific.

What can be learned when self-with-other representations are isolated from other sorts of ratings is discussed in the next major section of this chapter.

Session 4

In our research, we have intruded on the sacred line that generally separates "experimenters" from "subjects." We form investigative partnerships with our participants in such a way that the usual researcher–subject boundary nearly vanishes. We, as researchers, retain no secrets. In Session 4, for example, we rely on our participants to tell us what the results of our analyses of their data mean. We are the guides insofar as we walk them through the figures representing their ratings. They are the interpreters.

Our experiences with feedback dialogues in Session 4 have been, to understate the truth, rewarding. Most participants are surprised by the degree to which the methods we employ capture essential aspects of their lives, and are excited by their ability to recognize themselves in the structural representations they are given to review. One participant summarized the views of many when he said, "I had no idea where all that stuff you had me do was leading. All I did was type in a bunch of numbers into a computer, figuring that it wouldn't amount to much. But now that I see the results, I see *me!* It's beautiful, and it gives me a lot to think about." Another participant stated, "I already knew, in separate pieces, what is contained in these two figures. But this is the only opportunity I've had to see all the pieces together at one time. I'm amazed." Another indication that the partnership format is effective is the fact that 69 of the 71 individuals who began this study, including 8 individuals who had graduated from college the previous semester, returned 5 months after Session 4 to resume their work with us.

STRUCTURAL REPRESENTATIONS OF MATRICES

The displays we review with our participants in Session 4 are the results of performing hierarchical classes analyses on the matrices created in Sessions 2 and 3. The algorithm used in hierarchical classes analysis (henceforth abbreviated as HICLAS) was pioneered by DeBoeck and Rosenberg (1988). HICLAS has the unique ability to recover the contents of a two-way matrix by simultaneously computing subset–superset relationships contained in both the rows and columns of the matrix. That is, the algorithm alternates between the rows and columns (in this instance, targets and features) of a matrix, and locates the best-fitting row and column classes and their hierarchical relations. For readers familiar with modeling terminology, HICLAS is a set-theoretical model based on a modified iterative Boolean regression technique (Mickey, Mundle, & Engleman, 1983).

Clearly, this is not the place to describe HICLAS in any detail. Readers interested in comprehensive descriptions of HICLAS are referred to DeBoeck and Rosenberg (1988), Rosenberg (1988), and Gara (1990). Instead of elaborating any further on the algorithm per se, let us turn to an example of configuration (see Figure 14.1) that portrays the results of a HICLAS analysis of a young adult female's self-with-other representations.

Sarah's Self-with-Other Representations

Figure 14.1 contains a HICLAS-derived structure of a young adult's representations of herself-with-important-people in her life. We will call this person Sarah. She is a second-term junior in college.

Earlier, we have referred to a letter mailed to participants prior to Session 4. That letter invites project participants to bring to Session 4 any questions they have about themselves or their relationships that might be explored as part of the feedback portion of the session. In response to that invitation, Sarah has formulated a concern of hers in this way: "I think I am being too fussy about my relationships. When I see someone who I think may cause a problem for me, I don't bother with them. I am reeling from past hurts, and for that reason I don't want people to get too close to me." Sarah's interviewer has suggested that they both keep this issue in mind as they look over the results of her rating sessions.

The configuration reviewed by Sarah and her interviewer is reproduced in Figure 14.1. This figure, as noted above, contains a HICLAS-derived representation of the results of Sarah's Session 3 ratings of herself-with-important-people in her life. We now discuss this display in the same order in which Sarah and her interviewer explore its contents.

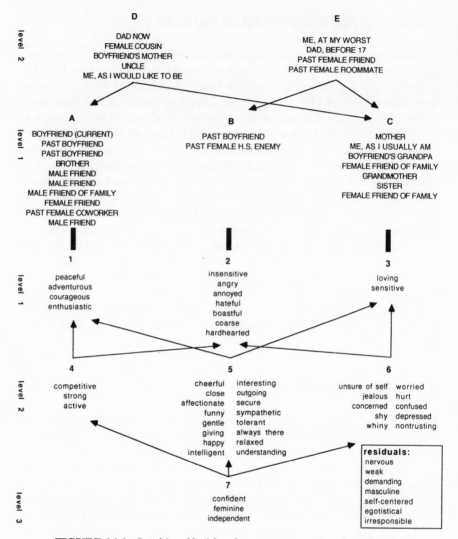

FIGURE 14.1. Sarah's self-with-others representational structure.

First, note the bold bars near the middle of the figure. These lines separate clusters of target people (top portion) from feature clusters (bottom portion). To facilitate "reading" the figure, target people clusters are labeled using the letters A through E, and feature clusters are numbered from 1 to 7.

HICLAS begins by identifying what are called Level 1 clusters of target people and features. Level 1 clusters appear in the rows just above and just below the bold bars (i.e., Clusters A, B, and C [target people] Clusters 1, 2, and 3 [features]). Beginning on the left-hand side, Cluster A contains the following individuals: Current Boyfriend, two Past Boyfriends, Brother, three Male Friends, a Male Friend of the Family, a Past Female Coworker, and a Female Friend.[5] With the exception of the last individual, who is in her 30s, all occupants of this cluster are in Sarah's age cohort. Feature Cluster 1 is most directly connected with Cluster A, and it comprises items that draw Cluster A away from other clusters of target people and make it a distinctive unit. This pattern shows that individuals in Cluster A share qualities enabling Sarah to experience herself as peaceful, adventurous, courageous, and enthusiastic. Although we soon loosen up our language so that we can speak of interlocking units, for now it is convenient to speak of features within a given cluster as defining the personal-attributes component of one of Sarah's self-with-other representational constellations. Thus, one representational unit contains the self experienced as peaceful, adventurous, courageous, and enthusiastic, and the individuals in Cluster A (mostly same age peers) are the people who most directly activate this unit of Sarah's internalized experiences.

Two people occupy Cluster B: an ex-boyfriend and a former high school female friend-turned-enemy. Sarah's story regarding her former boyfriend is simple and direct: "I can't stand him. He's despicable, and it would please me if great harm came to him." Her story about her former girlfriend is considerably more involved. In Session 1, Sarah has selected this individual (we will call her Jill) as a prototype of several females who were her pals during her first three semesters in high school, all of whom later became primary players in what Sarah refers to as "my primary hurt." She attended high school in a small rural town. Sarah was an excellent student and involved herself in a great number of school and community activities. She was one of the few students in her entire school interested in going to college. In the second semester of her sophomore year, Jill and Sarah's other close friends were "swept into sororities." These organizations became all-consuming. Jill and her friends pleaded with Sarah to become involved, but Sarah declined because of her college ambitions and other commitments. In reaction to Sarah's stand, Jill and the others accused her of being "uppity." Thereafter, Sarah was alternately shunned and physically bumped around in the school's hallways. Sarah surmises that a factor contributing to this rejection was "I was dating the male prize of the school, and I'm sure they were jealous." Despite whatever comfort her "prize" was able to offer, school became increasingly nightmarish. Finally, she went to her principal to discuss the problems she was having. "He told me to eat lots of raisins so I could get strong and defend myself." After that incident, Sarah's parents permitted her to transfer to a private school.

Partly as a result of these experiences, a self-with-other representation consisting of "insensitive," "angry," "annoyed," "hateful," "boastful," "coarse," and "hardhearted" has coalesced. Regarding Jill (and the others Jill stands for) and the Past Boyfriend in Cluster B, Sarah states, "I can hate them without the slightest guilt. They are bad people."

Cluster C, in addition to containing "Me, as I Usually Am," comprises Mother, Boyfriend's Grandpa, two Female Friends of the Family, Grandmother, and Sister. All of these individuals (including Sarah's 33-year-old sister) are considerably older than Sarah. They activate Sarah's self-with-other representation of being loving and sensitive. Sarah, recognizing that this cluster consists of older individuals, all of whom are female except for her boyfriend's grandfather, states, "I guess I feel safe with these people. I can be openly loving with them without any risk. Even my boyfriend's grandfather is like a woman. He is very gentle."

To summarize the Level 1 clusters, Sarah's self-with-others ratings have resulted in three distinct groupings of people with three corresponding feature clusters. Cluster A contains same-age peers with whom Sarah experiences enthusiasm and courage. Cluster B contains enemies who activate her annoyance and hate. Cluster C contains older individuals, primarily females (including Mother), who are the "others" in Sarah's self-with-other representational constellation of a loving and sensitive relationship.

Higher-order levels (i.e., Levels 2 and 3 in Figure 14.1) contain clusters of superset targets and features. A cluster is defined as a "superset" if it subsumes two or more subset groupings.

Clusters D and E appear at Level 2. Of all clusters, Cluster E and the feature clusters that define it provide information most relevant to the issue Sarah has brought with her to the session. The pattern of ratings she gives to "Me, at My Worst" brings that aspect of herself into Cluster E. Other "residents" of that cluster are Dad Before 17, and two Past Female Friends (one being her former roommate). In Session 1, Sarah has divided her father into "Dad Before [I was] 17" (Dad 1) and "Dad Now" (Dad 2). As she was growing up, Dad 1's occupation took him overseas for periods of 8 to 10 months a year. Sarah claims that "I must have loved him, but all I can really remember was how much I resented him when he was home. He got in the way of my relationship with Mom and got mad at me when I interfered. I got jealous. Also, I did not think he was sufficiently interested in me. He did nothing to convince me that he cared about me at all." Sarah's father retired when she was 17 years old, and since then, "I have been the light of his life."

As with Dad 1, it has been rough going with the two females in Cluster E. Recently, they have both turned against Sarah, and one has even accused her of a serious wrongdoing, an accusation Sarah considers to be untrue. In addressing herself to the question of why these individuals do not fall into Cluster B's grouping of enemies, Sarah makes the following observations: She is unable to decide simply that Cluster E people are "bad," giving herself a license to hate them. Rather, Cluster E people have the capacity of "making me feel that there is something wrong with me."

It is this feeling of not being a likable person that Sarah wants to avoid. She would prefer to think of herself as "good" and people who cause her misery as "bad." However, at least two present-day females in her life activate an earlier-formed internalized representation of interactions of "me-with-Dad." This is, of course, quite speculative, but given the fragments of Sarah's life history she has offered, it seems likely that her experiences of being unable to maintain the attention of her father have created within her some questions about her worthiness of affection.

One of the most reliable findings to date regarding HICLAS representations of self-with-others ratings is the following: When a Level 2 target cluster is a superset of two Level 1 target clusters, one of which is defined by a cluster of positive features and the other is defined by a cluster of negative features, the people in the superset cluster activate experiences of ambivalence. This phenomenon is clearly seen in Sarah's results. She both loves (Cluster 3) and hates (Cluster 2) Dad 1 and the two Female Friends who have turned against her, leading her to feel (from Cluster 6) unsure of herself, jealous, concerned, shy, whiny, worried, hurt, confused, depressed, and nontrusting. We drop down to Cluster 6 to obtain these features because, at the second level of features, it corresponds with Cluster E, and therefore, it plays a major role in identifying shared qualities that characterize Sarah in her relationships with people in Cluster E.

In summary, the portion of Sarah's HICLAS display we have just discussed probably contains an important key to understanding why she does not "want to get too close to people." The people she is particularly suspicious of are individuals whom she could love but who also have the capacity to turn against her, thereby activating a hurtful self-with-other representational configuration. She protects this from happening with the peers contained in Cluster A by prohibiting them from activating her loving and sensitive self.

However, some individuals in Sarah's life enable her to avoid this conflict when she envisions herself in interactions with them. These individuals are contained in Cluster D. They include Dad 2 ("always there for me these days"), a Female Cousin ("beautiful and terrific in every way"), her Boyfriend's Mother ("just the way a mother should be"), and a deceased, favorite Uncle. Cluster D also contains "Me, as I Would Like to Be"—Sarah's vision of her ideal self. Cluster D is a superset cluster of Clusters A and C. The arrows in Figure 14.1 show that Cluster D connects with Clusters 1 and 3, which in turn are both subsets of Cluster 5. Cluster

5 is a highly elaborated feature cluster containing positive affects such as "cheerful," "affectionate," and "happy"; comfortable feeling states such as "close," "secure," and "relaxed"; and admired qualities such as "giving," "intelligent," "outgoing," and "understanding." These features are prominently involved in Sarah's perceptions of herself-with-people in Cluster D. They also link up less directly with all other Target Clusters except for Cluster B's hated targets. Given Cluster 5's central, interconnective position in the structure, it is a major self-with-other representational constellation that is either fully or at least partially involved in nearly all of Sarah's relationships.

Another interlocking, superset component of Sarah's self-with-other subjective experiences appears in Cluster 4. Note that there is no target person cluster that directly corresponds to it. Rather, the features contained in it, "competitive," "strong," and "active," are activated in her relationships with individuals in Cluster A (primarily same-age peers) and Cluster B (enemies). In regard to this arrangement, Sarah says, "Yes, I am a very competitive person with my friends, and I guess with my enemies too. But it would be kind of pointless to be that way with older people [e.g., Cluster C], wouldn't it?"

Two more areas of Figure 14.1 need to be explained. In the lower right-hand corner is a list of personal attributes defined as "residuals." These are the features that Sarah either never uses or uses very infrequently to describe herself-with-others. As a consequence, they do not contribute to the structural space; in such instances, the HICLAS algorithm casts them aside as residuals. Thus, Sarah either seldom or never describes herself as "nervous," "weak," "demanding," "masculine," "self-centered," "egotistical," or "irresponsible." It would detract from our concentration on the self-with-other representational unit of analysis if we were to present a figure displaying Sarah's perceptions of others (Session 2 data); however, were we to do that, it would be seen that the features Sarah does not apply to herself are centrally involved in her characterizations of others. In other words, residual terms are personally meaningful to Sarah (i.e., she uses them systematically to describe others); they are simply not part of how she experiences herself in interpersonal relationships.

Finally, we turn to the features in Cluster 7. Unlike items listed as residuals, Cluster 7 features are those that Sarah *always* uses to describe herself no matter whom she imagines herself with. These features, "confident," "feminine," and "independent," are Sarah's "invariants." The prominence of these features in Sarah's self-with-others representational structure shows that Sarah has an abiding conviction that these vital ingredients of her past and present-day interactive experiences are activated by friends and enemies alike. They are the "constants," giving her a sense of self-continuity as she variously experiences courage, affection, annoyance, love, and even confusion and hurt.

We think of the contents of Cluster 7 as Sarah's fundamental beliefs about her social self. We would expect such attributes to be phenomenologically important to her. In addition, it is likely that these superset items are a major part of the glue that holds the overall self-with-others structure together (and thus may be analogous to central traits in impressions of others; Asch, 1946). Furthermore, these features are likely to be Sarah's "untouchables," in that she would strongly resist efforts to change them and deny evidence contradicting them.

We have devoted careful attention to Sarah's self-with-others representational structure in order to provide the reader with fairly detailed information about how such configurations are used in our research. We turn now to the self-with-others structure of another participant as an example of the variety of configurations seen at the level of the individual. In providing this second example, we will be less thorough and only address ourselves to some major aspects of the structure.

Arnold's Self-with-Other Representations

Arnold's "self-with-others" structure is considerably different from Sarah's. Arnold is a young adult male who is active in various college campus organizations. He considers most things to be going quite well for him. He is an excellent student in engineering, has a large number of male friends, and takes pride in his close relationships with family members. However, according to him, there is "a pocket of temporary emptiness" in his life. It has to do with the fact that he has no regular girlfriend. "There are two kinds of women," he proclaims. "One type will go to bed with you on a moment's notice, and who needs that? The other kind lead you on and then, just when things are beginning to heat up, just at the critical moment, they bail out, go back to their room, and leave you standing there like a fool."

Figure 14.2 displays the results of Arnold's ratings of himself-with-other-people. In comparison with Sarah's self-with-others structure, Arnold's is relatively simple. Yet, in its simplicity, it is quite informative. Cluster B in Arnold's configuration contains eight male friends and "Me, as I Usually Am." Features most strongly related to this grouping are contained in Cluster 2. They show that Arnold experiences himself as talkative, level-headed, sensible, practical, independent, sharing of interests, active, and talented when he is with these male companions. Note, however, what he is *not* when he is in their company. He neither "shows feelings" nor is warm, affectionate, or loving with them. These emotions are reserved for, and only activated by, family members. This can be seen in the figure by tracing the direction of the two arrows emanating from Cluster 5 that bypass Cluster 2 on their way to linking up with the remaining target person clusters, which contain, with one exception, all members of his immediate and extended family. Even the exception, Brother's Girlfriend (Cluster D), is no exception. She is the only female about his age

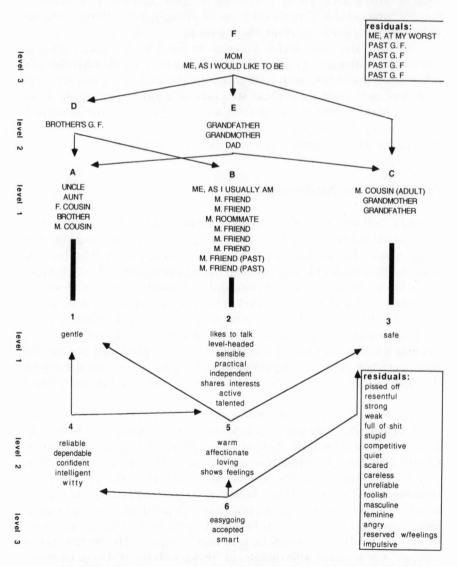

FIGURE 14.2. Arnold's self-with-others representational structure.

with whom he is close, and his brother is about to be married to her. Thus, she too, is considered "family."

In the main, everyone represented in the body of this display brings out either Arnold's level-headed or loving qualities. Two individuals, Mom and Brother's Girlfriend, activate both.

An important property of Arnold's self-with-others structure is the *absence* of negative qualities. All negative features, features he has liberally applied to others in his Session 2 ratings, appear as residuals. HICLAS recovers and represents convergent and contrasting, overlapping and nonoverlapping patterns contained in two-way matrices. It cannot recover nonexisting patterns. Features and self-with-other targets that cannot be structurally represented (because there is no structure *to* represent) become residuals. The diagram of Arnold's self-with-other relationships show that 5 targets and 16 features are not located in the body of the structural space. Instead, they are set aside as residuals.

Since Arnold does not wish to comment on the residual locations of his four ratings of himself-with-a-Past-Girlfriend and of "Me, at My Worst," speculations concerning what their location means is left to our interpretive judgments. Figure 14.2 clearly shows that Arnold rarely uses negative qualities in his ratings of himself-with-others. By "negative qualities," we are referring to residual features such as "resentful," "weak," "stupid," "scared," "careless," and "unreliable." He also does not apply to himself features that, on the surface, appear to be somewhat less "charged" (e.g., "quiet," "reserved with feelings," "feminine," and "masculine"). This pattern leads to the following two observations. First, explicit gender associations are not internalized as components of Arnold's self-with-other representations. This is particularly noteworthy, given that Arnold experiences himself quite differently with same-age males (Cluster B) than with same-age females (residuals). Second, Arnold "disavows" all negative qualities, insofar as there is no room for their appearance in his self-with-other subjective experiences. To acknowledge that negative affect is an aspect of his interactional history, as surely it must be, is too threatening to his overall sense of self. It appears that he handles such danger by disowning anger, resentment, and other negative feelings. Since he never (or very rarely) uses any of these terms to describe himself, we end up with an operationally defined list of "not-me" experiences.

The fact that Arnold's "Me, at My Worst" is a residual target supports this position. Its residual location means that he rates his "worst" with a pattern of 0's, 1's and 2's that prevents it from either entering into one of the existing target clusters or forming one of its own. Nor is there any recoverable consistency in any of his ratings of himself-with-a-Past-Girlfriend. We suspect that this result is based, in part, on Arnold's unwillingness or inability to integrate and "own" negative feelings as components of his internalized representations of interactions with others.

BEYOND CASE STUDIES: NOMOTHETIC PROSPECTS

At least on the basis of face validity and the enthusiastic response of our participants, it appears that self-with-other representational units, as analyzed by HICLAS, nicely capture heretofore unexplored aspects of individuals' social self-concepts. The manner in which HICLAS recovers individual units and locates them in the context of larger convergent and divergent, overlapping and nonoverlapping, subset and superset, interlocking categories offers inviting leverage for idiographic analyses. Although we consider our approach to be rich in its implications for conducting case studies, an important component of our overall investigation is to create suitable variables for making cross-person comparisons. Ultimately, we will assess the power of this research on the basis of our ability to move back and forth between idiographic and nomothetic levels of analyses.

Our nomothetic approach to these data will entail the identification of "shared" properties of self-with-other representational structures. That is, from each individual's HICLAS, we will calculate scores reflecting important underlying psychological variables and use these to make comparisons among participants. We now illustrate these nomothetic prospects by (1) describing two cognitive *structural* constructs, elaboration and rigidity; and (2) outlining preliminary efforts to index evaluative and gender-related *contents* of individuals' thinking about self in interpersonal relationships.

Elaboration and Rigidity of Self-with-Other Representational Structures

In their use of HICLAS to represent individuals' perceptions of self and others, Rosenberg and his colleagues (Rosenberg, 1988; Rosenberg & Gara, 1985; Robey et al., 1989) have identified the degree of elaboration as a significant aspect of such structures. Conceptually, "elaboration" refers to the extent to which an overall "cognitive structure" (in their work, the full set of one's multiple identities) is organized in a relatively simple versus complex manner. Elaboration has been operationalized by Rosenberg and his coworkers in several ways, including (1) number of clusters and (2) percentage of items (e.g., selves, other persons) in superordinate clusters. Evidence for the validity of the construct of elaboration is provided by Robey et al. (1989), who found that self-perception (but not person perception) structures of schizophrenics were less elaborated than those of "normals" and clinically depressed individuals.

In addition to assessing elaboration for each participant in our sample, we are experimenting with an index of rigidity. HICLAS computes a "goodness-of-fit" score for every target and feature that shows how well or how poorly any item belongs to its parent cluster. It also computes an overall goodness-of-fit score for the entire structure. A very high goodness-of-fit score for the overall structure can be taken to mean that the rater has rigidly assimilated each self-with-other relationship into existing mental units of representation. A lower overall goodness-of-fit score may be viewed either as an indication of structural flexibility or as an indication that the structure itself is in the process of accommodating to new or changing self-with-other experiences.[6] Here, our combined idiographic–nomothetic approach can come into play. That is, individuals with very high (or very low) goodness-of-fit scores in their self-with-other structures can be nomothetically identified and singled out for further intensive idiographic investigations, for the purpose of deepening our understanding of the meaning of scores on a particular index.

Evaluation and Gender in Self-with-Other Representational Structures

It is expected that a wide and diverse set of content issues will serve to organize individuals' self-with-other representational structures (e.g., dependence, trust, control). At the same time, however, evaluation and gender are two issues with which all individuals must come to grips. As a consequence, we have begun to develop indices of the evaluative (good–bad) and gender-related aspects of individuals' beliefs and feelings about self in relationships with important others.

Evaluation in Self-with-Other Structures

We have begun looking at the issue of evaluation by focusing on where "Me, as I Would Like to Be" and "Me, at My Worst" appear in each person's HICLAS depictions of the overall self-with-others structure. We take the latter as an example. Recall that Arnold's ratings of "Me, at My Worst" place it in the category of residuals. He is not unique in this regard. Other participants have rated their "worst" in a manner wherein HICLAS has located it in the overall self-with-others structure, but only as a stand-alone cluster containing one item—"Me, at My Worst." It has appeared as a subset unit with no connective superset target clusters. This pattern suggests that the rater is indicating, in effect, "I have a 'worst self,' but it plays no part in my relationships with the 25 most important people in my life." Other participants, like Sarah, have rated their "worst" state of interpersonal experience so that it is more completely integrated into their overall self-with-others structure. These three patterns ("Me, at My Worst" as a residual, as a stand-alone cluster, and as integrated into the structure) can be coded as 1, 2, and 3, respectively, and index the nomothetic property "Self at Worst Integration."

Some work similar to this line of thinking has already been done. One property, scored for all participants, was whether "Me, as I Usually Am" is located as a superset of "Me, at My Worst." This particular index of "Self at Worst Integration" separated 29 individuals from our sample of 71 participants and revealed a notable sex difference. Twenty-eight of a total sample of 49 females (i.e., 56%), and 1 of a total sample of 22 males (i.e., 4%) were identified as having rated "Me, at My Worst" in a manner that made it a subset of "Me, as I Usually Am" in their self-with-other representation structures. This pattern is consistent with sex differences discussed by Ogilvie and Clark (in press), wherein females are shown to be more likely than males to acknowledge negative emotion as an aspect of interpersonal relationships.

Gender and Self-with-Other Structures

We are beginning our exploration of how individuals incorporate gender into their self-with-other representations in a parallel fashion: We are assessing where the features "feminine" and "masculine" appear in each participant's HICLAS display. To take the former as an example, Sarah views herself as "feminine" in all her self-with-other relationships (i.e., it appears in Cluster 7 as one of her fundamental self-with-other beliefs). Sarah is not alone in this regard: 23 other females have included "feminine" in their most superordinate cluster. At the same time, 18 other females have placed it in a Level 2 grouping; 5 have put it in a Level 1 class; and, for 3 females, "feminine" is a residual. From these results, we can build a nomothetic property, "Feminine Self-with-Other Elaboration," arranging numbers as follows: 4 if Level 3 class, 3 if Level 2, 2 if Level 1, and 1 if residual. When that is done, the average score for females is 3.26 and the mean for males is 1.23. Although this overall gender difference serves as a partial validation of the index, it will be more important to explore how this measure covaries with other measures pertaining to perceptions of one's own femininity (e.g., Bem's [1974] Sex-Role Inventory) and with various styles of social interaction.

A BRIEF RECAPITULATION

We began this chapter by noting that our investigation of the self-with-other representation as a unit of analysis is part of a larger study of gender identity. Over the course of this longitudinal investigation, we are collecting a vast amount of information pertaining to the lives of our project participants. In addition to obtaining this information using open-ended interviews, a portion of nearly every session involves the collection of ratings using standardized formats. Using a variety of data reduction procedures, we are (and increasingly will be) in a position to address the causes, contents, and consequences of gender identity in great detail. Much of this work will be at the level of within-sample, nomothetic comparisons, and properties of self-with-other representational structures will be part of this endeavor. At the same time, as this chapter attempts to make clear, we are intent on preserving the individual as a unit of analysis. This will enable us not to lose sight of the fact that points of intersection in a table of aggregate results represent real people, who are organizing their relationships and their thoughts, feelings, and behaviors in unique—and in uniquely human—ways.

ACKNOWLEDGMENT

The preparation of this chapter and the research reported herein were supported by National Institute of Mental Health Grant No. MH40871-03/04.

NOTES

1. The term "representation" appears frequently in this chapter. Most often, we use the term in reference to individuals forming mental "representations" of self in interaction with (an)other person(s). In our model, each self-with-other representation is a separate unit of analysis. But the term is also used in another context. That is, we theorize that individuals' mental representations (i.e., first meaning) of self–other interactions are organized into larger units, and part of our research endeavor is to create "representations" (e.g., two-dimensional displays) that suggest how these larger units are structured. We mention this distinction here, hoping that an early warning will prevent later confusion regarding the two ways in which the term is used.

2. We refer here to the work concerned with self-as-known and efforts to explicate the content and structure of self-conceptions. Another large body of research and theory has dealt with self-as-knower and has explored various motives (e.g., self-consistency, self-presentations, self-esteem maintenance).

3. Procedures for reducing participants' important people lists to 25 names varied according to how many names the original lists contained. For example, a few participants brought with them lists of over 40 names. In such a case, the interviewer informed the participant early on that one of the goals of the session was to reduce the list to 25 names. Both the interviewer and the participant worked on that task throughout the interview. In other cases, participants were informed of the limitation of 25 names near the end of the interview, and the task became

one of selecting which of the remaining people on the list (i.e., people not yet described) were most significant. Finally, in some instances, the deletion of a few names was left in the hands of the interviewer because time had run out. That was done by reviewing the notes recorded on 3 × 5 cards during the interview and making "importance" judgments based on the participants' descriptions and comments about their relationships.

4. Hart (1988) is the only other researcher we are aware of who has done separate analyses of self-with-other units. In his study, he had adolescents rate themselves when "with" four (researcher-generated) others: mother, father, best friend, and "kids you don't know very well."

5. To protect Sarah's anonymity, people in Figure 14.1 are listed as Male Friend, Past Female Coworker, Boyfriend's Mother, and so on. It is crucial to keep in mind, however, that the display Sarah reviewed contained the names of specific individuals who were important to her.

6. It is also possible, of course, that relatively low goodness of fit reflects inability or unwillingness to do the rating task (e.g., random responding as a result of fatigue or lack of interest). We have, however, seen no evidence of such problems.

REFERENCES

Asch, S. E. (1946). Forming impressions of personality. *Journal of Abnormal and Social Psychology, 41,* 258–290.

Ashmore, R. D. (1990). Sex, gender, and the individual. In L. A. Pervin (Ed.), *Handbook of personality: Theory and research* (pp. 486–526). New York: Guilford Press.

Ashmore, R. D., & Del Boca, F. K. (1986). *The social psychology of female–male relations: A critical analysis of central concepts.* Orlando, FL: Academic Press.

Ashmore, R. D., & Ogilvie, D. M. (1989). *Gender identity, sex stereotypes, and social action.* Research proposal funded by the National Institute of Mental Health.

Atwood, G., & Stolorow, R. D. (1984). *Structures of subjectivity: Explorations in psychoanalytic phenomenology.* Hillsdale, NJ: Analytic Press.

Beebe, B., & Lachmann, F. (1988). The contribution of mother–infant mutual influence to the origins of self- and object representations. *Psychoanalytic Psychology, 5,* 305–337.

Bem, S. L. (1974). The measurement of psychological androgyny. *Journal of Consulting and Clinical Psychology, 42,* 165–172.

Cantor, N., & Kihlstrom, J. F. (1987). *Personality and social intelligence.* Englewood Cliffs, NJ: Prentice-Hall.

Carlson, R. (1988). Exemplary lives: The uses of psychobiography for theory development. *Journal of Personality, 56,* 105–138.

DeBoeck, P., & Rosenberg, S. (1988). Hierarchical classes: Model and data analysis. *Psychometrika, 53,* 361–381.

Freud, S. (1914). Remembering, repeating, and working through. *Collected Papers, 2,* 145–158.

Gara, M. (1990). A set theoretical model of person perception. *Multivariate Behavioral Research, 25,* 275–293.

Hart, D. (1988). The adolescent self-concept in social context. In D. K. Lapsley & F. C. Power (Eds.), *Self, ego, and identity: Integrative approaches* (pp. 71–90). New York: Springer-Verlag.

Higgins, E. T., Bond, R. N., Klein, R., & Strauman, T. (1986). Self-discrepancies and emotional vulnerability: How magnitude, accessibility, and type of discrepancy influence affect. *Journal of Personality and Social Psychology, 51,* 5–15.

Higgins, E. T., Klein, R., & Strauman, T. (1985). Self-concept discrepancy theory: A psychological model for distinguishing among different aspects of depression and anxiety. *Social Cognition, 3,* 51–76.

James, W. (1890). *Principles of psychology* (2 vols.) New York: Holt.

Kelly, G. A. (1955). *The psychology of personal constructs.* New York: Norton.

Kernberg, O. (1976). *Object relations theory and clinical psychoanalysis.* New York: Jason Aronson.

Kihlstrom, J. F., Cantor, N., Albright, T. S., Chew, B. R., Klein, S. B., & Niedenthal, P. M. (1988). Information processing and the study of the self. In L. Berkowitz (Ed.), *Advances in experimental social psychology* (Vol. 21, pp. 145–178). New York: Academic Press.

Kohut, H. (1977). *The restoration of the self.* New York: International Universities Press.

Kuhn, M. H., & McPartland, T. A. (1954). An empirical investigation of self-attitudes. *American Sociological Review, 19,* 68–76.

Linville, P. W. (1985). Self-complexity and affective extremity: Don't put all of your eggs in one cognitive basket. *Social Cognition, 3,* 94–120.

Markus, H. (1977). Self-schemata and processing information about the self. *Journal of Personality and Social Psychology, 35,* 63–78.

Markus, H. (1983). Self-knowledge: An expanded view. *Journal of Personality, 51,* 543–565.

Markus, H., & Nurius, P. (1986). Possible selves. *American Psychologist, 41,* 954–969.

Markus, H., & Wurf, E. (1987). The dynamic self-concept: A social psychological perspective. *Annual Review of Psychology, 38,* 299–337.

McGuire, W. J., & McGuire, C. V. (1988). Content and process in the experience of self. In L. Berkowitz (Ed.), *Advances in experimental social psychology* (Vol. 21, pp. 97–141). New York: Academic Press.

Mead, G. H. (1934). *Mind, self, and society.* Chicago: University of Chicago Press.

Mickey, M. R., Mundle, P., & Engleman, L. (1983). Boolean factor analysis. In W. J. Dixon (Ed.), *BMDP statistical software* (pp. 538–545, 692). Berkeley: University of California Press.

Mitchell, S. (1988). *Relational concepts in psychoanalysis.* Cambridge, MA: Harvard University Press.

Modell, A. (1984). *Psychoanalysis in a new context.* Madison, CT: International Universities Press.

Ogilvie, D. M. (1987a). Life satisfaction and identity structure in late middle-aged men and women. *Psychology and Aging, 2,* 217–224.

Ogilvie, D. M. (1987b). The undesired self: A neglected variable in personality research. *Journal of Personality and Social Psychology, 52,* 379–385.

Ogilvie, D. M., & Clark, M. D. (in press). The best and worst of it: Age and sex differences in self-discrepancy research. In R. P. Lipka & T. M. Brenthaupt (Eds.), *Self-perspectives across the lifespan* (Vol 2). Albany, NY: SUNY Press.

Robey, K. L., Cohen, B. D., & Gara, M. A. (1989). Self-structure in schizophrenia. *Journal of Abnormal Psychology, 98,* 436–442.

Rosenberg, S. (1977). New approaches to the analysis of personal constructs in person perception. In A. W. Landfield (Ed.), *Nebraska Symposium on Motivation* (Vol. 24, pp. 174–242). Lincoln: University of Nebraska Press.

Rosenberg, S. (1988). Self and others: Studies in social personality and autobiography. In L. Berkowitz (Ed.), *Advances in experimental social psychology* (Vol. 21, pp. 57–92). New York: Academic Press.

Rosenberg, S., & Gara, M. A. (1985). The multiplicity of personal identity. In P. Shaver (Ed.), *Review of personality and social psychology* (pp. 87–113). Beverly Hills, CA: Sage.

Stern, D. (1985). *The interpersonal world of the infant.* New York: Basic Books.

Stryker, S., & Serpe, R. T. (1982). Commitment, identity salience, and role behavior: Theory and research example. In W. Ickes & E. Knowles (Eds.), *Personality, roles, and social behavior* (pp. 199–218). New York: Springer-Verlag.

Sullivan, H. S. (1953). *The interpersonal theory of psychiatry.* New York: Norton.

Tomkins, S. S. (1987). Script theory. In J. Aronoff, A. I. Rabin, & R. A. Zucker (Eds.), *The emergence of personality* (pp. 147–216). New York: Springer.

Williams, J. E., & Best, D. L. (1982). *Measuring sex stereotypes: A thirty-nation study.* Beverly Hills, CA: Sage.

Wylie, R. C. (1974). *The self concept.* Lincoln: University of Nebraska Press.

Zurcher, L. A. (1977). *The mutable self: A self-concept for social change.* Beverly Hills, CA: Sage.

Index

Adaptation, 6, 7, 106, 107, 122
Affect, 19, 122, 138, 145–149, 183,
   196, 197, 200, 224, 225, 244,
   262, 271–273, 286, 287
  unintegrated, 1, 19,20
  attunement, 19, 20, 148, 149, 191
Alcohol, 240, 243, 250, 251
Anal stage, 11
Anxiety, 6, 7, 11, 132, 169, 173, 174,
   196, 287
  see also Affect
Arousal, 146, 271, 272
Attachment, 12, 24, 25, 144, 150, 186,
   197, 244
Attitudes, 37–58
  attitude involvement, 38
Attribution theory, 146
Autophotography, 35, 98, 103–106

B

Bandura, A., 69, 70, 198–200, 206
Binge eating; see Bulimia
Borderline personality disorder, 187
Bowlby, J., 12, 119, 150, 186, 197
Bulimia, 251, 252

C

Character, 3, 287
  character armor, 6
  character structure, 3

Cognitive dissonance, 197, 217, 218,
   257
Cognitive–experiential self-theory,
   111–136, 216
Collective self, 64
Commitment, 43, 45–47, 57, 98–
   101
Comparison, 69, 70, 72, 73, 211, 258,
   260, 277, 285, 291
  comparison processes, 260, 261,
   264–266
  see also Social comparison
Compulsive behavior, 5, 15
  Epstein's chapter, 131, 132, 134,
   135
  repetition compulsion, 215, 216
Consistency theory, 218
  evaluative consistency, 40, 41
Constructs; see Personal constructs
Cooley, C. H., 94
Countertransference, 23, 24, 29, 30,
   173, 223

D

Death, 29, 30
  death instinct, 11, 232, 233
Deconstruction, 246, 248, 249
Defense, 20
Defense mechanisms, 20, 21
Depression, 41, 144, 188, 189, 200,
   201, 220, 244, 273

E

Eastern philosophy, 151
  and the self, 109, 149, 150, 162,
    163, 174–176, 252
Eating; *see* Bulimia
Ecstasy, 238, 243, 252
Ego, 165–266, 216
  ego functions, 6
  ego involvement, 43–45, 47, 55, 56
  ego psychology 5–7
Ego-ideal, 172–174
Embarrassment, 241, 247
Emotion, 129, 144–146, 196, 242,
    271, 272
  see also Affect
Empathy, 140, 144, 148, 152, 161,
    166, 170, 178, 263, 266
Envy, 171
Erikson, E., 12, 169, 189, 191, 216
Escape from self, 238–253
Ethics, 173
Evaluative consistency, 40, 41
Experiential conceptual system, 109,
    111–136, 138, 150, 151
  evidence for, 124–128
  the feeling mind, 166

F

Fairbairn, W. R. O., 12, 119, 258
Festinger, L., 68, 70, 217, 262
Fixation, 11
Freud, S., 3–5, 11, 13, 17, 55, 112–
    117, 135, 149, 161, 162, 187,
    193, 213–216, 223, 232, 257,
    287

G

Gender, 282, 203, 291, 293, 297,
    308–310
Goals, 39, 43, 51–53, 58, 73, 79, 196–
    201, 218, 231, 232, 238, 239,
    241, 242, 252, 269
Guilt, 4, 9, 196, 239, 240

H

Heider, F., 218, 260, 261
Higgins, E. T., 39, 69, 195–197, 243,
    284, 286
Horney, K., 8, 121, 162, 214, 215
Hostility, 4, 28, 239

I

Id, 5, 38
  id psychology, 5
Idealization, 161, 170, 171, 211, 258,
    263, 264, 266, 267, 269, 276,
    277
Identification, 77, 291
Identity, 1, 12, 35, 42, 52, 56, 77–91,
    98, 148, 189–191, 205, 220,
    227, 247, 284, 297, 298
  and culture, 85, 86
  maintenance, 10–15
  negotiation, 190, 219
  social identity, 72, 77–80, 90, 91
  theme, 1, 12–15
  see also Gender
Impasse, 24–30
Impression management involvement,
    42, 43, 48–54
Information processing, 39
Interaction, 285, 303
Interdependence, 166
Internalization, 44, 149, 286, 289, 290
Interpersonal relationships; *see* Rela-
    tionships, social
Intersubjective approach, 1, 17, 30
  intersubjective context, 17, 22, 287
  intersubjective transactions, 289
Introspection, 275

J

James, W., 94, 185, 189, 194, 199,
    227, 257, 283
Jealousy, 272

Joining, 56
Jung, C., 111, 121, 122, 162, 212

K

Kelly, G. A., 111, 119, 285, 296
Kohut, H., 9, 17, 22, 25, 119, 161,
    187, 190, 198, 206, 211, 214,
    257, 258, 263–277, 287
Kernberg, O., 119, 167. 187, 287

L

Linville, P., 284
Loafing: see Social loafing
"Looking glass" self, 94
Love, 26, 29, 168, 238, 243

M

Mahler, M., 119, 258
Markus, H., 45, 87, 139, 186, 191,
    196, 257, 283, 285, 286
Masochism, 211, 238, 246–248, 253
McGuire, W., 85, 86, 142, 217, 283
Mead, G. H., 78, 94, 95, 283
Meditation, 238, 252, 253
Memory, 45, 105, 188, 293
Mirroring, 148, 161, 170, 171, 184,
    187, 211, 258, 263, 264–267,
    277
Mitchell, S., 17, 287, 288
Motivation, 19, 64, 67, 71, 73, 116,
    132, 168, 195–201
    unconscious, 5

N

Narcissism, 10, 188, 194, 263
    narcissistic decompensation, 10
    narcissistic personality disorder,
        110, 187, 188, 263

O

Object relations, 150, 161, 173, 258,
    263, 287, 290
Object representations; see
    Representations
Obsessive–compulsive personality, 1,
    4–14
    see also Compulsive behavior

P

Paradoxical techniques, 56, 225
Perception
    of others, 285, 286, 297, 304
    of self; see Self-perception
Personal constructs, 285
Persuasion, 35, 37–59
Piaget, J., 125, 126, 129
Preconscious, 112, 115, 129
Pride, 272
Private self, 35, 37, 41–44, 48, 53, 54,
    58, 64, 69, 166, 168
Psychoanalyst(s), 1, 19, 21, 22, 24, 25,
    111, 138, 150, 161, 164, 167,
    174, 186, 263
Psychopathology, 19, 24, 117, 120
Psychotherapy, 15, 26, 41, 46, 54, 56,
    134, 149, 167–169, 175–179,
    184, 188, 203, 211, 222–232,
    273, 287
Public self, 35, 36, 41–44, 46, 49, 50,
    53, 54, 64
Punishment, 240

R

Reflection, 258, 259, 260, 261, 263,
    265–276, 277
Reich, W., 6, 263
Relational model, 17, 21, 287, 288
Relationships
    hierarchical, 166, 168, 169, 171
    loss of, 194
    psychoanalytic, 160, 167, 170

Relationships *(continued)*
  social, 19, 55, 99, 100, 167, 173,
    176–178, 220, 221, 286, 295,
    304, 305
Repetition compulsion, 11, 116
Representations
  of interactions, 282, 289, 303,
    311
  of others, 18, 166, 186, 194, 195
  of self, 18, 166, 185, 186, 190, 193,
    194, 197, 201, 205, 212
  of self-with-others, 282–312
Resistance, 11, 12, 15, 24, 46, 47, 53,
    55, 117, 213, 215, 224, 232
RIGs (representations of interactions
    that have become generalized),
    288
Rogers, C., 113, 119, 121, 181, 191,
    197
Roles, 193
Rosenberg, M., 78, 81, 83, 188, 228,
    296, 297, 299, 308

S

Sadness; *see* Depression
Schemas, 16, 118, 131
Self, 1, 17, 18, 50, 94, 95, 109, 183–
    185, 238, 242–246, 257, 258
  cultural influences, 109, 160–178,
    181, 203–206, 245, 246
  expanding self, 109, 161–168, 177
  familial self, 109, 161–168, 177,
    291–299
  relational self, 165
  self-with-other, 211, 282, 286, 292
  self-with-other research paradigm,
    291–299
  social self, 282
  see also Private self; Public self
Self-assessment, 142–144, 147, 218
Self-awareness, 140, 141, 211, 238,
    242, 243, 245, 250
Self-complexity, 284
Self-concept, 35, 48, 78, 94–96, 98,
    99, 101, 102, 182, 184, 190,
    211, 213, 216, 219–222, 227,
    230, 290, 292
  social self-concept, 282, 308
Self-confirmation, 216, 219
Self-defeating behavior, 10, 11, 214,
    218, 222, 238–253
Self-enhancement, 188, 213–215, 217,
    221, 222, 233, 262, 263, 267
Self-efficacy, 37, 64, 69, 198–201, 206,
    257
Self-esteem, 45, 78, 119, 188, 196,
    217, 221, 226–230, 233, 257,
    259, 262, 311
  regulation, 7–10, 191
Self-evaluation, 35, 64–74, 140, 214,
    222, 228, 258, 259, 285
  maintenance, 191, 211, 258–277
Self-handicapping, 241
Self-ideal, 15, 278, 295
Self-image, 37, 39, 42–47, 55–58, 225,
    286
  see also Private self; Public self
Self-knowledge, 45, 48, 67, 68, 70–72,
    102, 138–154, 186, 206, 218,
    232, 284
Self-monitoring, 141, 142
Selfobject, 17, 18, 24, 166, 170, 171,
    263, 268, 287
Self-perception, 48, 143, 193, 283–
    285, 293, 308
Self-presentation, 38, 48, 50, 105, 278
Self psychology, 1, 9, 161, 211, 257,
    258, 275, 276, 289
Self-recognition, 140
Self-regulation, 18
  self-regulating other, 148, 149, 288
Self-representation; *see* Represen-
    tations, of self
Self-schema, 45, 182, 184, 186, 188–
    190, 192, 193, 195–201, 257
Self-theory, 176–179
Self-validation, 68
Self-verification, 86, 211, 213, 218–
    223
Self-view, 144, 211, 213–233
Separation, 27, 28, 109
  marital separation, 175

Sex, 174, 194, 243, 246–248
  see also Masochism
Shyness, 241
Social comparison, 35, 72
  see also Comparison
Social–ecological approach, 94–108
Social identity, 79, 80, 90, 91
Social loafing, 35, 64–74
Spiritual experiences, 14, 109, 135, 152, 153, 168, 171, 174–176
Stereotype; *see* Representations, of others
Stern, D., 18, 19, 148, 185, 288
Suicide, 169, 238, 246, 248–250, 253
Sullivan, H. S., 7, 8, 143, 214, 288
Superego, 172–174
Symbolism, 4, 6, 105
Suffering, 240

T

Therapy; *see* Psychotherapy
Transference, 23–25, 30, 171, 173, 223, 287
Twenty Statements Test, 283
Twinship, 277

U

Unconscious, 4, 5, 13, 14, 20, 22, 23, 25, 35, 42, 56, 109, 112, 114–117, 121, 133, 149, 150, 185–189, 190, 203, 286

W

Wachtel, P. L., 55, 193, 205, 215, 216, 221, 224, 225, 230, 231
We-self regard, 169–172
Winnicott, D. W., 149, 161, 191
Wylie, R. C., 282